# kinesiology

2nd Edition

# kinesiology

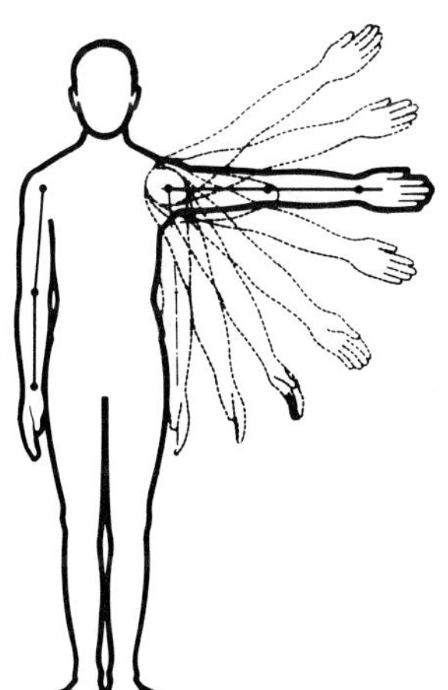

Marilyn M. Hinson
*Texas Woman's University*

Library of Congress Catalog Card Number: 80–68266

ISBN 0–697–07173–1



Printed in the United States of America
10 9 8 7 6 5 4 3

# Contents

# List of Illustrations

# Preface

This book is intended as a text for undergraduate courses in kinesiology. Its contents are based upon an underlying concept in which emphasis is placed on the importance of an anatomical basis as the pivotal point around which mechanical concepts can subsequently be formed. Toward that end, the book has been divided into two parts: Part I deals with anatomical aspects of kinesiology; Part II with mechanical aspects. The materials presented are believed to be sufficient for a full year's course; and by careful selection from among the several topics included, can be used equally well for a semester course.

This revision has been expanded significantly beyond the first edition. New materials have been included that relate to location of the total body center of mass by both the segmental and board with "knife-edge" methods. In addition, the determinations of average and instantaneous velocities and accelerations in both the linear and angular cases are explored. Existing sections on friction, leverage, projection, and fluids have all been lengthened to include additional concepts. A brief history of kinesiology has been provided as well as a review section on the physiology of muscular contraction.

Comprehensive bibliographies have been provided for both Parts I and II. The inquiring student would find them useful in the search for related and in-depth information.

It should be pointed out that the selection of terminology was made in order to agree, as much as possible, with the current literature. Two problems were encountered, however, which deserve mention. The first relates to the use of singular and plural suffixes. The suffix *ae* indicates the plural; as, for example, one *vertebra,* two *vertebrae.* Certain muscles carry this suffix in their names (levator scapulae, erector spinae, tensor fasciae latae), but are commonly used with a singular verb. It was decided to parallel that usage in this text, even though it is grammatically incorrect, because to do otherwise would be confusing. The *ae* suffix has been used to indicate the plural, when appropriate, only where muscle names are not concerned.

A second problem of contradiction arose from the lack of agreement in the literature as to whether the bones or the joints flex, extend, rotate, and so on. Certain authors state that a muscle flexes the forearm;

others stipulate that the muscle flexes the elbow joint; still others submit that it flexes the forearm at the elbow. The terminology selected for use in this text is that which indicates movement of the joint. Such phrases as "abduction of the hip joint" and "extension of the wrist joint" are typical of the phraseology employed.

Finally, it has been noted that pronunciations of muscle names are quite variable and sometimes confusing. To meet this problem, a pronunciation model has been included after the name of each muscle. The pronunciations are taken from *Dorland's Illustrated Medical Dictionary,* 24th edition, W. B. Saunders, 1965. In the case where traditional spellings have been preempted by more current terminology (i.e., *deltoid* instead of *deltoideus*), the pronunciation suggested is that of current usage.

Whereas the anatomical considerations of Part I are presented in a somewhat traditional manner, including origins, insertions, innervations, and actions, it will be noted that the many related discussions focus upon muscle location and angle of insertion as indicators of muscle action. The student is thereby invited to become acquainted with the logic of movement rather than the tedium of memorization.

In Part II, an attempt has been made to present the mechanical principles embodied by sport and dance in such a way that concepts can be built which will prepare the student to analyze movement. The major topics of stability, motion, Newton's Laws, spin and rebound, projection, and fluids have been kept as free of mathematical treatment as possible; where such treatment is included, it is presented to clarify the concepts discussed.

The chapters in Part I of the text conclude with summary remarks that are intended to help the student apply anatomical considerations to sport and dance rather than to consider them a nonintegrated, meaningless part of the kinesiology course. The chapters comprising Part II conclude with summaries which present, concisely, the principles discussed in the preceding pages. All chapters include suggested laboratory experiences which have, in the author's experience, proved to be of value in the achieving of a full understanding of the materials.

The final chapter of the book is one of a "recap" nature in which several movement problems from sport and dance are described and a decision is invited from the reader regarding the appropriateness, or inappropriateness, of the technique involved. Relevant anatomical and mechanical principles are then explored and a final solution is offered. The intent of the chapter is to bridge the gap between classroom theory and "in the field" experience.

The last movement problem is offered as an example of a kinesiological analysis that can easily be performed by the undergraduate student. It is based upon data acquisition by motion photography and addresses determinations of center of mass, force application, linear and angular velocities, and accelerations of a track start.

The author is indebted to many individuals for their invaluable help during the writing of the book. Particular acknowledgment is extended to Mary Johnson for her excellent illustrations. Appreciation is expressed also to Dr. Marjorie Wilson of the University of Minnesota, and to Dr. Aileene Lockhart of Texas Woman's University, for their continued encouragement; to Dr. Barbara Gench, Dr. Virginia Brewer, Judith Tate, and Dr. Claudine Sherrill for their critical reading of the manuscript, and to Evelyn Pack and Donna Ramsey for their tirelessness in the preparation of final copy. Finally, I would like to express my gratitude to William C. Brown Company Publishers for their aid in all phases of this manuscript's preparation.

*Marilyn M. Hinson*
Denton, Texas

**PART I**

# Anatomical Aspects of Human Motion

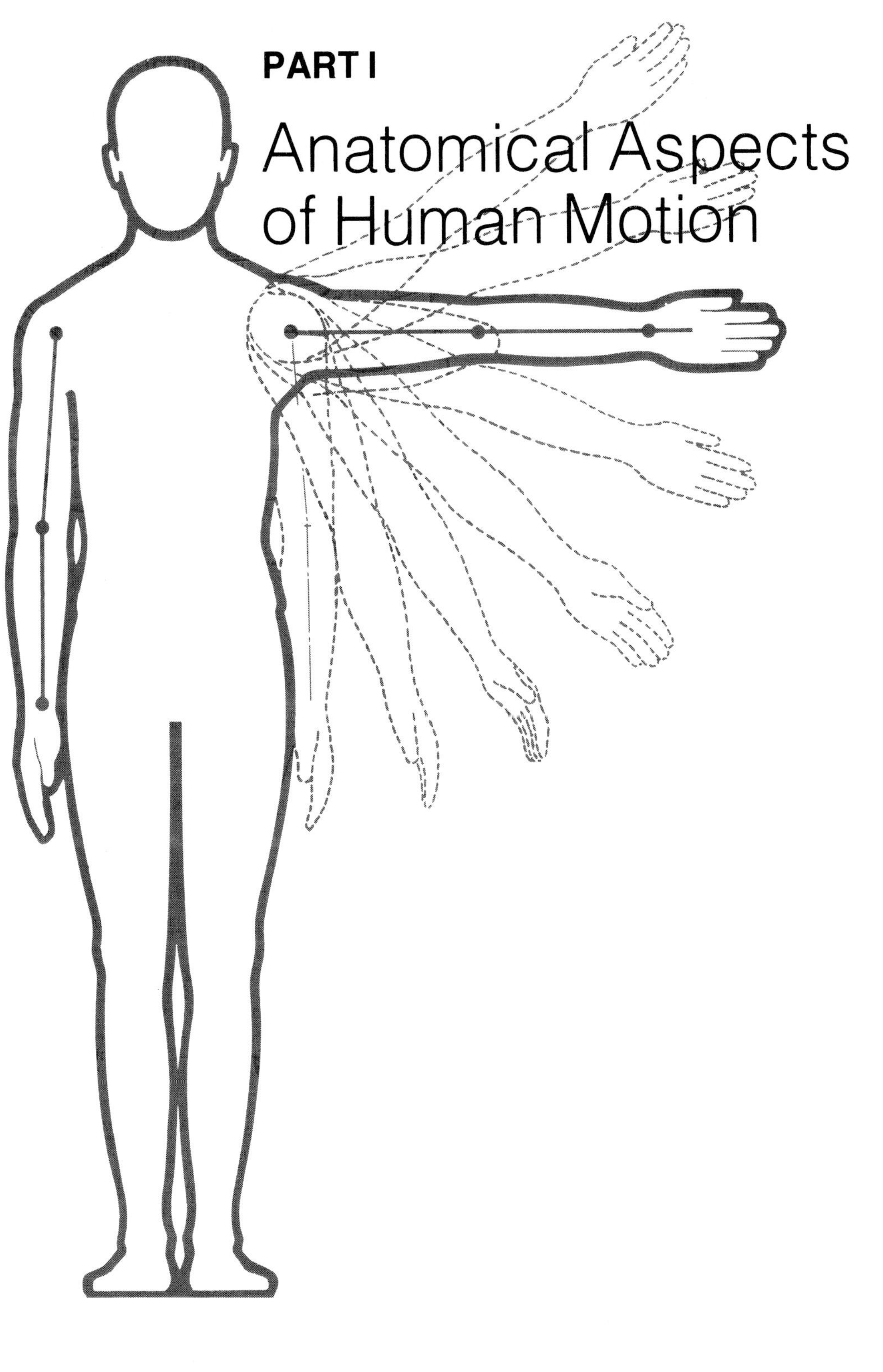

# The Beginning

# 1

## Introduction

Kinesiology has been widely accepted as an integral course in the undergraduate curriculum of those who will specialize in human movement. It is puzzling, therefore, that the meaning of the word *kinesiology* is not more commonly known. Taken literally, the word can be separated into its roots of *ology* (science of) and *kinein* (to move). Unfortunately, the resulting definition, "science of movement," is too broad to be useful, for to say that one is studying the science of movement could indicate anything from human anatomy to motor learning or exercise physiology. Certainly these disciplines are related to kinesiology—each shares a common object of study, the human being. Kinesiology is, however, uniquely different from all other movement sciences in that its focus is upon knowledge of the mechanics of movement which emerge from the blending of the knowledge of human anatomy with that knowledge basic to the study of physics. For example, in kinesiology, one learns to relate the facts of muscular origin and insertion of anatomy to such concepts as joint axis and angle of insertion in order to explain the actions of a given muscle. One learns, also, to relate muscle actions and joint positions to the demands of successful performance in sport and dance.

Kinesiology is seen, then, to be comprised of two subareas: the first is concerned with the production of movement, or lack of movement, by the muscles of the body—the second with events which result from the application of muscular force. The first subarea is known as *Anatomy of Human Motion*, and is so oriented as to answer such questions as "at what angle should the elbow be held to allow surrounding muscles to exert greatest strength?" or "why are the muscles of the thigh so important to the integrity of the knee joint?" The second subarea is referred to as *Mechanics of Human Motion*, and includes concepts designed to answer questions such as "at what angle should a shot be projected for longest distance?" and "what effect will top spin have on a forehand drive in tennis?"

In this text, Anatomy of Human Motion and Mechanics of Human Motion are treated as Parts One and Two, respectively. Each is introduced by a chapter comprised of basic concepts and terminology, and even though an attempt has been made to make a clean separation between the two parts, there is some inevitable overlap of the second part upon the first. It is urged, therefore, that the book be used in the sequence in which it is presented.

## A Brief History

The division of kinesiological materials into anatomical and mechanical subareas is not without some historical basis. Certainly Aristotle, who has been titled the Father of Kinesiology, was concerned not only with muscle actions but also with the influence of muscular activity upon the generation of force. It is remarkable and exciting that there was such keen interest in movement as was demonstrated by this Greek philosopher who lived more than 2000 years ago.

It was only some 100 years after Aristotle that Archimedes developed the principles of buoyancy that continue to be received as valid. It is unusual to find a kinesiology text that does not include his principles in its treatment of the mechanics of swimming.

Perhaps it was inevitable that man's curiosity about the basics of muscle contraction led Galen, a Roman who lived during the second century after Christ, to consider contractile properties of muscle. Although his explanation of the workings of nerves was more spiritual than scientific, he was nevertheless able to define agonism and antagonism with accuracy. He also coined the still-used terms of *diarthrosis* and *synarthrosis*, which relate to joint mobility.

Not until more than ten centuries after Galen did the works of Leonardo da Vinci begin. Best known as an artist, da Vinci was intrigued with the human body and its movement characteristics. Mechanics of posture, gait, and jumping all came under his careful scrutiny. His mechanical and engineering drawings are often seen today as logos of kinesiological societies, as cover designs of textbooks, and even on T-shirts.

What schoolchild has not heard of Galileo Galilie and the Leaning Tower of Pisa? Almost fairy-tale-like in the minds of many is the story of Galileo dropping various objects from the tower in the seventeenth century so he could prove that the pull of gravity is not selective: it exerts its influence to accelerate a falling body at the same rate regardless of the weight of the body. This important principle is used in many classrooms to explain phenomena related to such things as skydiving, projectile trajectory, and force absorption.

Sir Isaac Newton (1642-1727) is fondly associated with apples, for many would have it that he was observing apples fall from an apple tree when he discovered the laws of gravity, inertia, acceleration, and action-reaction. Be that as it may, his laws are considered basic to the study of the mechanics of movement, and are used universally to explain force resolution and composition, centripetal force, angle of projection, and virtually any other problem that confronts the movement scientist.

Approximately 140 years after Newton's death, Guillaume Duchenne returned the focus of interest to the basic study of muscle function. His work was based, to some extent, on that done previously by Luigi Galvani, who verified the presence of electrical potentials in muscle and nerve. Galvani's name is remembered often by those who study Galvanic Skin Response (GSR) in lie detector tests, tests of like and dislike, etc.

Duchenne built upon Galvani's work by developing a technique of stimulating the contraction of a muscle of the body and observing the reaction of the associated body parts. Even though Duchenne admitted that the contraction of a single muscle was not representative of the complicated interchange of muscle activity in movement, his work gave the kinesiologist a firmer base for analysis than did simple palpation.

During the same time period in which Duchenne was involved in his early electromyographic studies, Eadweard Muybridge (later known as Ed Weard) became interested in studying movement in a temporal manner. There are many legends about Muybridge. One of the most interesting has it that he visited a tavern that exhibited a painting of Napoleon on a galloping horse. The painting, as did all paintings of that era, depicted the horse with one hoof on the ground. Some discussion ensued and, as a result, Muybridge wagered a considerable sum that the artist was in error; that, in fact, horses at gallop did not always have one leg in contact with the ground. There was, rather, a period in each stride during which the horse was airborne. After considerable effort, expense, and consultation, Muybridge set several cameras along a horse track. As the horse passed each camera, a device was triggered so that each camera recorded the action in front of it. Muybridge won his bet! The photographic evidence proved that the horse was, indeed, airborne during part of the gallop stride. So dawned the era of motion photography as a tool for collection of movement data. Whether the manv legends about Eadweard Muybridge are true or not, credit must be given to him for his applications of photography to human movement. They remain classic to the sciences of kinesiology and biomechanics.

At approximately the same point in time, C. W. Braune and Otto Fisher, to be followed somewhat later by Rudolph Fick, completed basic research related to body segment weights, centers of gravity, and other parameters of importance to assessment of strength and center of gravity. Their works are classic in the sciences of kinesiology and biomechanics, and have been augmented by the findings of Dempster in his more current efforts.

In the middle 1900s, Arthur Steindler authored what has become a classic text in kinesiology entitled *Kinesiology of the Human Body under Normal and Pathological Conditions*. Because of the importance, past and present, of his manuscript, every serious student of kinesiology is urged to add it to his or her library at the earliest possible time.

## Nomenclature

We are now brought to the current day in our exploration of the historical events that have undergirded what we know as the science of kinesiology and/or biomechanics. It is of interest to note, at this point, that as our ability to analyze motion has progressed, so has our terminology. It is recognized that the many words used in conjunction with the study of human movement may be confusing to the student of the science—perhaps they are equally confusing to the professional. What *is* the difference between *kinesiology* and *biomechanics*? How do *statics, dynamics, kinetics,* and *kinematics* relate to the study of human movement? What are *electromyography and cinematography*? How does the study of *forces* relate to the science of movement? Let us answer the foregoing questions in order.

Regarding the difference between kinesiology and biomechanics, it was noted above that kinesiology can be defined broadly as the science of movement. It takes its base in a thorough knowledge of the anatomical and muscular structures of the human body. It is only when these have been mastered that mechanics of motion are introduced. Biomechanics, on the other hand, would appear to assume that its devotees already have a sound grasp of an anatomical and muscular knowledges and can proceed with an in-depth study of movement mechanics. There is, obviously, some overlap in the materials embodied by the titles of the two sciences. Whereas the kinesiologist is attentive to the mechanics of movement, he treats it somewhat superficially and only after anatomical considerations have been mastered. The biomechanist enters at this point, and with the kinesiologist's background, focuses upon the mechanics of movement and explores with all depth possible.

The terms *statics, dynamics, kinetics,* and *kinematics* have appeared since we began to use biomechanics as a scientific descriptor. Statics refers to that branch of biomechanics that is concerned with equilibrium—that is, *the sum of all moments must equal zero.* Such a concept may seem foreign to the uninitiated; it need not be so. The basic formula of statics translates simply that with a seesaw situation in which two children of equal weight are sitting at equal distances from the axis of the seesaw, no movement will occur. The seesaw is balanced. Equivalently, if the force of buoyancy equals the force of gravity, a body will neither sink nor rise. Also, any pull or push that is matched by one of the same force will yield no movement. In each of these examples, the sum of the moments of force is equal to zero. Said another way, each moment of force is neutralized by an equal and opposite moment. So it is with the subscience of statics.

Dynamics is the name of the biomechanical branch of interest that is concerned with movement and its velocity, acceleration, and associated forces. Subheadings of biomechanics are kinetics and kinematics. Kinetics includes that portion of dynamics that is concerned with body mass and with muscular forces that are applied to move that mass. To determine the position of the center of mass of a long jumper or to analyze the arm action of a high jumper is to study kinetics.

Students of kinematics do not concern themselves with the causes of motion but rather with the results of the causes. Projection paths of sports implements as well as of the body itself come under their close scrutiny. Spin and rebound are also of interest, as are the priniciples of aerodynamics.

Electromyography and cinematography are tools for the gathering of kinesiological and biomechanical data. Electromyographic records are taken, through special electrodes, of contracting or resting muscles. Determinations can be made regarding the strength of a muscle's contraction, the beginning and duration of contraction and, indeed, whether contraction is occurring at all.

Cinematographic data are film records made with motion picture cameras. The films are usually exposed at high speeds in order to yield a slow-motion quality when they are projected. Analysis of a sports movement is obviously enhanced because of the slowing of motion and also because the films provide a discrete and permanent record that can be restudied at will.

The study of forces is basic to the analysis of human movement. The gathering of force data is done through the use of special instrumentation that is sensitive to pushing or pulling. Peak forces as well as force profiles over time can be recorded to determine, for example, whether there is a difference in the grip strength of the right and left hands of highly skilled golfers, or to specify the amounts of force applied to the ground by a sprinter between heel-down and toe-off of the supporting foot.

It is hoped that this brief discussion of nomenclature has been clarifying and has dispelled any confusion. A note of caution is indicated, however. As of the date of the revision of this manuscript, no official terminology has been set forth that defines the various aspects of kinesiology and biomechanics. It is believed, nevertheless, that the definitions and explanations offered above are sound and reflect the thinking of the current leaders in the field.

# Terminology and Basic Concepts

# 2

The concepts presented in this chapter are considered to be basic to a study of the anatomical aspects of kinesiology. They are developed around a terminology that has been agreed upon by kinesiologists and that appears in most of the literature.

## Reference Positions

Two positions have been universally accepted as reference positions for joint movement (fig. 2.1). One, called the fundamental position, prescribes that the subject stand in upright posture with feet parallel and close, with the arms at the sides and the palms of the hands facing the body. The second reference position, the anatomical position, varies from the fundamental position only in that the palms face forward. Either position may be used to describe all joint movements of the body except those of the forearm during which the palm of the hand is turned inwardly and outwardly. The anatomical position must be used as reference for that motion.

The purpose of a reference position is to supply a starting point from which movement in any direction can be described. For example, a forward swing of the arm involves flexion of the shoulder joint; extension is defined as the joint movement which allows a downward and backward swing of the arm but only until the arm has returned to the reference position. Additional backward swing of the arm requires hypterextension of the shoulder joint. Since the muscles of the shoulder which cause extension are not necessarily the ones which cause hyperextension, the kinesiologist must be precise in describing the action of the arm in order to differentiate among the attendant activities of the surrounding muscles. The use of a reference position which has been universally accepted can provide for the required precision.

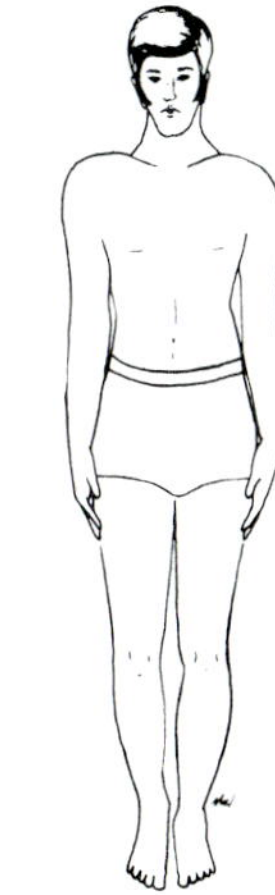

Fundamental position

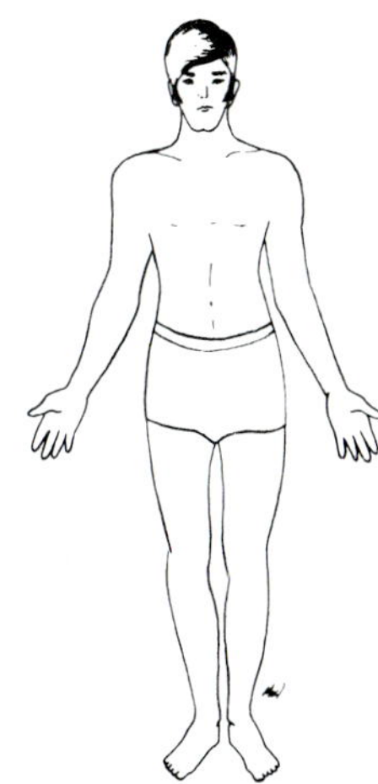

Anatomical position

**Figure 2.1. Reference positions**

## Types of Motion

The two types of motion referred to most frequently are linear or rectilinear, and angular. During linear motion, an object progresses in a straight line from one position to another with all of its parts moving in the same direction and at the same velocity. A boat, gliding through the water, is undergoing linear motion. The elevation and depression of the shoulder girdle when one shrugs the shoulders involves movement of the scapula which is linear in nature.

Angular motion, also called *rotary* or *rotatory motion*, is defined as motion in which all parts of an object move along the arc of a circle around a center or axis of rotation. A propeller exhibits angular motion with all of its parts moving along the arc of a complete circle, the center or axis of which is the hub. The forearm undergoes angular motion, also, when the elbow is bent and straightened as its parts follow the arc of a partial circle around an axis at the joint.

The varied movements of the human body as a whole are usually comprised of both angular and linear components. Walking, running, and jumping all combine the linear movement of the trunk with the angular movements of the limbs, and are referred to as combination movements involving both types of motion. When movements of only a portion of the body are described, however, they are referred to as being either linear or angular in nature, and small discrepancies are ignored. Even though the action of the scapula noted during shoulder shrugging is actually accompanied by a certain amount of angular motion, it is mainly linear and is described as such. Bending and straightening the elbow involves some gliding between the bones of that joint; however, the motion of the forearm is primarily angular and is so designated.

## Planes of Action

In order to facilitate the description and analysis of movements, kinesiologists have adopted the use of three anatomical reference planes. These planes, called *cardinal planes*, can be conceptualized as three large panes of glass. Each pane is oriented at right angles to the two remaining panes as they pass through the body.

The cardinal sagittal plane (fig. 2.2) progresses from the front to the back of the body, dividing it, by weight, into right and left halves. Movements are said to be occurring in the sagittal plane either when they are in the cardinal plane—nodding the head *yes*—or when they are in a plane parallel to the cardinal plane—a forward and backward swing of the arms. Joint actions which result in sagittal movements are called *flexion*, *extension*, and *hyperextension*.

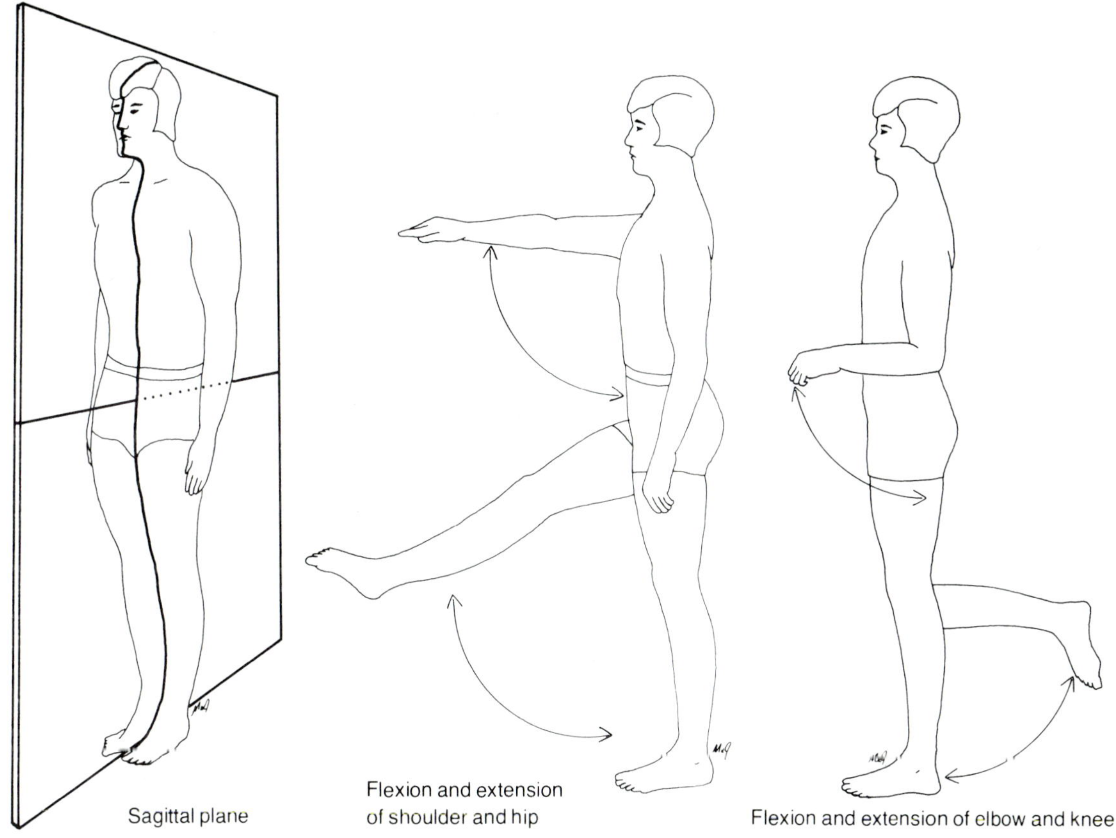


Figure 2.2. Sagittal plane and movements

The cardinal frontal plane (fig. 2.3) passes through the body from side to side, dividing it, by weight, into front and back halves. Almost all movements which occur in the frontal plane are in that cardinal plane and are exemplified by the sideward swings of the arms during the "jumping jack" exercise. Joint actions, which allow for angular movements in the frontal plane, are called *abduction* and *adduction* where the limbs are concerned and *lateral flexion* if the spine is involved.

The cardinal horizontal or transverse plane (fig. 2.4) divides the body, by weight, into a top half and a bottom half. It would be difficult to execute a movement in this cardinal plane since all motion would have to be localized in the hip region. The many movements of the body which are said to occur in the horizontal plane actually are in a plane parallel to the cardinal one. Turning the head to look from side to side, or turning the palms inwardly and outwardly are examples of movements in the horizontal plane. Joint actions which result in

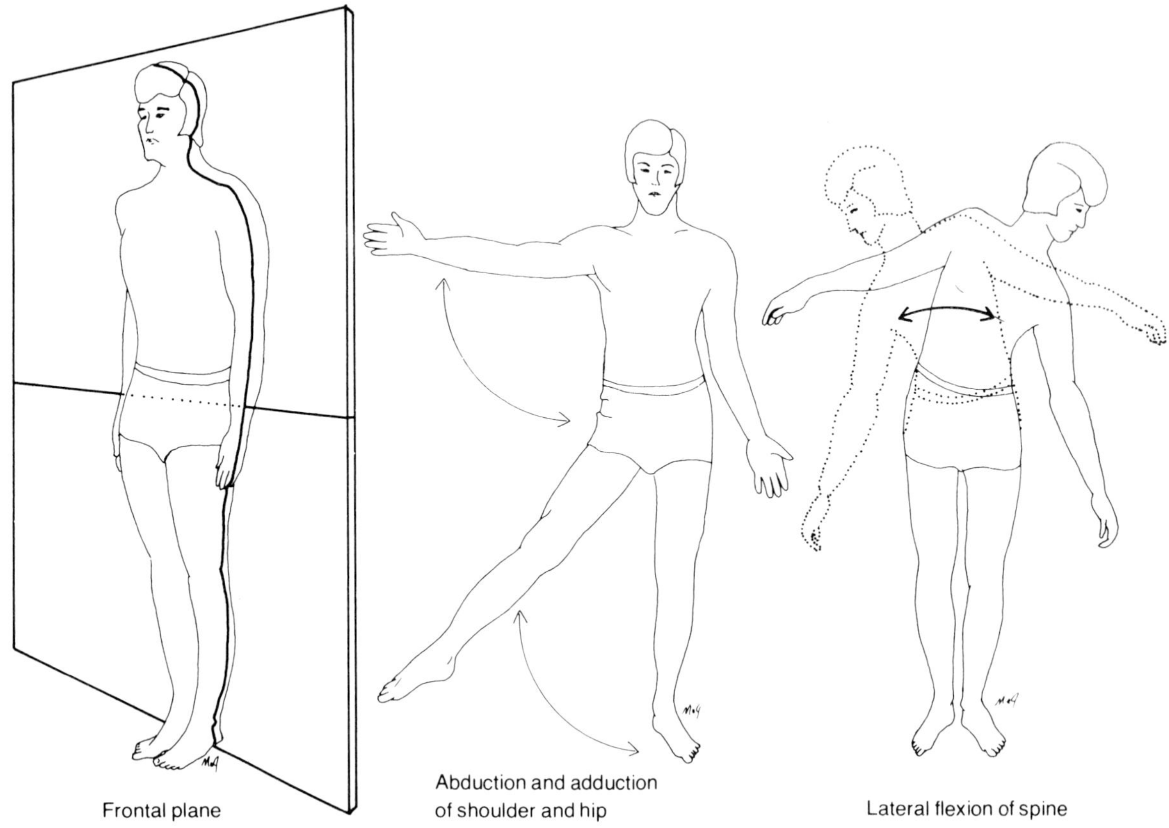


**Figure 2.3. Frontal plane and movements**

such movements are called *rotation,* and, where the limbs are concerned, are further described as being either inward or outward.

When the three cardinal planes are visualized as passing through the body simultaneously, it will be noted that there is a common point of intersection which is taken to be the center of mass, or as it is also called, the center of gravity.

## Axes

Movements occur in a plane and, if they are angular in nature, around an axis. Each of the three cardinal planes is conceptualized with an axis which is at right angles to it (fig. 2.5). An axis at right angles to the sagittal plane would be a horizontal one which is oriented from side to side. Because its orientation is the same as that of the frontal plane, this axis is called the *frontal axis.* An axis at right angles to the frontal plane is oriented from front to back as is the sagittal plane,

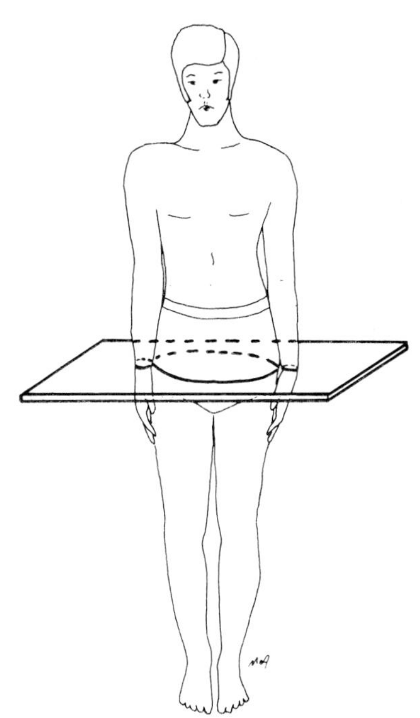


Horizontal plane

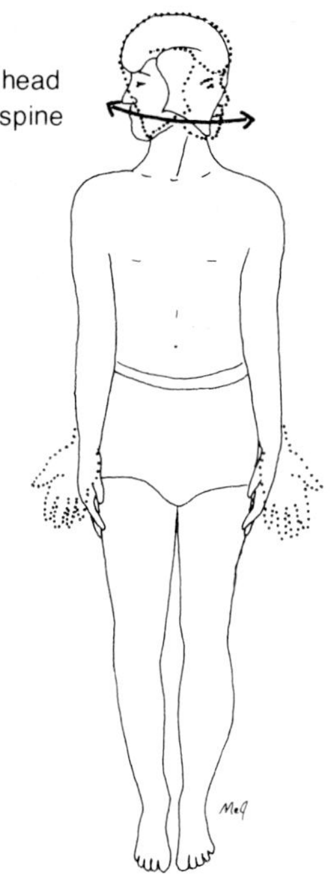


Pronation and supination of radius on ulna

**Figure 2.4. Horizontal plane and movements**

and is called, therefore, the *sagittal axis.* The axis at right angles to the horizontal plane is known as the *vertical axis* and passes downwardly through the top of the head.

Just as the three cardinal planes intersect at the center of mass, so do the three cardinal axes; however, since most angular movements of the skeleton occur in planes parallel to the cardinal planes, they consequently occur around axes parallel to the cardinal axes. The forward and backward swinging of the arm is said to occur around the frontal axis even though this particular axis passes through the body from side to side at shoulder level rather than at the level of the center of mass. Abduction and adduction of the leg is performed around a sagittal axis which passes through the hip; inward and outward rotation of the arm occurs around a vertical axis which passes downwardly through the top of the shoulder.

Planes and their axes are inseparable. Angular movements in the sagittal plane must occur around the frontal axis, just as angular movements in the frontal and horizontal planes must occur around the sagittal and vertical axes respectively.

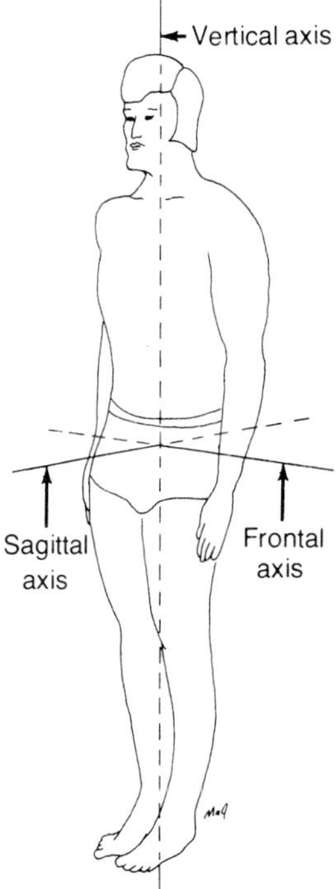


**Figure 2.5. Axes of rotation**

It is common for a kinesiologist to refer to the *long* or *longitudinal* axis of the body. This item of terminology appears to have stemmed from some confusion regarding those joints which provide for rotation. Inward and outward twisting of the arm while in anatomical position is occurring in the horizontal plane around a vertical axis; however, when exactly the same twisting motion is performed with the arm held in front of the body and at shoulder level, the plane is frontal and the axis is sagittal. To clarify any confusion, it has become practice to describe rotational movements of the spine and limbs as occurring around their long axes if these movements are not in the horizontal plane.

The use of both an axis and a plane is appropriate only if angular motions are being described. Since linear motion is defined as motion during which all parts of the object move in the same direction and at the same velocity, there can be no axis of rotation. Linear motion is described, then, as occurring simply in a plane; angular motion is described as occurring both in a plane and around an axis.

## Joint Mechanics

When two bones form a connection, the resulting articulation is called a *joint*. The purpose of most joints is to provide for movement of the bones of the skeleton; however, some joints are structured to yield strength or form to the skeleton.

### Fibrous Joints

In fibrous joints (fig. 2.6), the connecting bones are held in almost direct contact with each other, with only a thin layer of connective tissue separating them. These joints, exemplified in the human body only by the sutures of the skull, are immovable and are designed to give form and structural strength to the skull.

### Cartilaginous Joint

The cartilaginous joint (fig. 2.7) is formed by the union of bones with intervening discs of fibrocartilage which permit slight movement but great strength. The articulation between the two pubic bones as well as those between the vertebrae are examples.

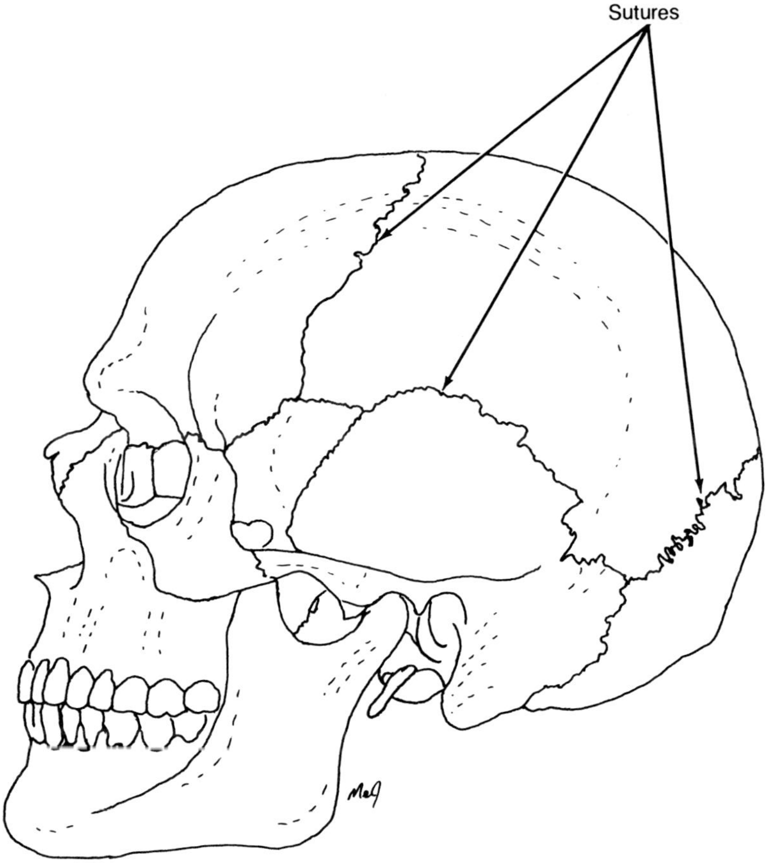

Sutures

**Figure 2.6. Fibrous joints of the skull**

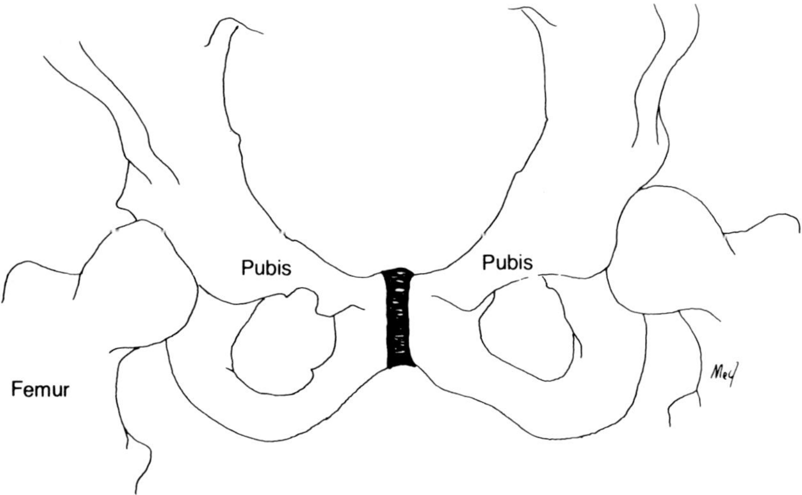


**Figure 2.7. Cartilaginous joint between pubic bones**

## Synovial Joints

Synovial or diarthrodial joints are freely movable and are characterized by the presence of a space between the articulating surfaces of the bones (fig. 2.8). The ends of the bones which make up the joint are typically flared and are covered with cartilage. The entire joint is wrapped with fibrous tissue—the synovial membrane—from which is secreted the lubricant, synovial fluid. Ligaments course between the bones to provide strength.

The synovial joint, because of its freedom of movement, is of utmost importance to the study of kinesiology. Such joints are categorized according to the number of axes around which the articulating bones can rotate. The anatomical reference position will be assumed for the discussion that follows.

**Nonaxial Joint** If the movement of articulating bones is linear rather than angular, the joint is nonaxial and displays gliding rather than angular motion. The amount of motion between the bones is limited either by ligaments or bony processes which surround the articulation. Examples of the gliding joints can be found between most of the carpal bones (fig. 2.9). Palpation of one of these gliding joints is shown in figure 2.10, wherein the pisiform bone is shown as a fist is made. The hand is then relaxed and pressure is applied with the fingers of the other hand to move the pisiform from side to side.

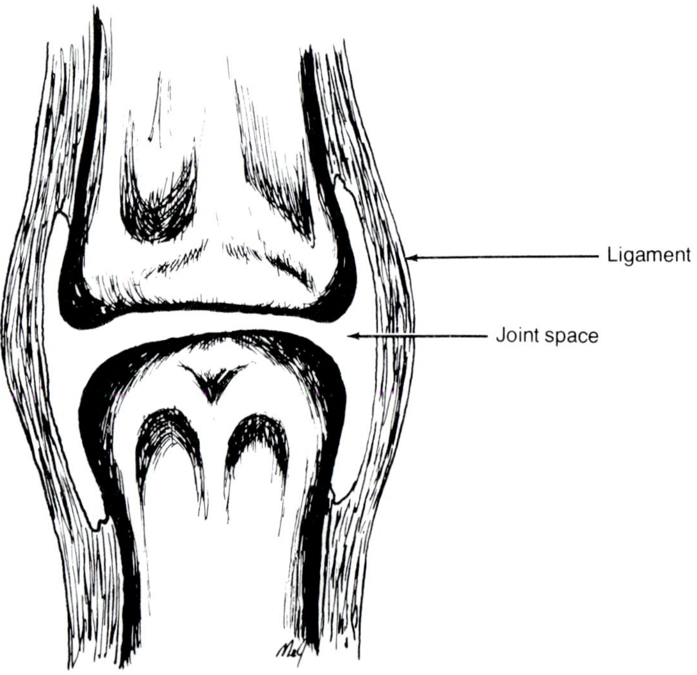


Figure 2.8. A synovial joint

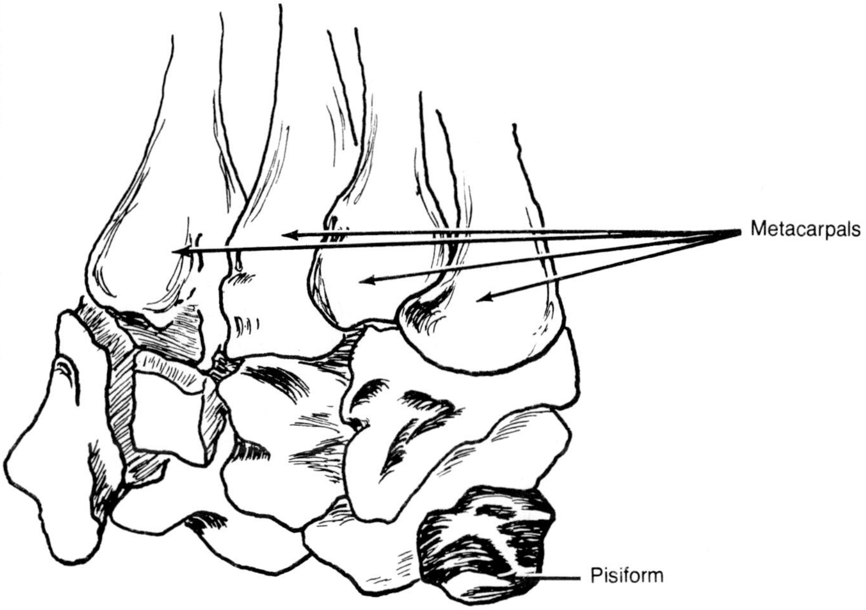

Metacarpals

Pisiform

Figure 2.9. Gliding joints of carpal bones

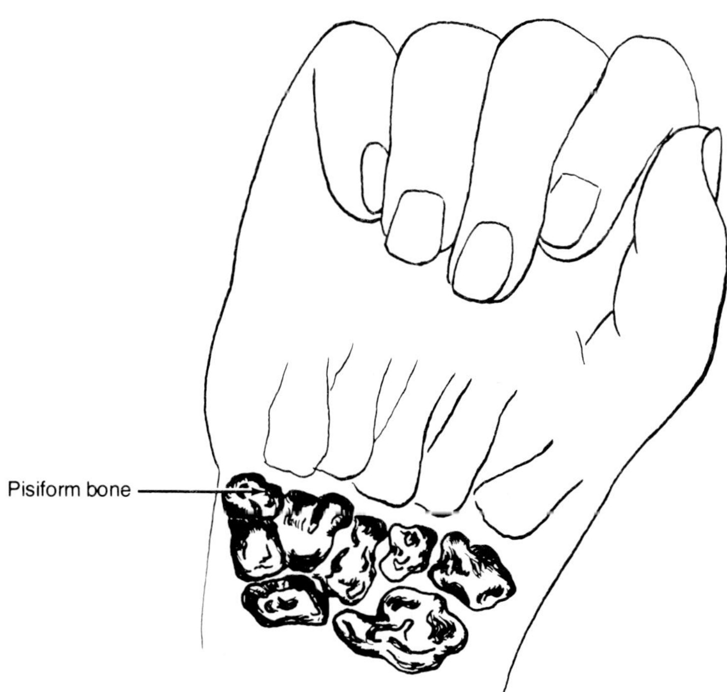


Figure 2.10. Palpation of pisiform bone

**Uniaxial Joint** A joint which permits angular motion around a single axis is called a *uniaxial joint.* The elbow joint, a hinge joint, allows rotation only around a frontal axis as the elbow is flexed and extended (fig. 2.11). The proximal radioulnar joint, a pivot joint (fig. 2.12), allows rotation only around a vertical axis as the forearm is pronated and supinated (inwardly and outwardly rotated).

**Biaxial Joint** If a bone is permitted, by the articulation it forms with another bone, to rotate around two perpendicular axes, its articulation is biaxial. The wrist joint, a condyloid joint, is formed by the oval surface of the lunate and navicular bones of the wrist and the elliptical cavity of the radius and articular disc (fig. 2.13). This arrangement provides for rotation of the hand around a frontal axis as the wrist is flexed and extended, and around a sagittal axis as the wrist is radially and ulnarly deviated (abducted and adducted). Because the joint is elongated rather than round, no motion is allowed around a vertical axis.

**Figure 2.11. Hinge joint of the elbow**

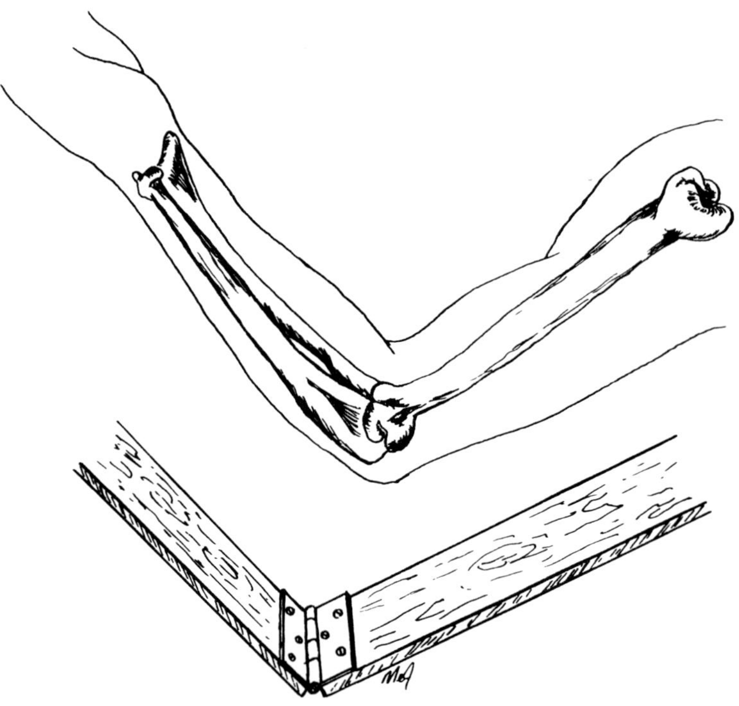

Humerus
Radio-ulnar joint

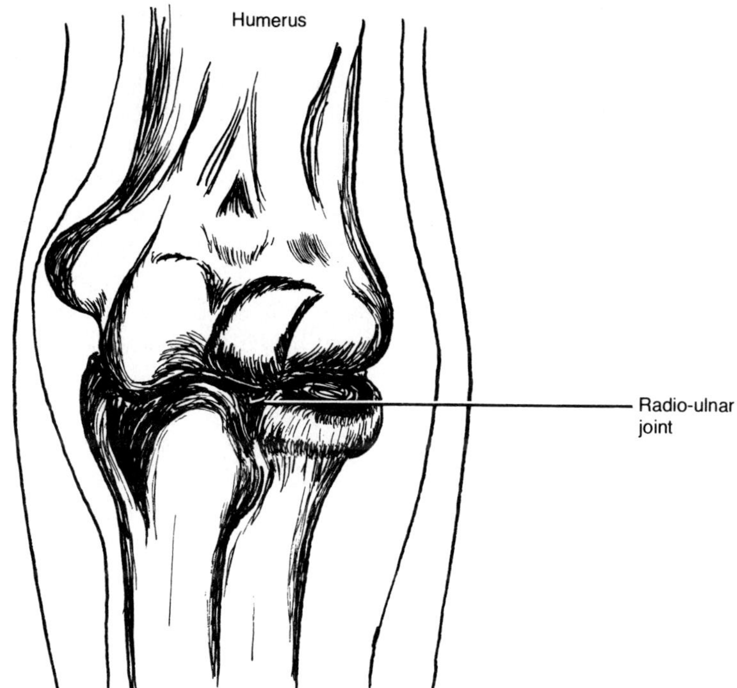

**Figure 2.12. Pivot joint between radius and ulna**

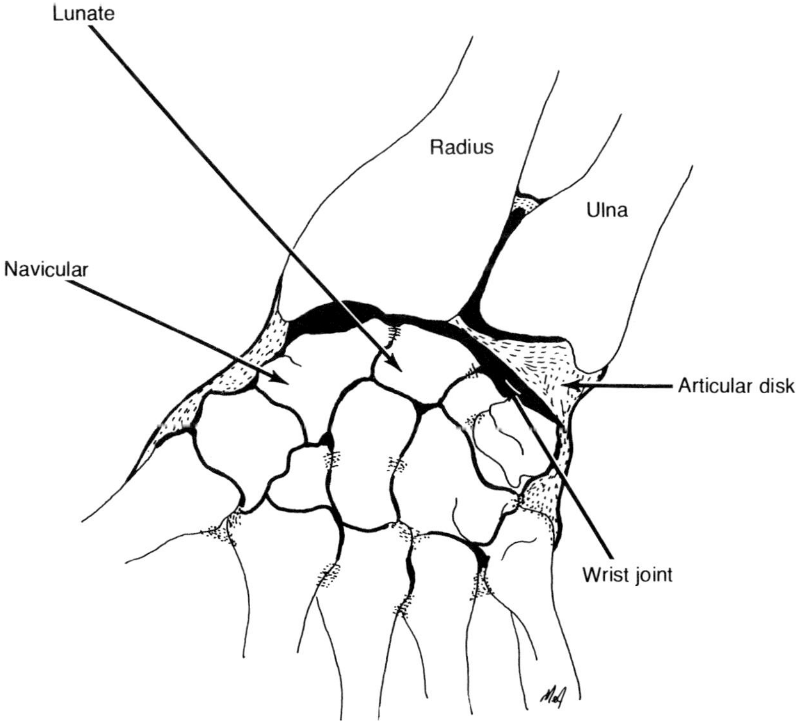

Lunate
Radius
Ulna
Navicular
Articular disk
Wrist joint

**Figure 2.13. Condyloid joint of the wrist**

Condyloid joints, by allowing for both flexion-extension and abduction-adduction movements, are capable, also, of permitting circumduction. Using the wrist joint again as an example, it will be noted that the hand can be made to circumscribe a cone, the apex of which is at the wirst. The base of the cone is traced by the fingertips. Circumduction is a combination movement and can be performed at any joint which comprises both flexion-extension and abduction-adduction capabilities. Other examples of these joints are the metacarpophalangeal joints of the fingers.

A second variety of the biaxial joint is the saddle joint in which the opposing surfaces of the bones are shaped reciprocally in a concave and convex manner. The joint resembles a rider in a saddle and is exemplified by the carpometacarpal joint of the thumb (fig. 2.14). The metacarpal of the thumb is the rider and the multangulus major is the saddle. The saddle joint allows for a flexion-extension type of motion (the rider rocking forward and backward in the saddle), for an abduction-adduction type of motion (the rider slipping from side to side in the saddle), and for circumduction.

**Triaxial Joint** The triaxial joint permits freedom of movement around the sagittal, frontal, and vertical axes. These joints, known as *ball-and-socket joints,* are formed by the reception of the globe-shaped head of one bone into the round concavity of the second bone. The best examples of the ball-and-socket joints are those of the hip and shoulder in which the three rotational axes can be easily imagined as the limb is flexed, extended, abducted, adducted, rotated, and circumducted (fig. 2.15).

**Figure 2.14. Saddle joint of thumb**

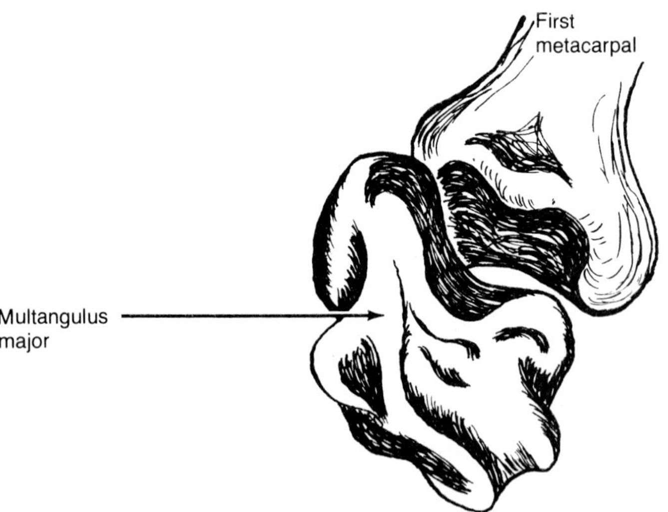

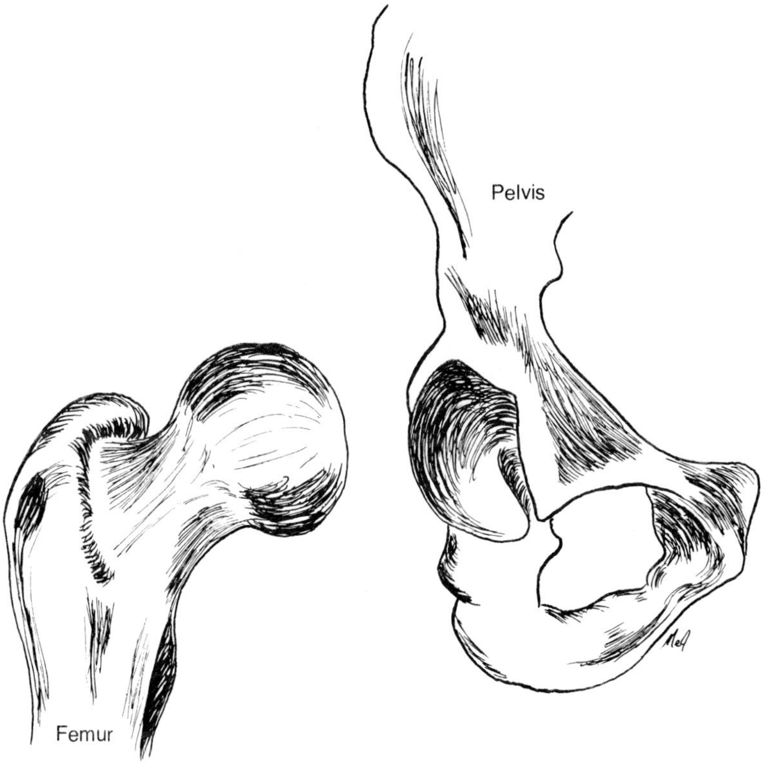

Figure 2.15. Ball-and-socket joint of hip

One may wonder, at this point, why such importance is attached to the axial nature of the respective synovial joints. In order to fully appreciate, rather than simply memorize, the actions of muscles, the muscles must be envisioned with respect to the axes of rotation of the joint they surround. For example, the axis of rotation of the hinge joint at the elbow passes through the two bony prominences at the distal end of the humerus (fig. 2.16). Any muscle which crosses the elbow joint and is anterior to the axis will flex the joint and move the lower arm forward and upward in the sagittal plane. Conversely, any muscle crossing the joint posterior to the axis will extend the joint, causing the lower arm to move downwardly and backward in the sagittal plane.

The axes of rotation of the specific joints will be discussed fully in the chapters devoted to the respective portions of the body, and the muscles will be described with regard to their locations about the axes. The tedium of memorizing muscle actions can then be replaced, in part at least, by logical deduction.

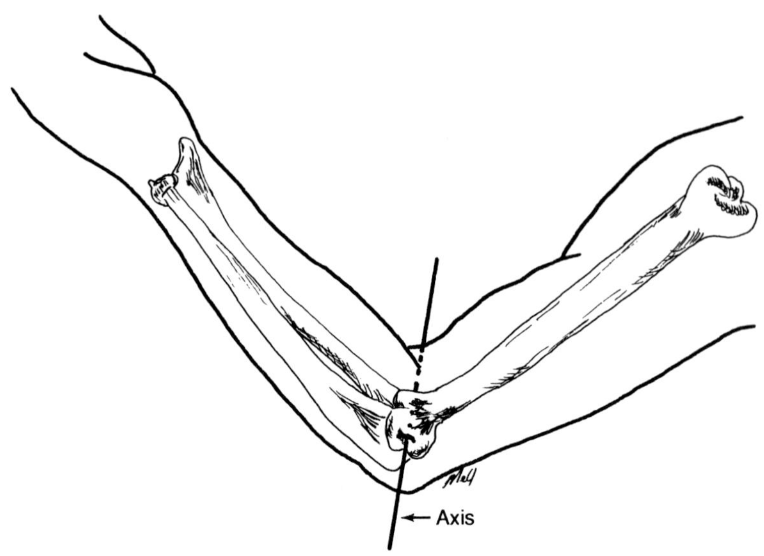


Figure 2.16. Axis of rotation of elbow joint

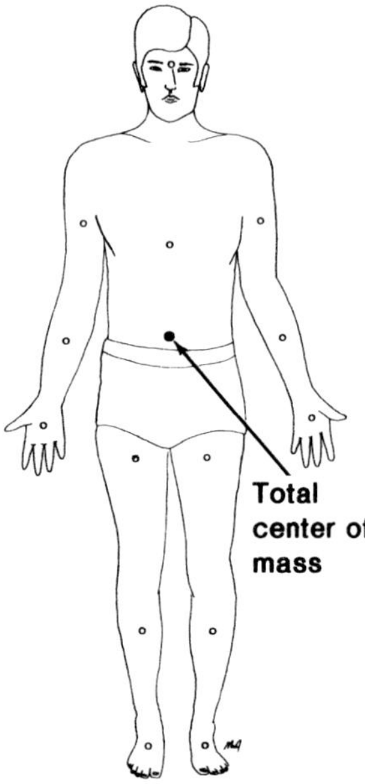

Total center of mass

Figure 2.17. Total and segmental centers of mass

## Center of Mass of the Human Body and Its Segments

The point in the human body at which its mass is concentrated is the total body center of mass. The location of this point depends upon the posture of the body—standing, sitting, arms raised, trunk flexed—as well as upon the build of the body—narrow shoulders, wide hips, heavy thighs—but for purposes of this discussion, it will suffice to assume the standing position, and locate the total body center of mass in the middle of the pelvis, at or about the level of the upper sacrum.

The point in a segment of the human body at which its mass is concentrated is the segmental center of mass. Figure 2.17 illustrates the approximate locations of these centers, as well as that of the total body center of mass.

The importance of the various centers of mass to kinesiology lies primarily in the fact that as segments of the body are moved against the force of gravity, their weights are considered to be localized at their centers of mass. As will be seen in the following discussion on leverage, the location of the weight of a segment can dictate whether that segment will be capable of generating speed or force. Principles relating center of mass to stability and equilibrium are discussed in Part II, "Mechanical Aspects of Human Motion."

## Levers of the Human Body

A lever is a rigid bar that has an axis of rotation *(A)*, a point at which force is applied *(F)*, and a resistance which must be balanced or overcome *(R)*. The three types of levers are designated according to which of their three components, axis, force, or resistance, is between the other two components.

In a first class lever, the axis of rotation is located somewhere between the point of force application and the resistance (fig. 2.18). In the second class lever, the resistance is between the force and the axis (fig. 2.19). The third class lever is distinguished by the locations of the axis and resistance on the ends of the lever with the force application between them (fig. 2.20).

All levers can be divided into two segments known as the *moment arm,* which is the perpendicular distance between the line of force application and the axis, and the *resistance arm,* which is the perpendicular distance between the line of resistance and the axis. When the moment arm is equal to the resistance arm, the lever has a mechanical advantage of one; that is, for every unit of weight the resistance represents, an equivalent unit of force will be required to balance the

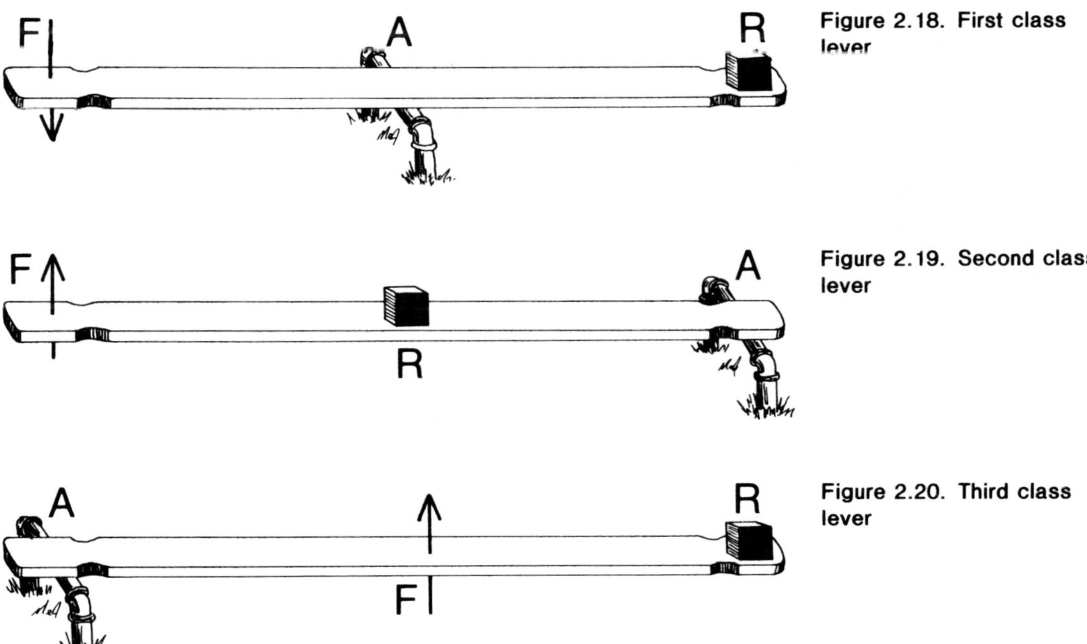


Figure 2.18. First class lever

Figure 2.19. Second class lever

Figure 2.20. Third class lever

Figure 2.21. Moment arm and resistance arm of a first class lever

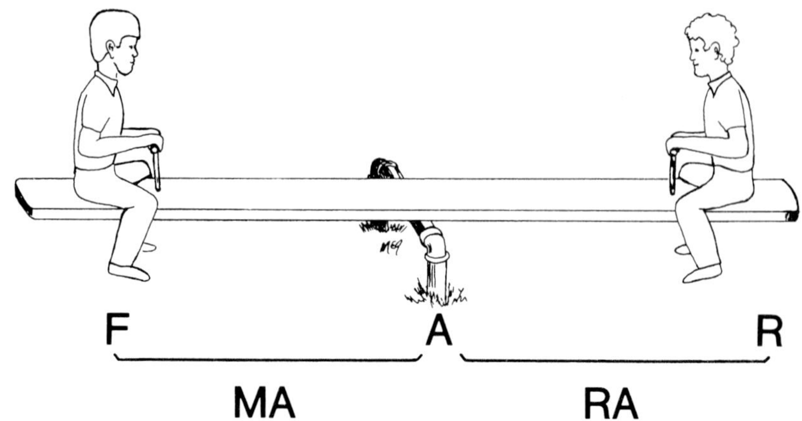


lever. In the case of the seesaw shown in figure 2.21, the moment arm and the resistance arm are equal. If the child on the right weighs 25 kilograms, the child on the left must also weigh 25 kilograms if the seesaw is to balance.

The use of a screw driver to pry open a paint can, although still a first class lever, yields a different mechanical advantage (fig. 2.22). If the resistance arm is 2 centimeters long and the moment arm is 20 centimeters long, the mechanical advantage is 10. For every ten units of resistance with which the can is capped, only one unit of force is required to balance the lever.

It can be seen that mechanical advantage is equal to the moment arm divided by the resistance arm—$MA/RA$. It will be noted, also, that depending upon the location of the axis between the force application and the point of resistance, the mechanical advantage of a first class lever can range from less than one (axis located close to force point) to infinity (axis located close to resistance). The greater the mechanical advantage, the greater the resistance that can be balanced by a given force.

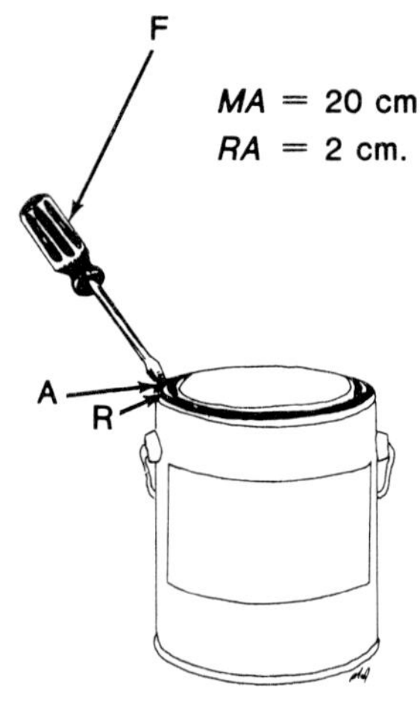


Figure 2.22. First class lever with mechanical advantage of ten

Application of the concept of mechanical advantage to the second class lever indicates that, regardless of the placement of the resistance along the lever, the moment arm will always be longer than the resistance arm. The mechanical advantage must always be, then, greater than one and can range, again, to infinity as the resistance is placed closer and closer to the axis.

The third class lever, conversely, yields a mechanical advantage which is always less than one. Regardless of the point at which the force is applied, the resistance arm will always be longer than the moment arm.

Using mechanical advantage as the criterion, it is possible to rank the three lever types with regard to their capacity to balance and overcome resistance. The second class lever, with its mechanical advantage of one or more, has greatest capacity, and the third class lever, with its mechanical advantage of less than one has the weakest capacity.

The student may question the phrase "balance the lever" used in the foregoing discussion since levers are employed usually not to balance resistance, but rather to overcome it. All considerations regarding leverage are based upon force requirements to balance resistances. If the balancing force is known, it is known, also, that any increment in force, no matter how small, will cause the lever to move and thus overcome the resistance.

The levers of the human body are the bony segments of the skeleton. Axes of the levers are the joints; points of force application are the insertions of the muscles; and resistances are the centers of mass of the bony segments to be moved, whether they are additionally weighted by some object to be lifted, or whether they offer only the resistance of their own weights.

In the human body, first and second class levers are seldom found. Examples of a first class lever are the triceps brachii, acting on the forearm when it is positioned above the head (see p. 89, fig. 4.12), and the neck extensors pulling downwardly on the back of the head to balance its weight across the first vertebra. A second class lever is exemplified by the forearm and the brachioradialis. Since the center of mass of the forearm is between the elbow and the insertion of the brachioradialis (see p. 84, fig. 4.7), a second class system is formed.

Third class levers predominate in the human body, being found almost totally throughout the upper and lower extremities. This may seem paradoxical in view of the relatively heavy weights or resistances which we are able to lift and move. The paradox disappears, however, when we consider that our muscles are capable of exerting forces far in excess of any resistance we overcome. The quadriceps, the anterior muscles of the upper leg, are able to apply a force of 200 to 300 kilograms. A visit to the weight room will show that the maximum weight (resistance) which can be lifted by extending the knee is probably between 20 and 40 kilograms. It is clear that the human body is handicapped in its strength capability by the adverse mechanical advantage of third class levers.

One may wonder why the human body has not evolved as a system of forceful second class levers rather than weak third class levers. The reason appears to be in the fact that third class levers are capable of generating great speed. Their predominance in the human body

Figure 2.23. Third class lever with mechanical advantage of one-fourth

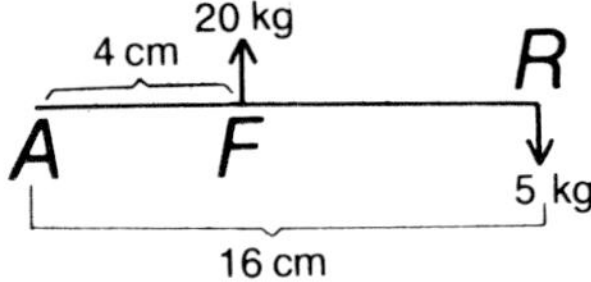


allows us to perform throwing and kicking tasks at incredible speeds rather than having to overcome great resistances with the ponderousness of the second class lever.

Leverage calculations are relatively simple and are derived from the formula $F \cdot MA = R \cdot RA$. This is a mathematical statement of balanced levers in which $F$ is force, $MA$ is the moment arm, $R$ is resistance, and $RA$ is resistance arm. Figure 2.23 illustrates a third class lever with a moment arm of 4 and a resistance arm of 16. The resistance to be balanced is 5 kilograms. By rearranging the formula to $F = R \cdot RA/MA$ and substituting, force is found to be 20 kilograms. Any force in excess of 20 kilograms will overcome a resistance of 5 kilograms if the lever has a mechanical advantage of one-fourth.

A second example of a leverage calculation is shown in figure 2.24. The mechanical advantage is 7/35 or 1/5, and the force being applied is 40 kilograms. Since $R = F \cdot MA/RA$, it can be found that a resistance of 8 kilograms will be balanced. A force of 40 kilograms is required to hold a lower leg weighing 8 kilograms in full extension.

## Composition of Forces

Force is a vector quantity. It has both magnitude (kilograms, pounds, grams) and direction (horizontal, vertical, diagonal). Because it is a vector, force can be represented by a line the length of which is scaled to the units of the force, and direction of which is indicated by an

Figure 2.24. Third class lever with mechanical advantage of one-fifth

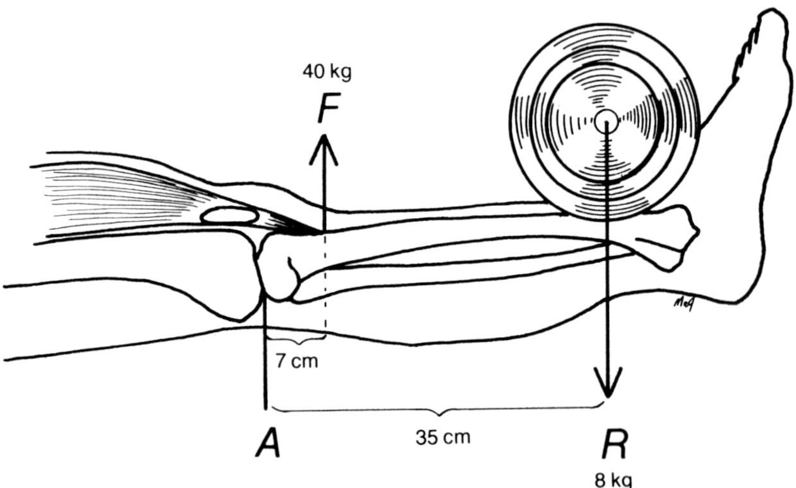

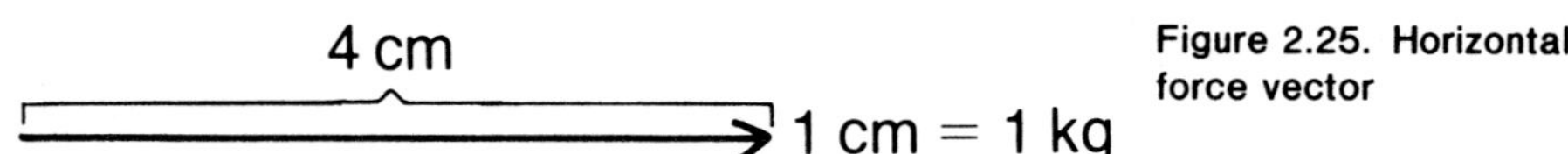


Figure 2.25. Horizontal force vector

arrow at the end of the line. Figure 2.25 is a horizontal force vector which is 4 centimeters long. It has been scaled so that 1 centimeter of length equals 1 kilogram of force. The vector represents, therefore, 4 kilograms of force directed horizontally and to the right.

In figure 2.26, two forces ($F_1$ and $F_2$), each of 4 kilograms, are being applied simultaneously to an object. Their total effect, that is, their resultant ($F$), is 8 kilograms and is directed to the right.

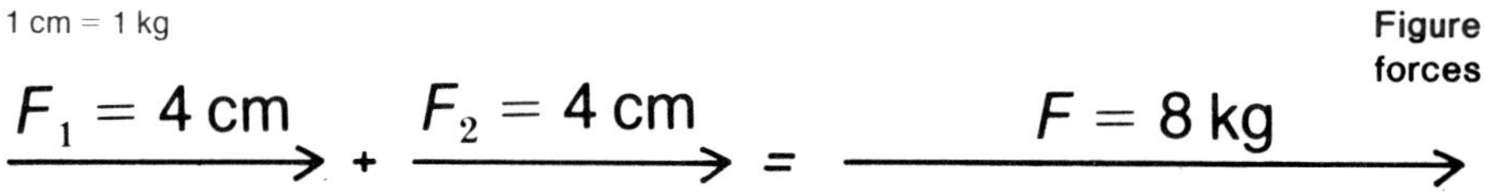

1 cm = 1 kg

$F_1 = 4$ cm $\rightarrow$ + $F_2 = 4$ cm $\rightarrow$ = $F = 8$ kg $\rightarrow$

Figure 2.26. Summing of forces

Figure 2.27 shows two forces of different magnitudes and opposite directions being applied simultaneously to an object. The resultant of these forces is 2 kilograms directed to the left.

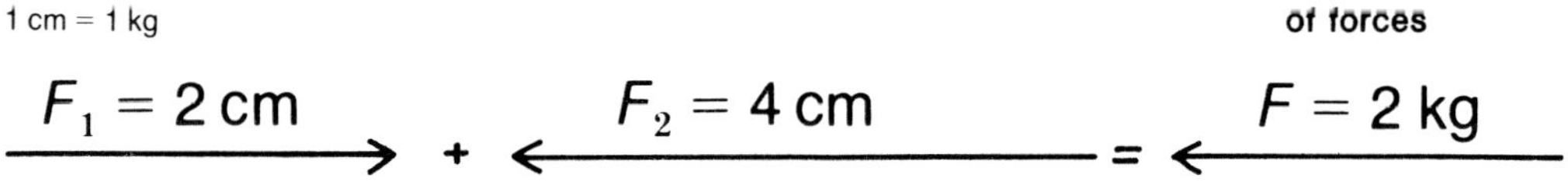

1 cm = 1 kg

$F_1 = 2$ cm $\rightarrow$ + $\leftarrow$ $F_2 = 4$ cm = $\leftarrow$ $F = 2$ kg

Figure 2.27. Subtraction of forces

Figure 2.28 depicts several forces being applied to the scapula by the simultaneous contraction of surrounding musculature. The resultant of these forces is two units in magnitude and is directed vertically. Under the conditions shown in the illustration, the scapula will be elevated with two units of force.

From the above discussion, a general statement can be made: If two or more forces are applied simultaneously and along a common direction, their resultant is the algebraic sum of the forces. The direction of the resultant will be that of the remaining algebraic sign.

When forces act at an angle to each other rather than along a directional line, their resultant must be found by other means. If $F_1$ and $F_2$ (figure 2.29) are acting at right angles to each other, their resultant, $F$, will be the diagonal of a parallelogram constructed around them. The magnitude of the resultant is calculated as shown in the figure. The direction of the resultant is traditionally reported as the

Figure 2.28. Summation of forces

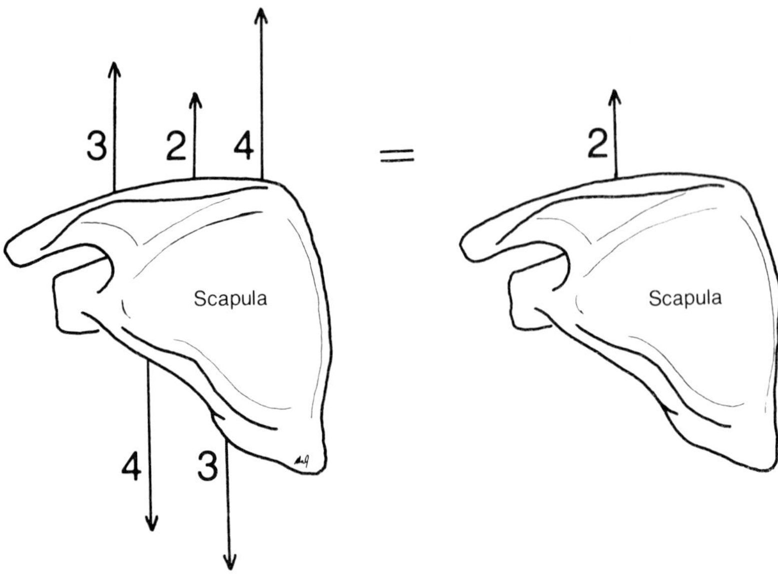


Figure 2.29. Determination of the resultant force, $F$

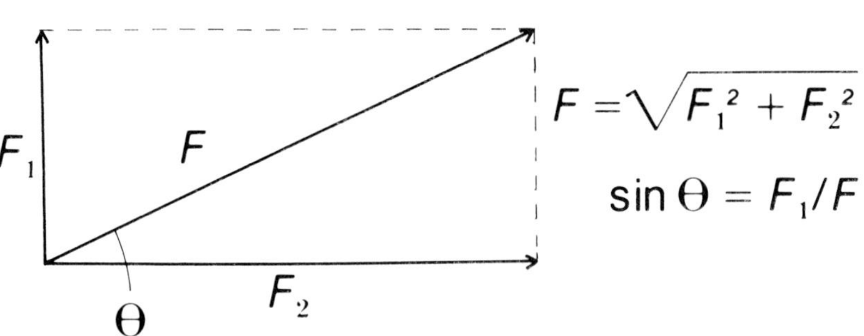


angle it makes, in a counterclockwise direction, with the horizontal. This angle can be found easily through the use of trigonometric functions.

If $F_1$ and $F_2$ are not at right angles to each other (figure 2.30), their resultant will still be the diagonal of a parallelogram; however, the magnitude and direction of the resultant must be calculated by use of the trigonometric law of cosines.

For the purposes of this text, resultants will be incorporated in the narrative in a conceptual rather than mathematical way. The student who is interested in exploring further the mathematics of force composition is urged to refer to the several biomechanic texts which are currently available.

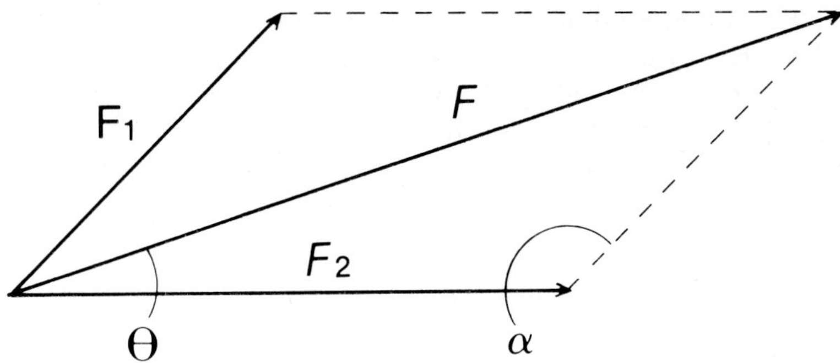


Figure 2.30. Determination of resultant, $F$, from the two forces, $F_1$ and $F_2$.

$$F = \sqrt{F_1{}^2 + F_2{}^2 - 2\,F_1F_2 \cos \alpha}$$

$$\cos \alpha = \frac{F_1{}^2 + F_2{}^2 - F^2}{2\,F_1F_2}$$

$$\text{and } \cos \Theta = \frac{F^2 + F_2{}^2 - F_1{}^2}{2\,F F_2}$$

## Resolution of Forces

Force resolution is the converse of force composition. To resolve a force is to separate it into two forces, the directions of which are known. Only diagonal forces such as those illustrated in figure 2.31 will be considered; such forces will be resolved into two component forces which are at right angles to each other.

The procedure of resolution will be enhanced if two rules are followed:

1. The two components of a diagonal force will be at right angles to each other and will include the diagonal force vector between them.
2. The lengths of the two component force vectors will be such that when the tips of the two component vectors are connected to the tip of the diagonal vector, a rectangle will result.

Figure 2.31 illustrates the procedure of force resolution. From the end of the diagonal force vector *F*, two vectors are drawn at right angles and on either side of *F*. When the tips of the three arrows are connected, a rectangle is formed.

Figure 2.32 shows the application of force resolution to a problem in kinesiology. A diagonal force representing a muscle is seen to attach to the scapula. By resolving the diagonal vector, it can be observed that the muscle in question moves the scapula diagonally because of its tendency to pull the scapula toward the spine and toward the head.

Force resolution is exemplified again in figure 2.33, in which the biceps brachii is illustrated as attached diagonally to the forearm. Resolution of the force vector of the biceps brachii is accomplished by drawing, from the end of the diagonal force vector, an arrow along the forearm and one at right angles to the forearm. The appropriate length of the two component vectors has been achieved when a rectangle results from the connection of the three arrow tips.

The case of force resolution of diagonal muscle pull against bony levers such as the forearm is a special one. The two component vectors are always envisioned as being along or parallel to the bone and perpendicular to the bone. The vector which is directed along the bone and toward the joint acts to press the articulating surfaces of the bones together; this component is called, therefore, the *stabilizing component*. The vector at right angles to the bone is the component which causes the bone to rotate about the joint axis and is called the *angular component*. Comparison of the relative lengths of the angular and

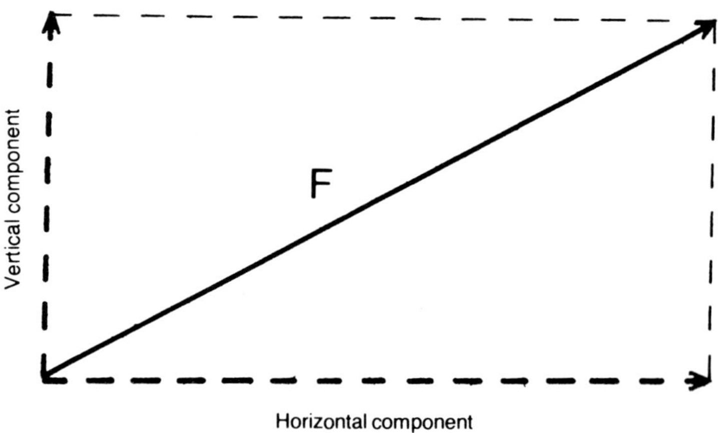


**Figure 2.31.** Resolution of the force, *F* into its vertical and horizontal components

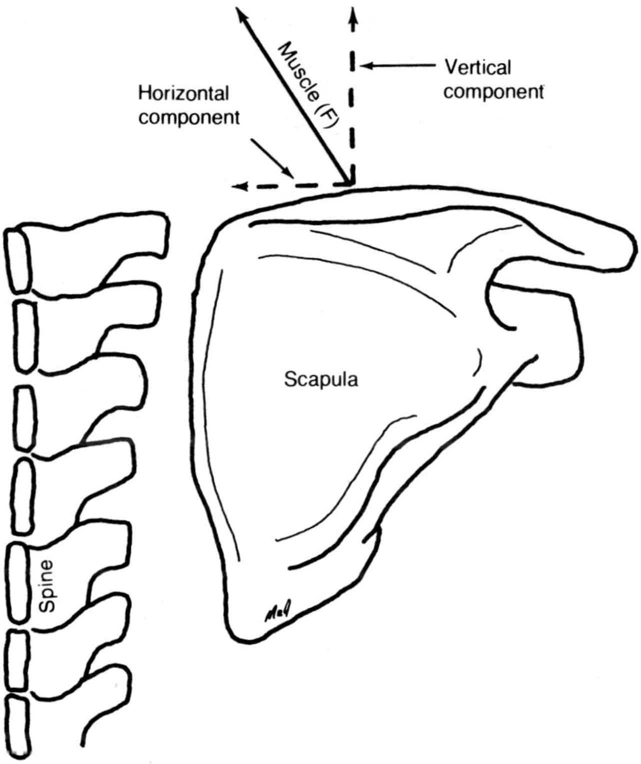

Muscle (F)
Vertical component
Horizontal component
Scapula
Spine

**Figure 2.32. Resolution of a diagonal force, *F***

Angular force component
10 kg
Stabilizing force component

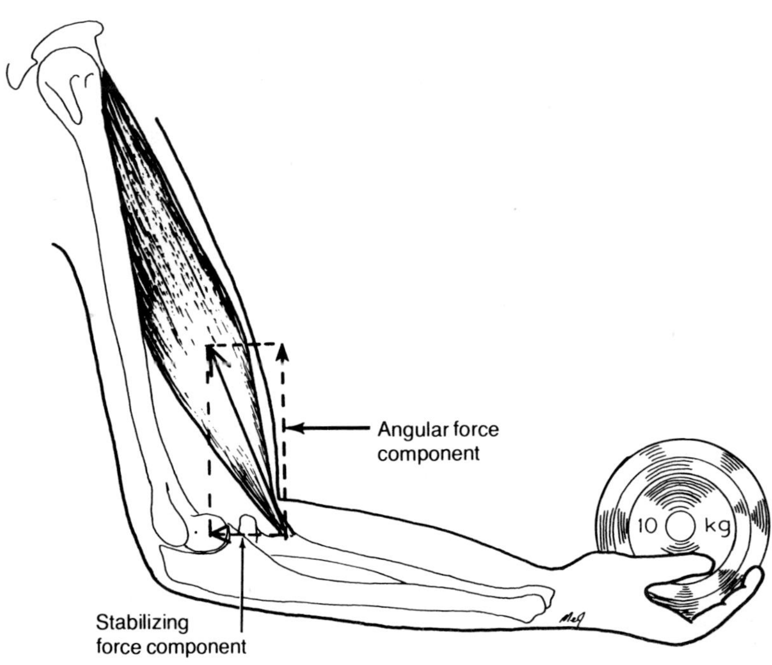

**Figure 2.33. Force resolution of the pull of the biceps brachii**

stabilizing vectors will lead to conclusions regarding the effectiveness of a muscle to move the joint it crosses. The longer the angular component is in relationship to the stabilizing component, the more effectively the muscle can cause movement and the less effectively it can stabilize the joint.

Several joints of the body are crossed by muscles which, according to the position of the joint, have changeable angles of insertion. The elbow, knee, and hip joints are examples, and to illustrate this discussion, the elbow will be chosen as it is crossed by the biceps brachii.

If the elbow is held in full extension, the angle between the tendon of the biceps and the radius is small. Resolution of the biceps' force yields a long stabilizing component and a comparatively short angular component—the biceps is relatively ineffective as a mover of the forearm when the elbow is extended. As the elbow is flexed, however, the angle between the tendon and the radius gradually becomes larger; the accompanying resolution comprises angular components which are lengthening as the stabilizing components are becoming shorter. The biceps is thus becoming more and more effective as a mover and less and less effective as a stabilizer.

When the elbow joint reaches a point of flexion in which the angle between the tendon of the biceps and the radius is 90 degrees, the only component of force is the angular one. At this joint position, the biceps will be at its peak effectiveness as a mover but will apply no stabilizing force to the joint.

Continued flexion of the elbow causes the angle between the tendon and the radius to become greater than 90 degrees. Resolution of the biceps' force will again yield two components, one the angular component, and the other a component directed along the bone but away from the joint. The latter component is acting to pull the joint apart and is called the *dislocating component.* The dislocating component of the biceps' force gradually elongates as the elbow joint flexes to full range; the angular component simultaneously shortens and indicates a decreasing effectiveness of the biceps as the elbow nears full flexion.

The biceps brachii, as well as any other muscle which can be made to insert through a range of angles, will be mechanically at its optimum to provide strength when it attaches at 90 degrees. The farther from the perpendicular the angle of insertion becomes, the weaker the muscle will be as a joint mover.

## Muscle Attachments

In its simplest form, a muscle has two bony attachments and crosses a single joint. When the muscle contracts, it shortens, causing its two attachments to become closer together as permitted by the joint. Typically, one attachment is on a bone which moves easily; the other attachment is on a bone more difficult to move. It is to be expected that contraction of the muscle will cause motion of the bone which is the freer of the two to move. When the body is in anatomical or fundamental reference position, one can predict very accurately which bone will move with contraction of an attaching muscle. For example, a muscle which attaches to the ribs and to the upper arm will cause the arm to move rather than the ribs; a muscle which courses from a bone in the forearm to a bone in the hand will cause the hand to move rather than the forearm. Because of the predictability of action, it is possible to distinguish between the two attachments according to which will be stable and which will move. The origin of a muscle is the attachment on the more stable of the two bones; the insertion is the attachment on the bone freer to move.

In the performance of sports and dance techniques, the position of the body or the movement task to be performed may require the origin and insertion to alternate. The brachialis, an elbow flexor which attaches to the humerus and the ulna, usually acts to pull the forearm (insertion) toward the humerus (origin) when it contracts. If the forearm is stabilized, however, as it would be during the performance of the chinning exercise, contraction of the brachialis will flex the elbow by pulling the humerus toward the forearm. The origin and insertion have reversed themselves to satisfy the requirements of the task. A second example can be seen in the rectus abdominis. It is listed as a flexor of the spine, with its origin at the pubis and its insertion on the ribs. It is to be expected, therefore, that contraction of this muscle will cause the spine to bow and the shoulders and trunk to bend forward toward the hips. This expectation will be correct if the body is in anatomical position, because the bearing of weight precludes significant movement of the hips toward the torso. If the upper body is held stable, however, contraction of the rectus abdominis will rotate the pubic crest upwardly around the hip joints for upward tilt of the pelvis. Origin and insertion have, thus, been reversed.

One school of kinesiological thought recommends the use of *proximal* and *distal* or *medial* and *lateral* to describe muscle attachments. According to this terminology, the brachialis would be depicted as a muscle with proximal attachment on the humerus and distal attachment of the ulna. Whereas this terminology has the advantage of consistency (proximal seldom becomes distal, etc.), it does not inform the reader of the true nature of the movement to be caused. To know that a muscle that attaches to the scapula and to the back of the head is contracting with an origin on the scapula is to know that muscular effort is being spent to move the head, not the scapula. Knowing only that the muscle attaches proximally on the head and distally to the scapula does nothing to describe the type of movement to be expected.

Physiologically, a muscle is comprised of a contractile portion and one or more cordlike structures called *tendons.* The type of muscle envisioned most frequently is that shown in figure 2.34. The contractile portion in the center rounds smoothly to form a *belly* and then becomes tendinous on each end. The biceps brachii is an example of such a muscle. Through its tendons, it attaches to bony prominences on the scapula and radius (see p. 72, fig. 3.26). Not all muscles have such typical characteristics, however. Some do not originate with a tendinous attachment, but rather make attachment through the sheaths of the contractile fibers, themselves. Examples are the muscles that attach to the scapula (see chapter 3). The reason for the different structures would appear to stem from the size of the surface area of

**Figure 2.34. Relative lengths of a typical muscle during stretch, contraction, and rest**

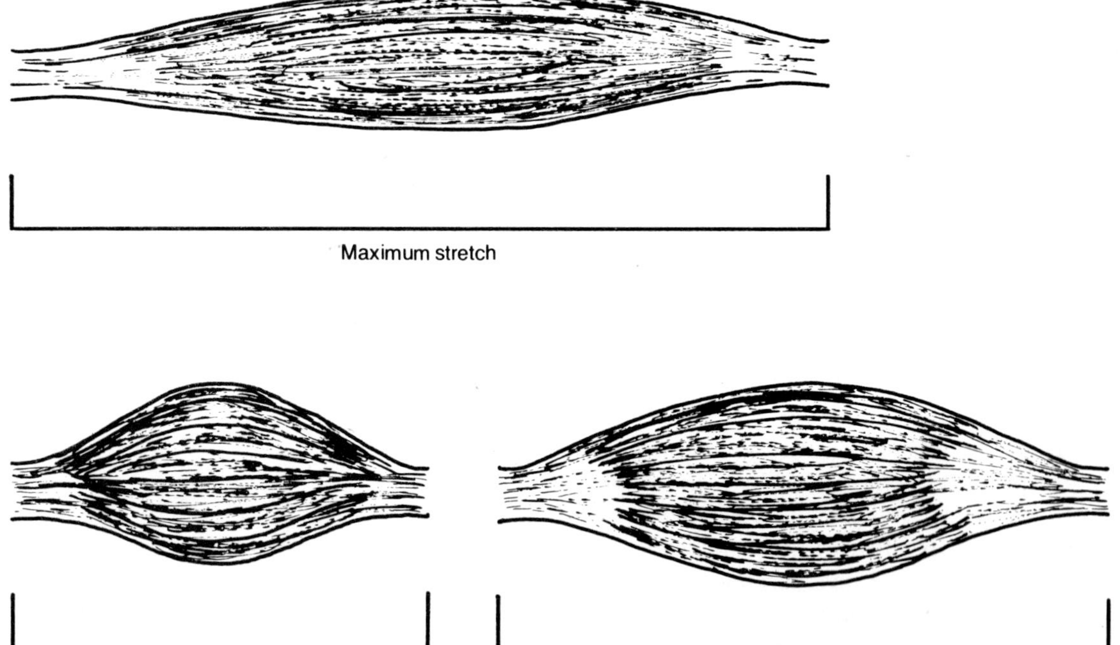

attachment. If the area is large, contraction force can be spread sufficiently to allow attachment via the fiber sheaths. If the area is small, the muscle must terminate in strong tendons that can transmit large amounts of force to their respective bony prominences.

## Excursion Ratio

Muscle tissue is characterized by the properties of extensibility, elasticity, and contractility. Its extensibility property allows it to stretch; its elasticity permits it to return from stretch to its resting length; its ability to contract allows it to shorten from the resting length. In figure 2.34, a typical muscle is depicted at its resting, stretched, and contracted length. The ratio of stretched length to contracted length is referred to as the *excursion ratio of the muscle.* For the muscle illustrated, the excursion ratio is 2:1; that is, the muscle is capable of stretching to a length twice as long as it can shorten. A ratio of 2:1 is considered average for muscles of the human body, and is, for the most part, adequate to allow joints to move through their full ranges. Where muscles cross several joints, however, their excursion ratios may be inadequate to allow either for simultaneous extension or flexion of the several joints involved. This is exemplified by the muscle which extends the fingers. It is a multiple-joint muscle, crossing some five joints between its origin above the elbow and its insertion on the third phalanx of each finger. When an attempt is made to hold the wrist and fingers in full extension, it will be noted that the wrist is limited in its range. If the fingers are allowed to curl, the wrist can extend farther—evidence that the contractile ability of the muscle is not sufficient to move all of the joints it crosses through their full ranges of extension. Similarly, the extensibility of the muscle will not allow all the joints to flex simultaneously. It is impossible to maintain a firm fist while also flexing the wrist because the muscle is incapable of stretching to that extent.

## Muscle Fiber Arrangement

Muscle fibers are arranged according to two basic patterns, longitudinal and penniform (fig. 2.35). Included under the longitudinal arrangement are strap, rhomboidal, triangular, and fusiform muscles. These are exemplified in the human body by the sartorius, pronator quadratus, pectoralis major, and biceps brachii, respectively, and have in common an above average excursion ratio, but are somewhat limited, when compared to penniform muscles, in strength. Penniform muscles are subcategorized as single penniform, bipenniform, and

Figure 2.35. Fiber structure of human muscles

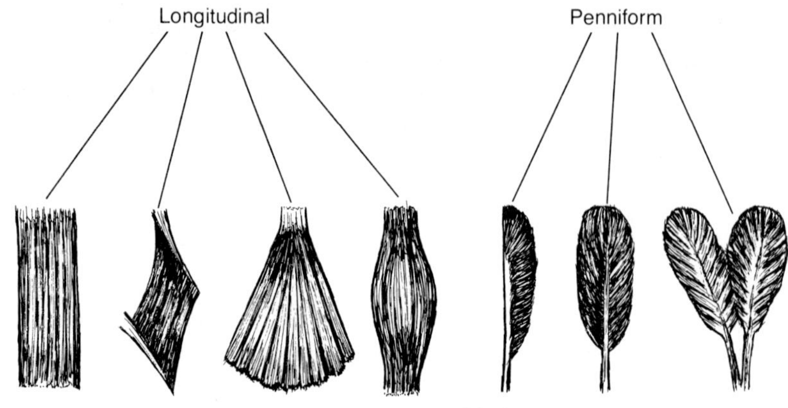


multipenniform. The flexor digitorum longus, rectus femoris, and deltoid are examples of these arrangements and, together with all other penniform muscles, offer comparatively low excursion ratios but are extremely strong.

Knowledge of the fiber arrangements of the many muscles of the body can be of help to the kinesiologist as he seeks to explain a specific muscle's contribution to movement. Muscles which are required for strength of movement are, in general, penniform; it is not surprising that many of the muscles of the lower limb are of that arrangement. Muscles of the upper limb are more of the longitudinal type demanded for range of movement.

## The Anatomy of Contraction: An Overview

Whereas an intense treatment of neuroanatomy is beyond the scope of this book, it may be helpful to provide a brief overview of the structure of the nervous system and the physiology of muscle contraction. Remarks will be limited to the central and peripheral nervous systems and to contraction mechanics of striated muscle; they should be considered only as a review of more basic material.

The structural unit of the nervous system is a neuron. It is composed of a cell body and processes called axons and dendrites. Nerve impulses are conducted to the cell body by dendrites and away from it by axons. Through this basic structure and its combination with other neurons, impulses are passed from the central nervous system to the peripheral nervous system and also returned to it. It is the combination of many axon fibers, which makes up the nerve.

The majority of axon fibers are surrounded by a myelin sheath, which is laid down by Schwann cells. These cells engulf the axon and rotate around it several times, adding a layer of myelin with each rotation, until the sheath is complete. The purpose of the sheath is to prevent significant flow of ions between the extracellular spaces and the axon. The sheath acts, therefore, much as an electrical insulation.

At intervals along the axon, the sheath is interrupted, exposing uninsulated areas called the nodes of Ranvier. Ions flow with ease through the nodes and allow a nerve impulse to jump from node to node rather than to be conducted continuously through the fiber. Such *saltatory* progress of the impulse is thought to contribute to the higher velocities of nerve transmission of myelinated fibers as compared to their unmyelinated counterparts.

It can be seen that a nerve is a complex structure comprised of myelinated and unmyelinated axons, which carry nerve impulses throughout the body. Axons vary considerably in length, some are less than a centimeter long, whereas others extend for over a meter. Even with such variation, however, it is necessary for axons to junction or synapse either with the cell body at their originations and/or with dendrites at their ends.

In its simplest form, a synapse is a narrow gap between the flared end of an axon and the cell body or a dendrite of another cell body. At the flared termination of the axon are vesicles containing an excitatory substance that is secreted by the arrival of a stimulus and increases the permeability of the postsynaptic membrane to sodium ions. Sodium ions, carrying their electropositive charge, rush through the membrane and reverse the normal negative charge that is characteristic of the resting state of the membrane. Depolarization is now complete and the impulse has been transmitted across the synapse.

Almost immediately after depolarization occurs, the membrane once again becomes impermeable to sodium ions. Not only is further inward movement blocked but also is any outward flow. The membrane is, however, permeable to potassium ions, which are attracted from inside the membrane to the outside because of the electronegative state created there by depolarization. This rapid diffusion of the potassium ions returns the membrane to its resting voltage and repolarization has begun. It cannot be complete, however, until the sodium and potassium ions are returned to their original locations outside and inside the membrane. This process is accomplished by the sodium and potassium pumps—a relatively slow and energy consuming process. When the ions have been returned, repolarization is complete and the membrane has reestablished its true resting state.

Depolarization and repolarization do not occur only in the area of the synapse, as might be supposed from the foregoing discussion. Rather, depolarization, followed closely by repolarization, travels in wavelike fashion along the length of an axon. It will be recalled that the wave of movement along myelinated fibers is saltatory in nature, whereas it occurs through the entire length of unmyelinated fibers. It is the wave of depolarization that is thought of as the transmission of a nerve impulse.

Any interruption in the wave of depolarization will, of course, block nerve transmission. Among such interruptions are trauma, nutritional imbalance, and local anesthetics. Local anesthetics have been developed expressly to prevent the secretion of excitatory transmitters by the vesicles of the axons. Nutritional imbalances of potassium, sodium, and calcium can impede the processes of depolarization and repolarization and can result in increased or decreased excitability of the membrane.

Trauma to nerve tissues ranges generally from first to fifth degree in severity. First-degree trauma is characterized by the presence of pressure extreme enough to block transmission but not cause degeneration of tissue. Numbness in the feet after sitting on hard surfaces for long periods of time may be indicative of the exertion of pressure on the sciatic nerve.

Fifth-degree trauma involves the complete severance of a nerve trunk with accompanying loss of sensation and muscular paralysis. Surgerv involving the rejoining of the severed ends or of uniting them by grafts is often indicated for these types of trauma. Under satisfactory conditions, regeneration of axons can occur at the rate of 1 to 2 mm per day. Not all regenerating axons find their original paths, however. Some may find their way to the wrong end organ. Examples of such misdirection can be felt when rubbing a scar causes pricks of sensation on the opposite side of the trauma.

Just as the neuron is the structural unit of the nervous system, the muscle fiber (or cell) is the basic unit of the muscular system. Muscle fibers are typically arranged in parallel fashion throughout the muscle, although they may or may not be parallel to the length of the muscle. Various arrangements are possible and are discussed later in this chapter. It should be noted, however, that when a muscle fiber contracts, it does so by applying a force through its length.

The transmission of a nervous impulse to a muscle fiber is basically the same as has been discovered above regarding neural synapses. The synapse between an axon and muscle fiber is called the neuromuscular junction (also called a myoneural synapse). The appearance of the neuromuscular junction differs from that of the neural synapse in that the axon that terminates at a muscle fiber does so by branching into a rootlike structure called sole feet or endplate feet. These invaginate to the muscle fiber; however, they do not enter the fiber membrane and, therefore, require the same synaptic mechanism discussed above to transmit impulses. Excitatory transmitter is released in the presence of a stimulus and initiates the wave of depolarization over the synapse and through the muscle fiber. Perhaps the major distinction between nerve and muscle fiber depolarization is that whereas depolarization down a nerve is accomplished for the sole reason of propagating an impulse to an end organ, depolarization of the muscle fiber—itself an end organ—is to provide for its contraction. Accepting, therefore, that the concepts of waves of depolarization and repolarization are as viable for muscle fiber as they are for nerve fiber, we can turn to a review of the current theory of the mechanics of contraction.

It has been noted that the basic unit of a muscle is the muscle fiber. Most muscle fibers extend the length of the muscle itself and are innervated by a single neuromuscular junction located in the middle of the fiber. Within the fiber, numerous myofibrils are organized in parallel with the length of the fiber and comprise, in turn, myosin and actin filaments, which are also arranged in parallel with the fiber length. The actin (light) and myosin (dark) filaments interdigitate somewhat to give rise to the appearance of microscopic bands of color called I (light or isotropic) and A (dark or anisotropic). Z-bands attach the myofibrils together at their ends and provide the structure that requires all filaments to be side by side. Since actin filaments are shorter than myosin filaments, they are capable of closing and opening on each other in a sliding sort of way to provide for shortening and lengthening of the myofibril, the muscle fiber, and, therefore, the muscle itself.

Myofibrils form an intracellular matrix called the sarcoplasm, which provides a special organization of tubules that communicate to extracellular spaces and, therefore, to extracellular fluids. This so-called T-system allows the action potential of depolarization to reach the interior of the fiber.

It is important to recall that a single axon may, at its termination, branch to innervate as many as 1000 muscle fibers and as few as 10. Regardless of the number of fibers with which an axon communicates, all of them (a motor unit) will respond to a nerve impulse transmitted along the axon. Their simultaneous response is called a twitch and will differ from other twitches within the muscle in terms of speed of contraction, the frequency of contraction, and the strength of contraction.

Speed of contraction is related both to the diameter of the axon, the thickness of the myelin sheath and to the physiologic properties of the innervated fibers. Large, well-myelinated axons can transmit impulses at speeds exceeding 100 meters per second. Small, unmyelinated fibers are capable of transmitting at the considerably slower speeds of only centimeters per second. These axon characteristics, coupled with *fast-twitch* and *slow-twitch* muscle fibers, provide for almost infinite possibilities within the range of contraction speeds.

Frequency of contraction is related to the refractory period of both the transmitting axon and the contracting fibers. Long refractory periods slow contraction frequency, just as short refractory periods increase contraction frequency. Another aspect that may relate to contraction frequency is that of endurance of motor units. It could be postulated that refractory periods in concert with ability of the fibers to resist fatigue may further contribute to our ability to perform motor skills with coordination and efficiency.

Contraction strength is related to the size of the fiber and the innervating axon. The larger these are, the stronger will be the contraction. In contrast to popular belief, the strength of the nerve impulse has no effect; if the stimulus is strong enough to cause transmission, it will produce maximum contraction of the motor unit—the *all-or-nothing* law.

In summary, the design of the neural and muscular systems of the human body can be likened to a multiwire cable linking the central nervous system to the musculature of the skeleton. Within the cable are myelinated wires capable of transmitting to the muscle (motor) as well as wires that can transmit back to the central nervous system (sensory). Speed of transmission within the cable varies according to thickness and myelination of the wires. The wires branch as they approach the muscle and invaginate, randomly, a number of fibers. Through the process of depolarization and repolarization, the fiber and its subparts—the myofibril and actin and myosin filaments—provide for shortening and lengthening of the muscle as a whole.

## Types of Muscular Force

The two general modes of contraction of muscle are static and dynamic. During static contraction, a muscle does not change its length. There is, therefore, no observable motion in the joint over which the muscle crosses. Such contractions may or may not be maximal depending upon the requirements of the task. When a dancer holds the arms in second position to execute a pose, the muscles of the shoulder must contract statically to neutralize the pull of gravity—but the contraction is only a partial one. When a firm fist is made, both the extensors and flexors contract statically, each to neutralize the tendency of the other to move the wrist joint. The firmer the fist, the more the contraction approaches maximum. When static contractions are embodied in strength-gaining programs, they are referred to as *isometric contractions* and are usually characterized by maximum effort. Forceful pressing of the hands together in front of the chest is an example of an isometric exercise involving static contraction.

Dynamic contractions are accompanied by changes in muscle length. When the muscle shortens, the contraction is said to be concentric and the joint crossed by the muscle will be made to move according to action with which the muscle is credited. For example, the biceps brachii is an elbow flexor; when it contracts concentrically it shortens, causing the elbow to flex. The contraction may be partial or maximal; however, when such contractions are performed for the purpose of strength gain, they are typically of a maximal level. Concentric contractions can be of two types, isotonic or isokinetic. Isotonic contractions are those required when a given weight is moved through a range of joint motion. Bench presses, and arm curls with barbells are common weight-lifting examples of isotonic contractions against the resistance of weights, whereas pushups, sit-ups, and chin-ups exemplify isotonic contractions during which the body is the resistance.

Isokinetic contractions differ from their isotonic counterparts in that the muscle must shorten at a certain rate of velocity to ensure a constant rate of limb movement. Specially geared isokinetic exercisers are used to ensure not only appropriate contraction rates but also that the muscle can contract maximally, if desired, through the complete range of motion.

Dynamic contractions need not always involve shortening of the muscle. Suppose the right elbow is flexed to a 90-degree angle and in the hand has been placed a five-kilogram weight. If the musculature of the elbow is of sufficient strength, the weight can be held in position (static contraction of the elbow flexors), or even brought toward the shoulder by flexing the elbow farther (concentric contraction). If the musculature is weak, however, the weight in the hand will gradually extend the elbow regardless of voluntary effort to resist. The elbow flexors are vigorously active, but are being forced to lengthen by the "too-heavy" weight. Such contractions are eccentric contractions and are as much a part of human movement as are concentric contractions. Without the muscle's ability to lengthen as it contracts, we would not be able to lower resistances after we have lifted them. A forward elevation of the arm is accomplished by concentric contraction of the flexor muscles of the shoulder. Lowering of the arm to the side of the body is accomplished by eccentric contraction of the same muscles; otherwise the arm would fall, uncontrolled, in response to the pull of gravity. It may seem surprising that the opposite muscles, the shoulder extensors, are not involved in returning the arm to the side; however, when it is remembered that the function of a muscle is to pull against a bone, it will follow that the extensors will be recruited only if it is desired that the arm be returned to the side with a force greater than that naturally afforded by gravity.

## Roles of the Muscular System

The muscles of the human body can assume various responsibilities as they carry out movement tasks. These responsibilities, or roles, are those of agonist, antagonist, stabilizer, and neutralizer.

A muscle acts as an agonist when it is directly involved in causing a given joint action. The influence of an agonist upon a joint action may be either a primary one or an assistive one, depending upon its size, angle of insertion, and force arm to the joint's axis of rotation.

An antagonist is a muscle on the opposite side of the joint axis from the agonist and, as such, causes the opposite joint action. Antagonists can also be primary or assistive in their involvement, and are important to muscular control in two ways: (1) antagonists must relax to some degree in order to allow agonists to move the joint of concern; (2) antagonists must function to protect the joint structure from injury during powerful movement patterns. During knee extension against resistance, for example, the quadriceps are the agonists and the hamstrings are the antagonists; however, the quadriceps can affect extension only if the hamstrings relax and allow the knee joint to move. If knee extension is performed powerfully the hamstrings, after their initial relaxation, must contract against the momentum of the lower leg to prevent a tearing of the ligaments and other soft tissues of the joint. Since contraction of the antagonists typically applies stabilizing force, the centrifugal force developed by the lower leg is neutralized. It should be noted, at this point, that when the knee is flexed against resistance, the quadriceps reverse roles to become antagonists while the hamstrings become the agonists.

Stabilizers are muscles which act, during a particular movement task, to support a body part or to make that body part firm against the influence of some force. The deltoid stabilizes the humerus by supporting it in the transverse plane while the archer is at full draw; and the abdominal muscles stabilize the pelvis to make it a firm base upon which the legs may execute the flutter kick during the freestyle in swimming.

Neutralizers are muscles which contract to prevent unwanted actions which occur as a result of the contraction of other muscles. Several examples of neutralizers can be found among the muscles which move the scapula. For example, the rhomboids lie between the spine and the scapula. Their line of pull dictates that when they contract, they will pull the scapula both upwardly (elevation) and toward the spine (adduction). Suppose the movement pattern being attempted requires the scapula to elevate only; some other muscle (an abductor) must be recruited which will, when it contracts, neutralize the adducting force of the rhomboids.

## Spurt and Shunt Muscles

The terms *spurt* and *shunt* occurred originally in engineering terminology; however, they are being used with increasing frequence in kinesiology to describe the relationship of muscular origins and insertions to the joints these muscles cross. A shunt muscle is one which originates closer to a joint it crosses than it inserts. The brachioradialis is an excellent example of a shunt muscle at the elbow joint. A spurt muscle is one which originates farther from the joint than it inserts and is exemplified at the elbow joint by the brachialis.

Several muscles of the human body cross more than one joint and, as they do so, have characteristics of both shunt and spurt muscles depending upon the joint being regarded. The biceps brachii, hamstrings, and quadriceps are all examples of such muscles and display shunt characteristics at the shoulder or hip joint but are spurt muscles at the elbow or knee.

Shunt muscles are notable in that resolution of their lines of pull result in longer stabilizing vectors than angular vectors. Spurt muscles, on the other hand, provide for longer angular vectors than stabilizing vectors. The hamstrings and quadriceps, then, are mainly effective as stabilizers of the hip joint and movers of the knee joint. Similarly, the gastrocnemius is a stabilizer of the knee joint and a mover of the ankle joint.

There is some controversy among kinesiologists regarding the validity of the spurt-shunt theory. Some researchers insist that the qualities of spurt and shunt muscles are due simply to the fact that their respective force arms have different lengths. Others offer that any differences noted are caused by the ratios of length of contractile tissue to length of tendinous material of the various muscles. Regardless of the viewpoint, however, the concept appears to be much the same.

# 3 The Shoulder

When man became a biped, he began the long, slow, and purposeful journey in evolution required to meet the demands of upright posture. Among the pertinent developmental changes were those of the shoulder complex. With the elimination of its weight-bearing responsibilities, the shoulder has become admirably adapted to its new purpose of providing mobility of the upper limb.

## Bones of the Shoulder

The bones which comprise the shoulder complex are the scapula, the clavicle, and the humerus. The scapula, a broad, long bone, acts as a platform on which movements of the humerus are based. The clavicle holds the scapula and humerus away from the body for more freedom of movement of the arm, and the humerus represents the first link in the chain of bony levers of the upper limb.

The scapula, clavicle, and humerus exhibit an intricate interplay of action toward the goal of aligning the glenoid fossa in a favorable direction for movement of the humerus, as hardly any action of the humerus can take place without associated and supplementary actions of the scapula. Throughout the entire range of motion of the humerus in the frontal and sagittal planes, approximately one-third of the mobility is the contribution of scapular movement; the remaining two-thirds of the mobility occurs at the ball-and-socket joint of the shoulder. It follows, then, that without the "free swinging" nature of the scapula, the humerus would be severely limited in its range of motion.

## Bone Markings

Figures 3.1 and 3.2 are offered as reviews of the anatomical landmarks of the clavicle, scapula, and humerus. All bone markings which will be used in the discussion of muscular attachments are noted.

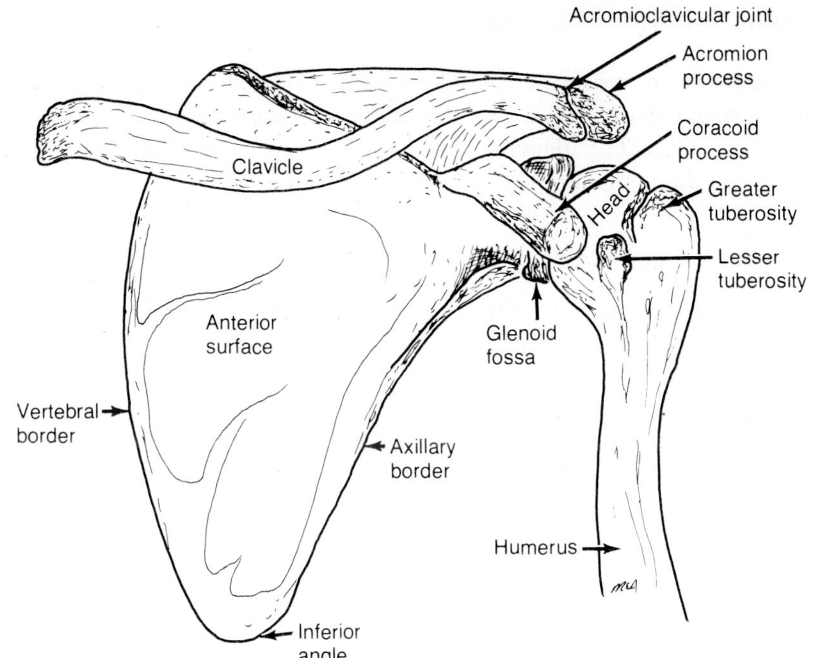


**Figure 3.1. Left scapula, clavicle and humerus, anterior view**

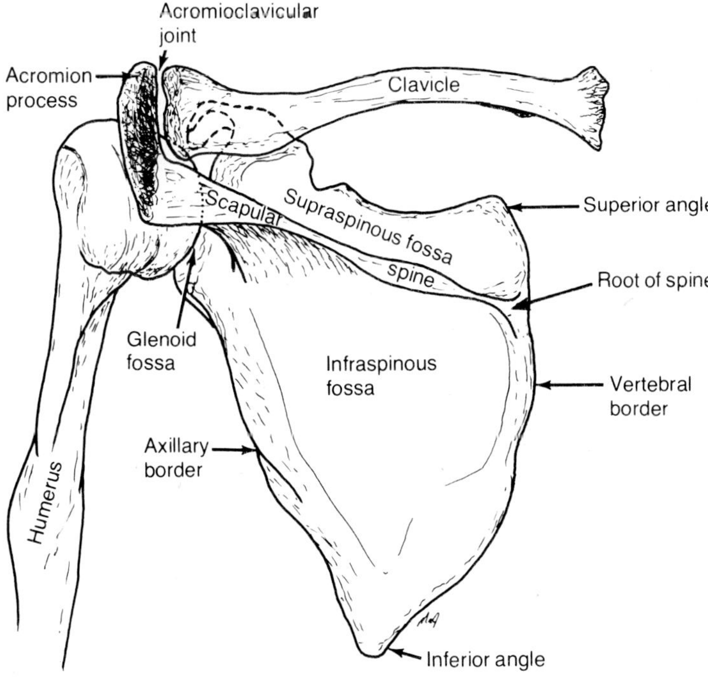


**Figure 3.2. Left scapula, clavicle and humerus, posterior view**

## Joints of the Shoulder

Three joints comprise the shoulder complex. The sternoclavicular and acromioclavicular joints allow the scapula to glide along the surface of the rib cage. The glenohumeral joint comprises the articulation between the humerus and the scapula.

### Sternoclavicular Joint

The sternoclavicular joint (fig. 3.3) joins the sternum and the clavicle, and is the only bony anticulation between the upper limb and the torso. The clavicle is well anchored to the sternum through this joint and surrounding ligaments. Even under unusually severe applications of force, the joint tends to maintain its integrity. The joint is synovial, and is a modification of the ball-and-socket structure with three axes of rotation which allow for elevation and depression (sagittal axis), horizontal flexion and extension (vertical axis), and upward and downward rotation (frontal axis) of the clavicle (fig. 3.4).

The actions of the scapula which result from movement of the clavicle include abduction and adduction and elevation and depression. These movements are more linear than angular in nature with scapular abduction/adduction resulting from horizontal flexion and extension of the clavicle, and scapular elevation/depression resulting from elevation and depression of the clavicle. Both pairs of actions of the scapula are accompanied by a gliding of the clavicle on the acromion process.

**Figure 3.3. Sternoclavicular joints**

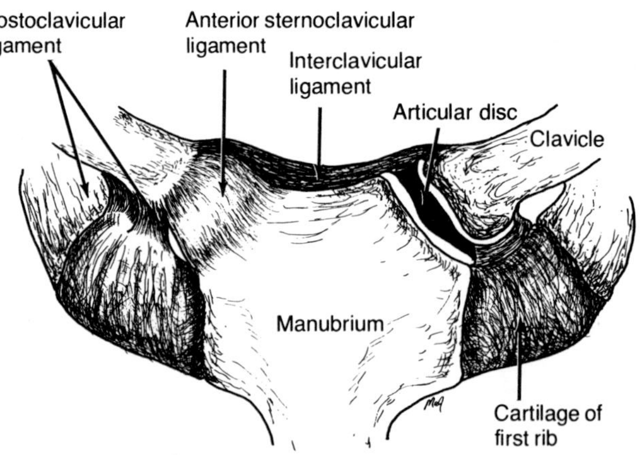

**Figure 3.4. Axes of sternoclavicular joint and accompanying scapular actions**

Sagittal axis

Vertical axis

Frontal axis

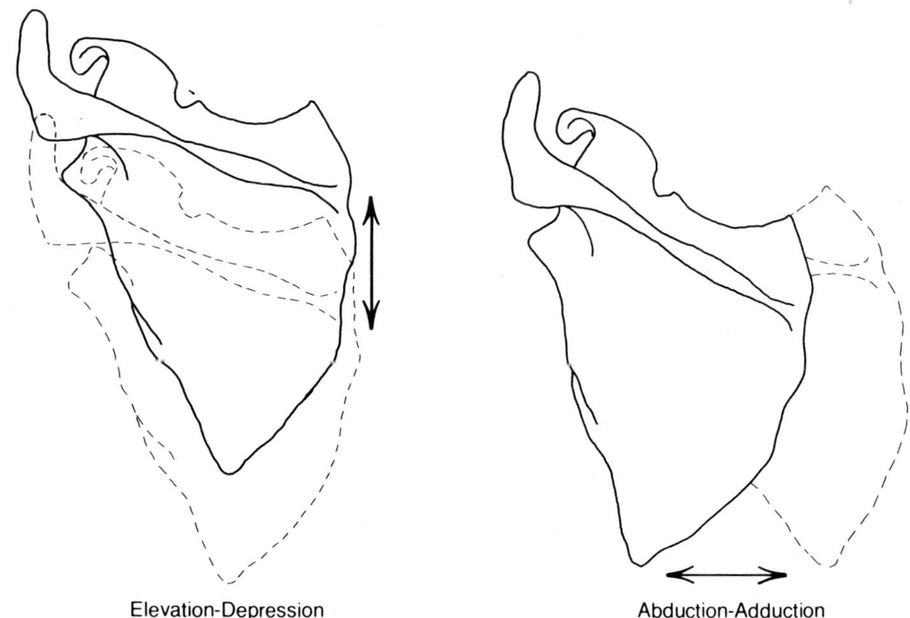

The ligaments surrounding the sternoclavicular joint are the interclavicular, costoclavicular, and anterior and posterior sternoclavicular ligaments. Not only do these ligaments bind the clavicle to the first rib and sternum; they also blend with the joint capsule to reinforce it.

### Acromioclavicular Joint

The acromioclavicular joint (fig. 3.5) is the articulation of the clavicle with the acromion process of the scapula. The joint is a triaxial synovial joint which also permits a certain amount of gliding or linear motion. Its three axes of rotation allow scapular action as indicated in figure 3.6 and comprise upward and downward tilt about a frontal axis; upward and downward rotation about a sagittal axis; and "winging" of the scapula about a vertical axis.

**Figure 3.5. Acromioclavicular joint, anterior view**

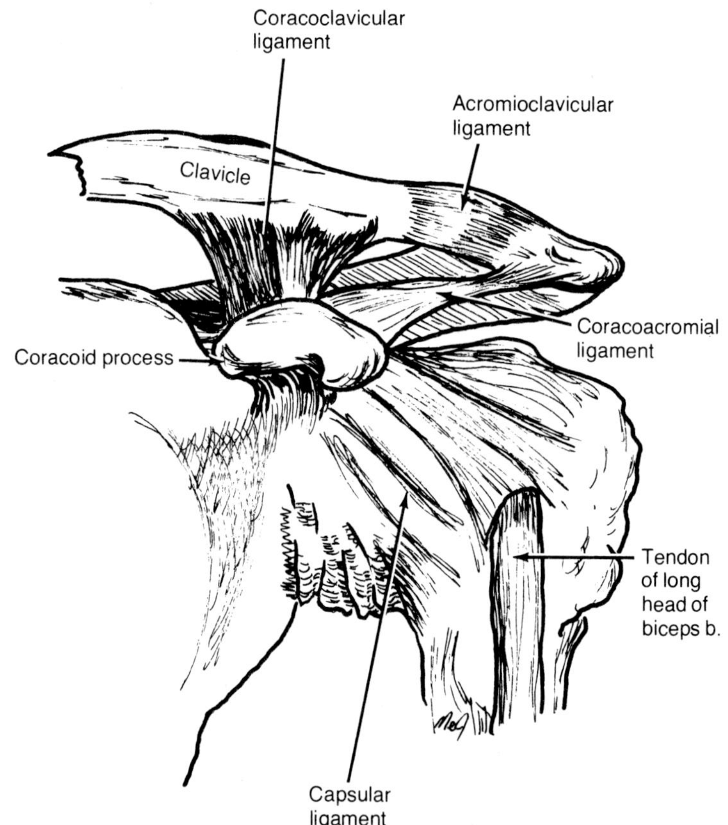

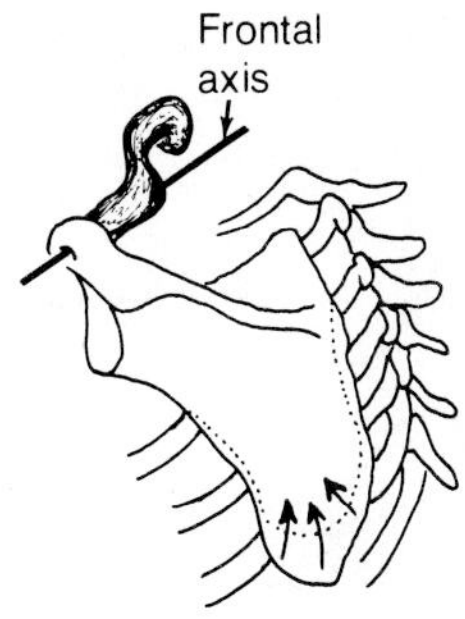

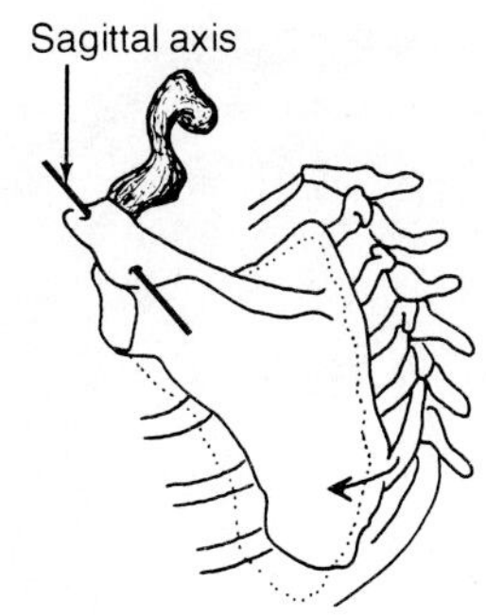

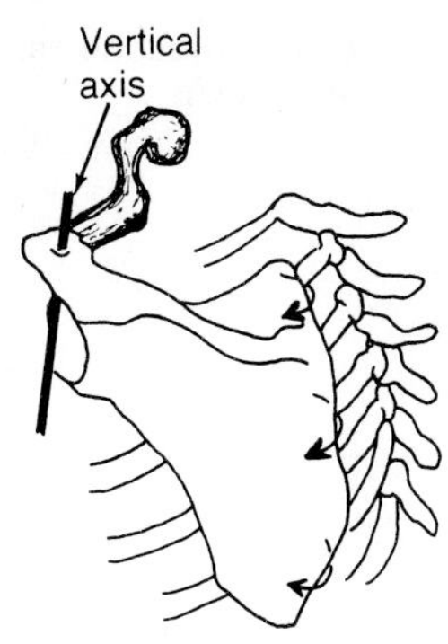


**Figure 3.6. Axes of the acromioclavicular joint**

The capsule of the acromioclavicular joint is weaker and looser than that of the sternoclavicular joint, and thus the integrity of the joint is largely dependent on the ligaments. The major ligaments are the superior and inferior acromioclavicular ligaments and the coracoclavicular ligament. The two acromioclavicular ligaments bind the clavicle to the acromion process and help prevent upward dislocation of the joint. The coracoclavicular ligament binds the clavicle to the coracoid process to not only provide stability to the joint, but also to act as the major force in connecting the clavicle to the scapula.

As mentioned before, the acromioclavicular joint is weaker than the sternoclavicular joint. Forces, such as those incurred by falling on the outstretched arm or on the tip of the shoulder, will be transmitted to the clavicle and will tend to either dislocate the clavicle from its two attachments or to fracture it. Since the sternoclavicular joint is the strongest link in the clavicular chain, dislocations of the medial head of the clavicle are seldom seen. In children, the clavicle itself appears to be the weakest link, for it is not unusual to see fractured "collar bones" after falls from trees or fences. In adulthood, however, the acromioclavicular joints tend to be the weakest link; dislocations at this joint, called *shoulder separations,* are all-too-common among athletes who engage in contact sports. A contributing factor to the high incidence of shoulder separations among football players may well be their pregame drill of standing slightly off-center to each other and vigorously bumping shoulders. The forceful contact can cause severe stretching of the coracoacromial ligament and thus disable it as a stabilizer of the acromioclavicular joint.

## Glenohumeral Joint (Shoulder Joint)

The glenohumeral joint (fig. 3.7), a synovial ball-and-socket joint, is the freest joint of the body. It is formed by the large globular head of the humerus and the glenoid fossa of the scapula. The glenoid

Figure 3.7. Glenohumeral (shoulder) joint

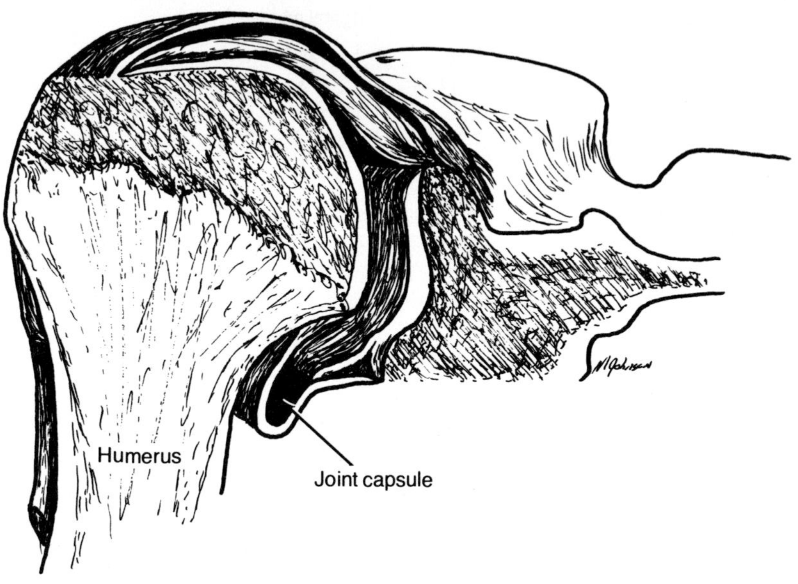


fossa is small and shallow and contacts only about one-third of the head of the humerus at a given time. This arrangement makes possible the extensive mobility of the joint; however, stability is minimal, being provided by the joint capsule and surrounding muscles rather than by the structure of the joint itself.

The glenohumeral joint permits rotation about three axes, all three of which pass through the head of the humerus (fig. 3.8). Flexion, extension, and hyperextension of the joint move the humerus about a frontal axis; abduction and adduction move the humerus about a sagittal axis; and inward and outward rotation move the humerus around a vertical axis. In addition, the joint can allow horizontal adduction and abduction (figure 3.9) which comprise the movement of the humerus in a horizontal plane from in front of the body to the side (horizontal abduction), or from the side of the body to the front (horizontal adduction). Neither horizontal abduction nor horizontal adduction can occur from anatomical reference position. They must be preceded either by flexion or by abduction of the joint and are, therefore, regarded as combination movements. It should be noted, however, that when the actions of a given muscle include horizontal abduction or adduction, the required preliminary flexion or abduction movement is disregarded in movement analysis.

The coracohumeral ligament is the ligament of greatest importance to the integrity of the shoulder joint. It limits outward rotation

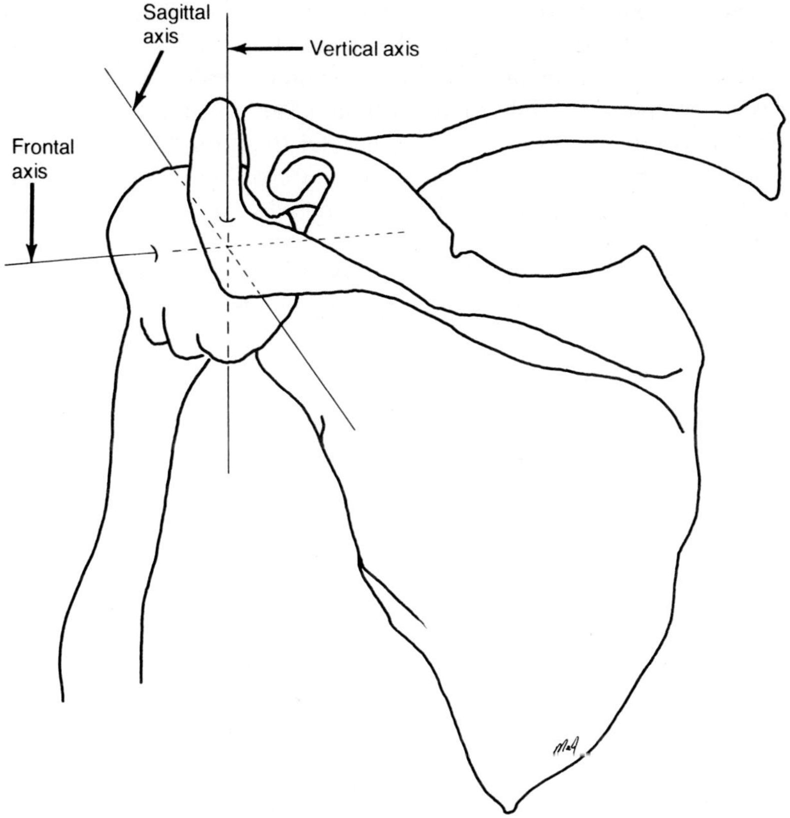

Figure 3.8. Axes of glenohumeral (shoulder) joint

around the long axis of the humerus and thus prevents dislocations which might otherwise occur during such actions as the overhead throw pattern.

A considerable amount of motion accompanies humeral rotation at the shoulder joint, and consequently there is a build-up of friction within the joint, between bones and tendons, and between muscle layers. The synovial fluid secreted within the joint capsule minimizes the joint friction, and fibrous pockets known as *bursae* act to decrease the irritating effects of friction between the other anatomical structures. These bursae are lined with a synovial membrane similar to that of the joint, and contain a lubricating fluid which allows their inner surfaces to slip easily on each other. The overall result is much like holding a bag of water between the palms of the hands and moving them back and forth. Friction is negligible when compared to that which results from the same movement of the hands when the palms are allowed to contact each other.

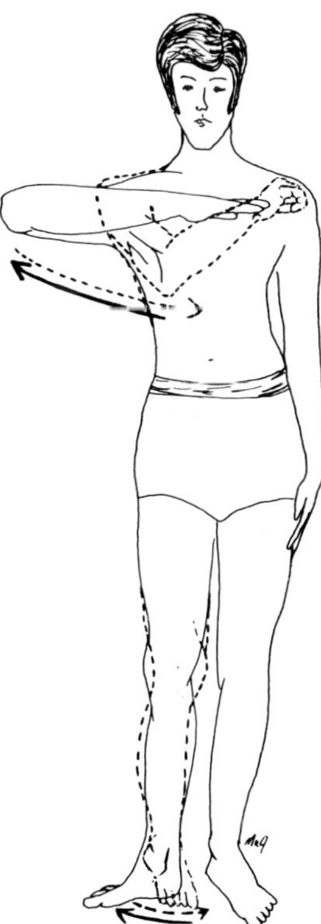

Figure 3.9. Horizontal adduction and abduction of glenohumeral (shoulder) joint

Several bursae are located around the shoulder joint. Some cushion the capsule against pressure from muscles and the bony prominence of the coracoid process; some surround tendons of the larger muscles in the area; and others are found between layers of muscles which move in opposition to each other. Of these bursae, the subacromion bursae is of greatest interest. It separates the deltoid and teres major muscles from the underlying muscles of the rotator cuff. Normally, the membrane of the bursa is loose and thin; however, it tends to thicken with age and become filled with scar tissue from previous injuries. Inflammation and swelling frequently accompany the degeneration, and the bursa is then no longer able to separate the two muscle groups as they glide over each other. Elevation of the arm allows contact between the muscles and is, therefore, accompanied by acute pain—a condition known as *bursitis.*

## Musculature

The musculature of the shoulder is divided into two groups. Group 1 is comprised of the muscles which move or stabilize the scapula, and Group 2 is comprised of the muscles which move the humerus.

### Group 1: Scapula Movers

The muscles which stabilize or move the scapula are the trapezius, rhomboids, levator scapulae, serratus anterior, pectoralis minor, and subclavius. All of these muscles except the subclavius have dual actions; however, only their actions on the scapula will be considered here.

**Trapezius** (trape'zius) The trapezius (fig. 3.10) is a flat triangular muscle located superficially on the upper back. It is subdivided into four parts which are easily palpated between the spine and scapula.

*Origin*

Part 1: Occipital bone.
Part 2: Ligamentum nuchae.
Part 3: Spinous processes of the seventh cervical and first three thoracic vertebrae.
Part 4: Spinous processes of the fourth through twelfth thoracic vertebrae.

Figure 3.10. Trapezius, posterior view

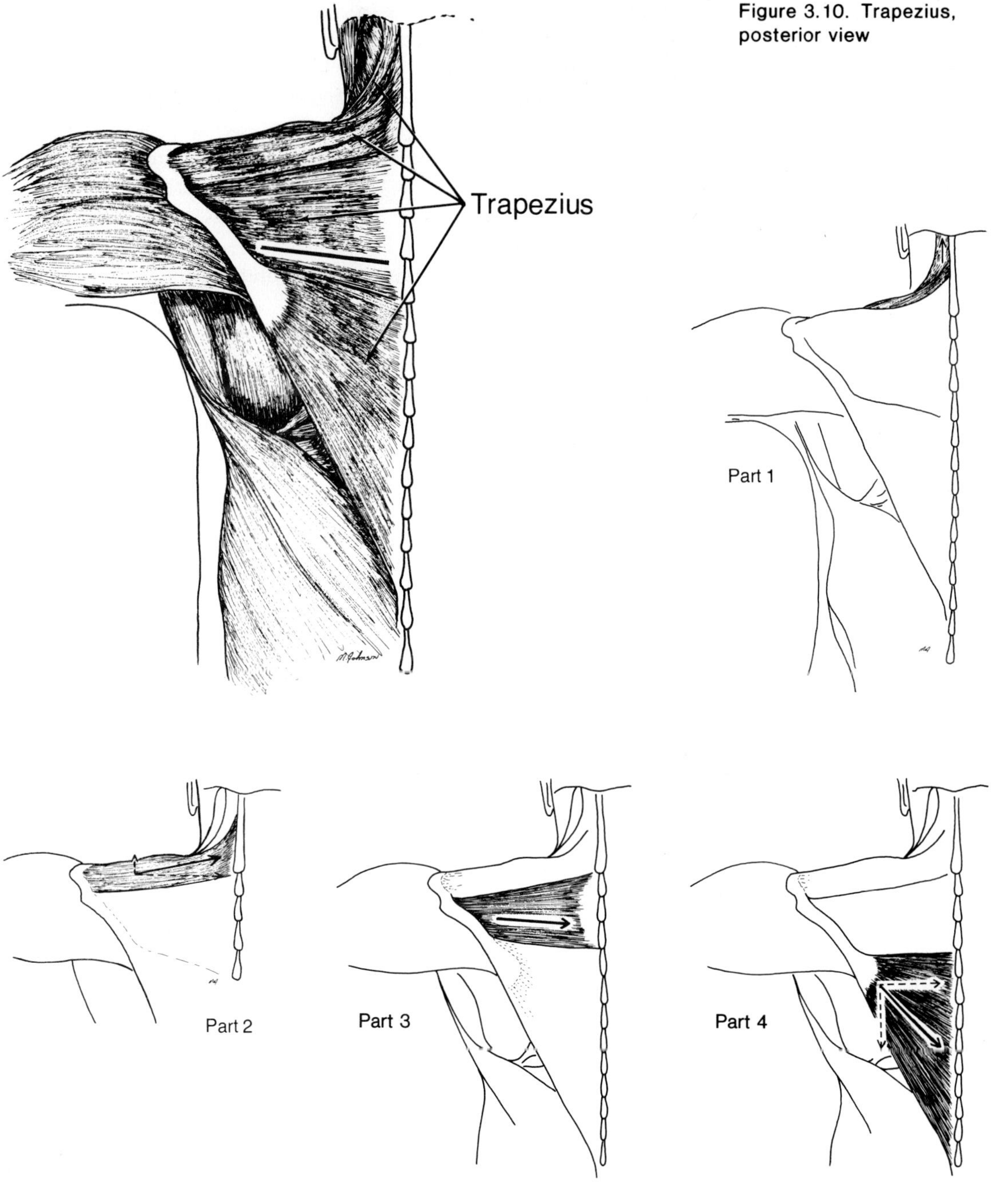

Trapezius

Part 1

Part 2

Part 3

Part 4

*Insertion*
Part 1: Outer third of clavicle.
Part 2: Acromion process.
Part 3: Scapular spine.
Part 4: Root of scapular spine.

*Innervation* Spinal accessory nerve and third and fourth cervical nerves.

*Action*
Part 1: Elevation.
Part 2: Elevation, adduction, upward rotation.
Part 3: Adduction.
Part 4: Depression, adduction, upward rotation.

Since the trapezius lies primarily in the frontal plane, its contraction causes frontal plane movements of the scapula. Part 1, with its attachments on the base of the skull and clavicle, will pull upwardly on the clavicle when it contracts. The force on the clavicle is transferred to the scapula via the acromioclavicular joint to elevate the scapula.

Part 2 has a diagonal fiber direction—its origin being slightly higher than its insertion. Resolution of the line of pull yields two component forces, of which one is directed toward the head (elevation) and one directed toward the spine (adduction). The third action of Part 2, upward rotation, occurs because the muscle crosses the acromioclavicular joint superior to the sagittal axis of that joint and, during contraction, pulls the acromion toward the neck by pivoting the scapula around its articulation with the clavicle.

The third part of the trapezius courses horizontally between the spine and scapula. Its only action is, therefore, adduction.

Part 4, like Part 2, represents a diagonal force vector; however, its origin is lower than its distal attachment. The two component forces for this portion of the trapezius are directed downwardly (depression) and toward the spine (adduction). Because Part 4 attaches medial to the acromioclavicular joint and approaches that attachment from below, it upwardly rotates the scapula by pulling downwardly on the root of the scapular spine.

By comparing the actions of the four parts of the trapezius, both agonism and antagonism can be seen. Parts 1 and 2 are agonistic to each other in elevation, but are antagonistic to the depressive action of Part 4. Parts 2 and 4 are agonists during upward rotation, and Parts 2, 3, and 4 are agonists during adduction.

**Levator Scapulae** (leva'tor scap'ulae) The levator scapulae (fig. 3.11) is located on the lateral and posterior aspect of the neck. It lies beneath Part 1 of the trapezius and cannot be palpated except through that muscle portion.

*Origin* Transverse processes of the first four cervical vertebrae.

*Insertion* Vertebral border of the scapula, between the superior angle and the root of the scapular spine.

*Innervation* Third and fourth cervical nerves, and a branch of the dorsal scapular nerve.

*Action* Elevation, adduction, downward rotation of the scapula.

The line of pull of the levator scapulae is a diagonal one which, when resolved, yields a long vertical component and a comparatively short horizontal component. Its function as an elevator is, therefore, better than its function as an adductor. Downward rotation of the scapula is accomplished by pulling upwardly on the vertebral border of the scapula in order to lower the inferior angle. The rotation action is more easily visualized when it is remembered that downward rotation

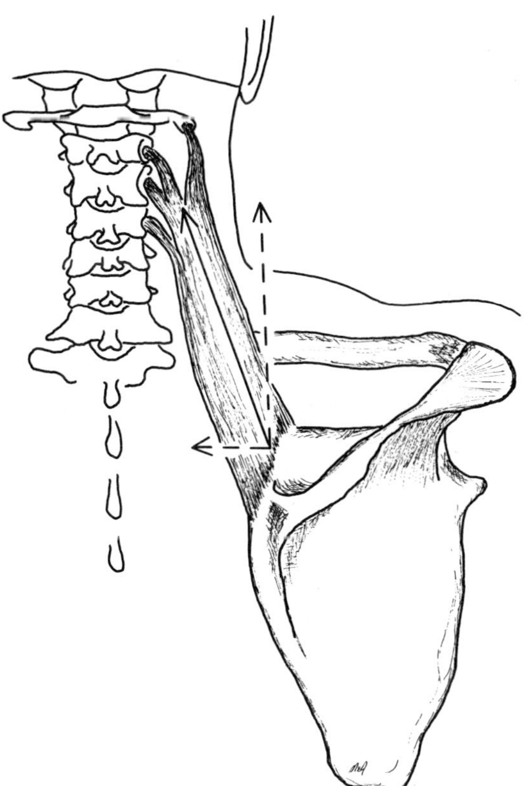

Figure 3.11. Levator scapulae, posterior view

is the return of upward rotation; the levator scapulae downwardly rotates only if the scapula is already rotated upwardly to some degree.

The levator scapulae is important to the support and stability of the scapula during regular upright posture and when weights are carried on the shoulder or in the hand. Not only do weights tend to depress the shoulder, they also cause the center of mass to shift in their directions. To compensate for both conditions, the shoulder is elevated by contracting the levator and Parts 1 and 2 of the trapezius.

**Rhomboids** (rhom'boids) The rhomboids (fig. 3.12) are located beneath Part 3 and the uppermost portion of Part 4 of the trapezius. The rhomboids are divided into rhomboid major and rhomboid minor. Functionally, however, they may be considered a single muscle. The rhomboids cannot be palpated directly.

*Origin* Spinous processes of the seventh cervical and first five thoracic vertebrae.

*Insertion* Vertebral border of scapula from the scapular spine to the inferior angle.

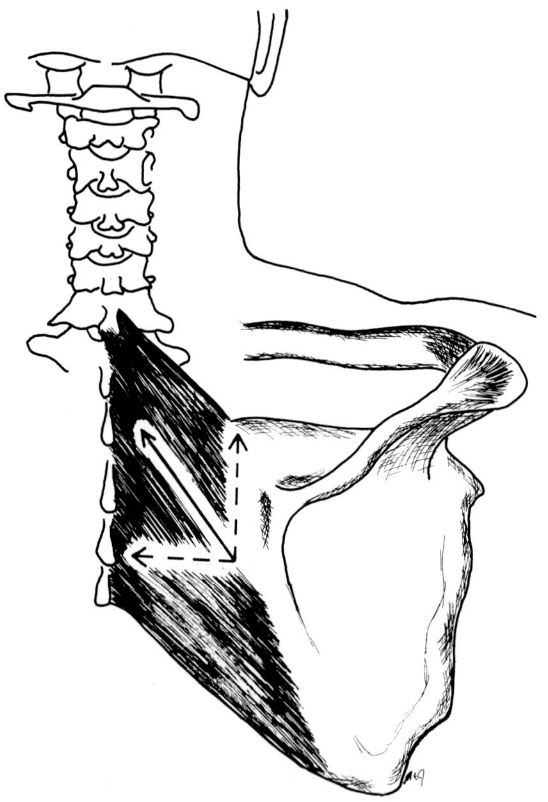

Figure 3.12. Rhomboids, posterior view

*Innervation* Dorsal scapular nerve.

*Action* Elevation, adduction, downward rotation of the scapula.

Resolution of the diagonal line of pull of the rhomboids produces the two components which explain the elevation and adduction action of the muscles. The downward rotation action is provided particularly by the lower fibers, which contract to pull medially and upwardly on the inferior angle of the scapula. The rhomboids are active also in maintaining normal posture as they prevent extreme upward rotation of the scapula and hold the inferior angle close to the rib cage. The latter function may be illustrated by asking a partner to place his hand against the small of his back. The examiner can easily insert a finger beneath the vertebral border of the scapula, because the trapezius and rhomboids are relaxed. When the subject is instructed to lift his hand off the back, the rhomboids will contract strongly to pull the scapula to the ribs and will force the examiner's fingers out from underneath the scapula.

**Serratus Anterior** (serra'tus ante'rior) The serratus anterior (fig. 3.13) takes its name from the saw-toothed fashion with which it attaches to the ribs. The muscle lies beneath the scapula and courses along the surface of the ribs to attach to the front of the rib cage underneath the pectoralis major. The muscle may be palpated in the area below the axilla as the arm is raised overhead against resistance.

*Origin* Upper nine ribs at the side of the chest.

*Insertion* Vertebral border of scapula between the superior and inferior angles.

*Innervation* Long thoracic nerve.

*Action* Abduction and upward rotation of the scapula.

The direction of the fibers of the serratus is very nearly horizontal to make the muscle quite effective as a scapular abductor. The lower fibers are effective as upward rotators since they are in a position to exert a lateral pull on the inferior angle as Part 4 of the trapezius pulls downwardly on the root of the scapular spine. In these two actions—scapular abduction and upward rotation—the serratus is considered to be one of the most important muscles of the shoulder. Loss of the serratus seriously impairs ability to reach forward with the arm since that action must be accompanied by abduction of the scapula to align the glenoid fossa in a forward direction. Similarly, subjects who have suffered paralysis of the serratus are typically unable to raise the arm overhead because of muscular insufficiency in upward rotation. The serratus also acts with the rhomboids to prevent winging of the scapula by holding the scapula close to the rib cage.

Figure 3.13. Serratus anterior, lateral view

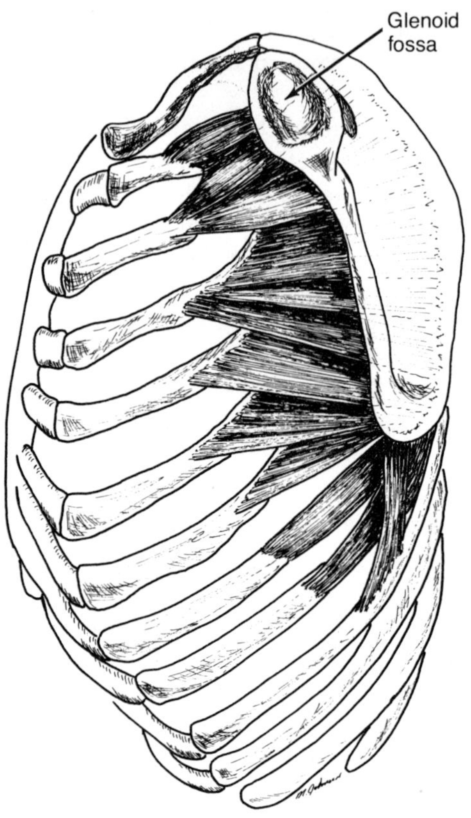


**Pectoralis Minor** (pectora'lis mi'nor) The pectoralis minor (fig. 3.14) is located on the front of the chest. It is covered by the pectoralis major and, though it cannot be palpated directly, it can be examined on a subject who has placed the hand on the small of the back. If the pectoralis major is relaxed, the coracoid can be located, and the proximal portion of the pectoralis minor can be felt contracting as the subject lifts the hand off the back.

*Origin* Third, fourth, and fifth ribs just lateral to their costal cartilages.

*Insertion* Coracoid process of the scapula.

*Innervation* Medial anterior thoracic nerve.

*Action* Abduction, depression, downward rotation, upward tilt of the scapula.

The fibers of the pectoralis minor are directed downward, inward, and forward from their attachment on the coracoid. The ability of this muscle to depress the scapula is easily recognized as a function of its downward direction; however, at first glance, its abduction, tilt, and

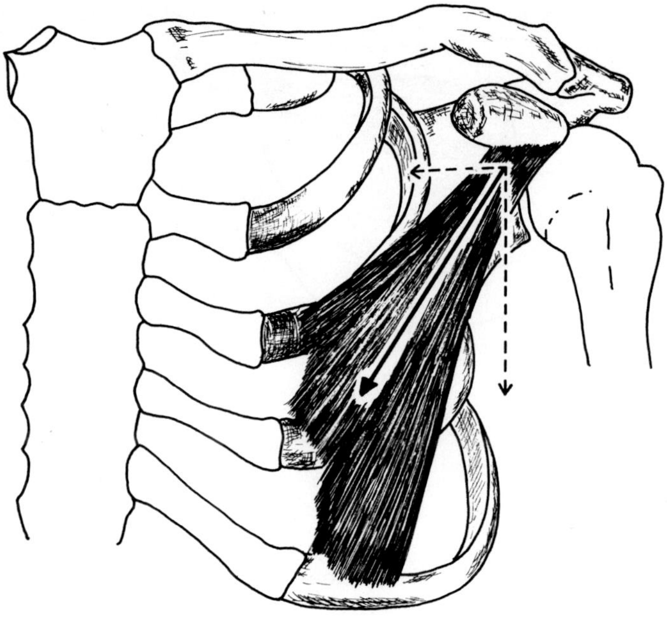

Figure 3.14. Pectoralis minor, anterior view

downward rotation actions are not so clearly envisioned. To abduct, the pectoralis minor pulls the coracoid medially around the rigid brace supplied by the clavicle, consequently, the scapula glides laterally along the rib cage and the acromion glides forward against the distal end of the clavicle. To tilt the scapula, the pectoralis minor pulls downwardly on the coracoid to rotate the scapula around the frontal axis of the acromioclavicular joint. The downward rotation function of this muscle is a result of the downward pull on the end of the coracoid which returns the scapula to anatomical position.

**Subclavius** (subcla'vius) The subclavius (fig. 3.15) is located underneath the clavicle and is covered by the pectoralis major. It cannot be palpated directly.

*Origin* Cartilaginous junction of the first rib.

*Insertion* Inferior surface of middle half of clavicle.

*Innervation* Fibers of the fifth and sixth cervical nerves.

*Action* Stabilizes sternoclavicular joint; weak depressor of clavicle.

Resolution of the line of pull of the subclavious yields the two component vectors shown in figure 3.15. The relative length of the components, when compared to each other, infers that the muscle is effective in pulling the clavicle toward the sternum to stabilize the sternoclavicular joint but is lacking in ability to depress the clavicle.

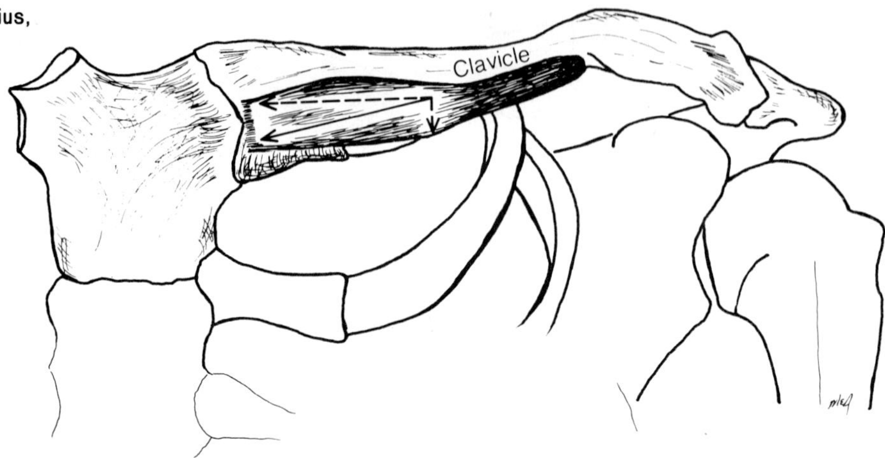


Figure 3.15. Subclavius, anterior view

## Comments

Figure 3.16 illustrates directions of scapular movement in the frontal plane. The muscles which provide for the movements are noted in conjunction with the directional arrows. Thus it can be seen, for example, that the levator scapulae, Parts 1 and 2 of the trapezius, and the rhomboids all have some ability to elevate the scapula. Similarly, depressors, adductors, abductors, and upward and downward rotators can be noted at a glance. Mention was made earlier that the muscles which move the scapula are also the muscles which stabilize the scapula. In general, mobility of the scapula is desired if the task to be accomplished is based upon extended range of the humerus. Reaching forward, upward, or backward with the arm during backswing or wind-up patterns is dependent upon scapular mobility. Conversely, stability of the scapula is desired when force is being applied by or to the arm. Hanging from a high bar in preparation for chinning oneself applies an upward force to the arm which is transmitted to the scapula causing it to elevate. In order to moderate the elevation, the scapular depressors contract and the scapula is made firm. In golf, softball, or tennis, the scapula must be stabilized at the moment of impact of the ball with the club, bat, or racket if force is to be applied firmly and effectively. In swimming, a firm scapula during the pull phase of the stroke results in greater efficiency.

Of all athletes, it is perhaps the dancer who best knows the value of mobilizing and stabilizing the scapulae. From lifts in pas de deux to the performance of forward falls, the ability to moderate degrees of scapular firmness is requisite to success. Indeed it appears that scapular placement is of such importance to the dancer that the accepted stage posture of the dancer includes the depressed scapula.

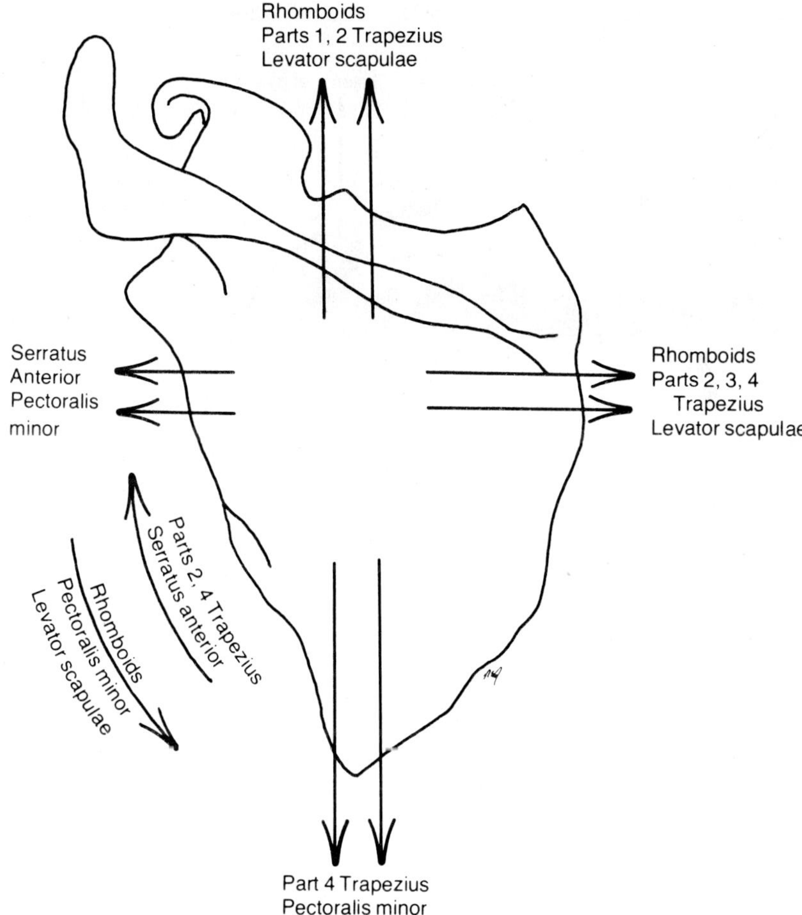


**Figure 3.16. Scapula movers, posterior view**

## Group 2: Muscles Which Move the Humerus

Muscles of Group 2 are the deltoid, pectoralis major, latissimus dorsi, teres major, infraspinatus-teres minor, subscapularis, supraspinatus, biceps brachii, coracobrachialis, and the long head of the triceps brachii. Their actions on the humerus depend upon their relationships to the three axes of rotation of the glenohumeral joint and include flexion-extension-hyperextension, abduction-adduction, horizontal abduction-adduction, inward-outward rotation, and circumduction.

**Deltoid** (del'toid) The deltoid (fig. 3.17) is a superficial muscle comprised of three portions located on the point of the shoulder and the upper arm; the muscle is comparatively large in man and is penniform in structure. All portions of the muscle may be directly palpated and observed.

Figure 3.17. Deltoid, posterior view

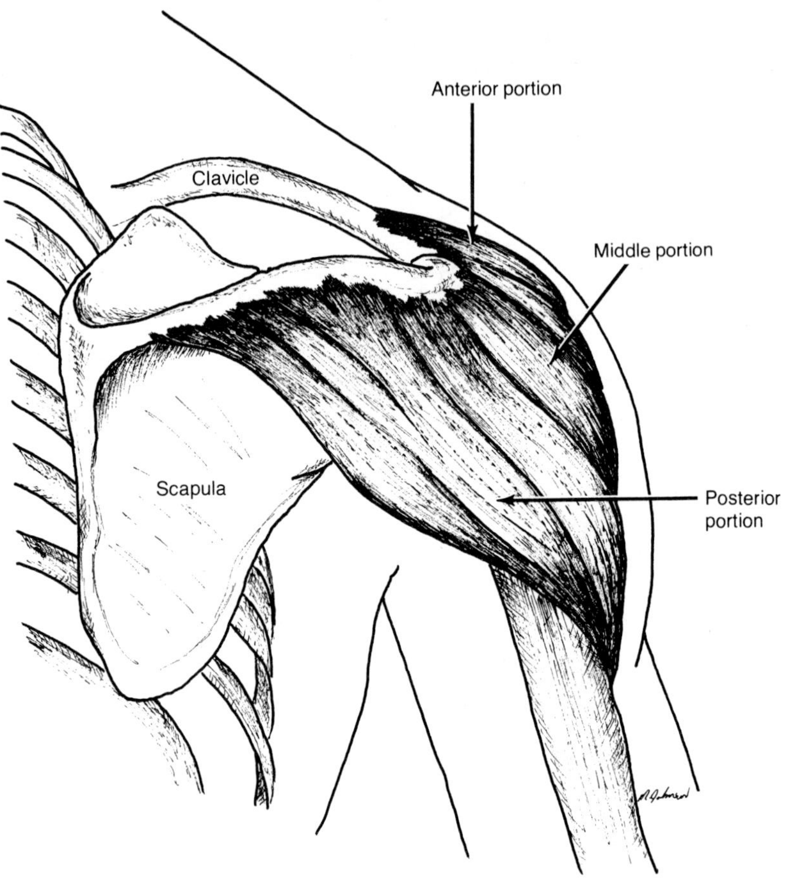


*Origin* Outer third of the clavicle, top of the acromion process, and scapular spine.

*Insertion* Midpoint of the humerus on the lateral aspect.

*Innervation* Axillary nerve.

*Action* As a whole the deltoid acts to abduct the glenohumeral joint. The fibers most important to this action are those of the middle portion. The anterior portion acts in flexion, horizontal adduction, and inward rotation of the glenohumeral joint; the posterior portion causes extension, horizontal abduction, and outward rotation of that joint.

The actions of the deltoid can be clarified if they are studied with respect to the three axes of the shoulder joint. The muscle as a whole courses lateral to the sagittal axis and, therefore, performs the abduction movement. It will be seen, however, that the most anterior and posterior fibers are very close to this axis, and will have limited effectiveness in abduction. In some individuals, these fibers will be directly aligned with the axis and consequently will be inactive during any frontal plane movement. In others, these fibers may even pass medial to the axis to become weak adductors.

The location of the deltoid with respect to the frontal axis indicates that some fibers pass anterior to this axis and will flex at the joint; other fibers are posterior to the axis and will extend at the joint. The fibers farthest from the axis will be most effective in these actions.

When the humerus is envisioned in the transverse plane during horizontal adduction and abduction, a portion of the deltoid is seen to be located anterior to the axis and will horizontally adduct; the portion located posterior to the axis will horizontally abduct. The effectiveness of the respective fibers increases with their distances from the vertical axis. Inward and outward rotation are performed also by the anterior and posterior portions, respectively. Since fibers of the middle portion cross the vertical axis, they will have no function either in rotation or in horizontal abduction/adduction.

**Supraspinatus** (supraspina'tus) The supraspinatus (fig. 3.18) is a powerful muscle located, as its name implies, in the supraspinous fossa of the scapula. It is covered by Part 2 of the trapezius and cannot be palpated directly. The muscle is a member of the rotator cuff.

*Origin* Supraspinous fossa.

*Insertion* Top of the greater tuberosity of the humerus.

*Innervation* Suprascapular nerve.

*Action* Abduction, outward rotation of the glenohumeral joint.

The supraspinatus is primarily effective as an abductor of the shoulder joint (fig. 3.18). Not only does it course well superior to the sagittal axis, but it is also in a position to pull the head of the humerus

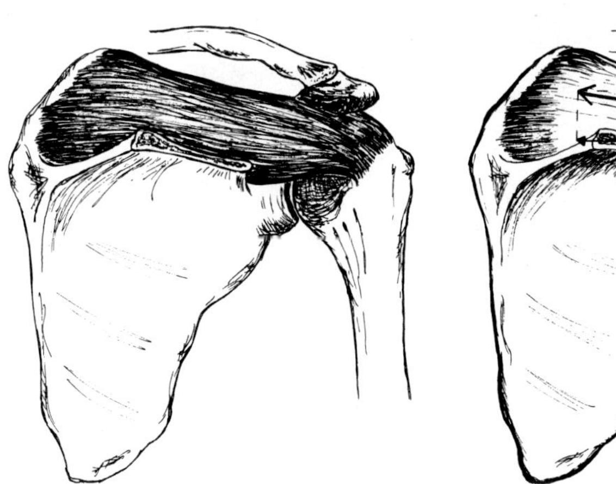

**Figure 3.18. Supraspinatus, posterior view**

into the glenoid fossa. In this latter action, it complements the pull of the deltoid during abduction (see "Rotator Cuff," this chapter).

The outward rotation function of the supraspinatus is accomplished because its distal attachment is on the posterior portion of the greater tuberosity. The line of pull of the muscle is, therefore, slightly posterior to the vertical axis of the shoulder joint.

**Pectoralis Major** (pectora'lis ma'jor) The pectoralis major (fig. 3.19) is the large muscle on the front of the chest. It is superficial and may be palpated directly. The muscle is divided into a clavicular portion and a sternal portion.

*Origin* Clavicular portion: Medial two-thirds of the clavicle. Sternal portion: Anterior aspect of the sternum, cartilages of the first six ribs.

*Insertion* Both portions: Lateral aspect of the humerus, just below the head for a distance of some five centimeters.

*Innervation* Medial anterior thoracic and lateral anterior thoracic nerves.

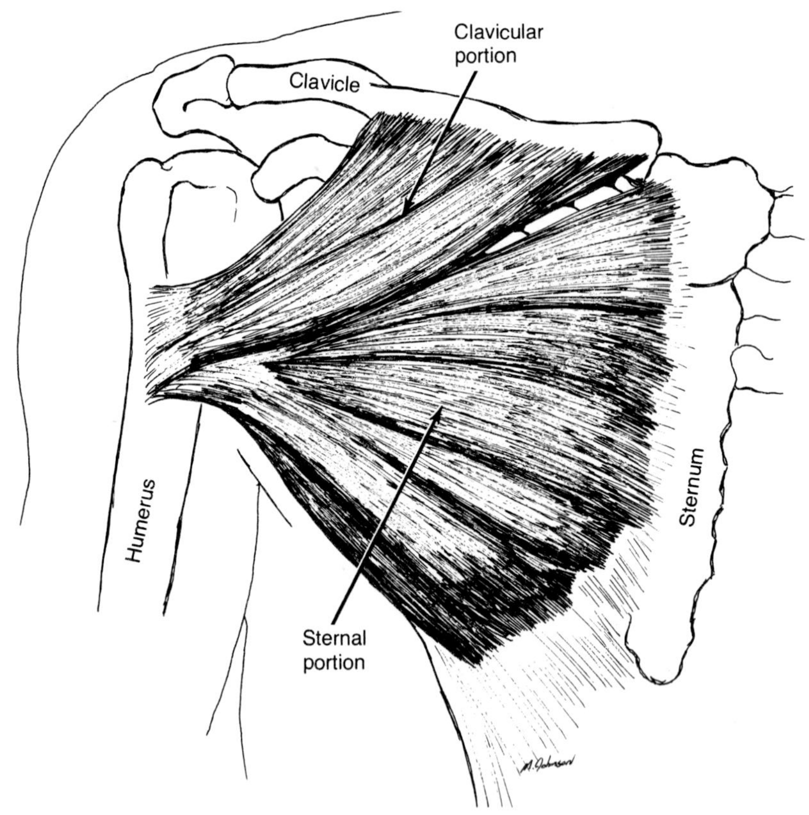


**Figure 3.19. Pectoralis major, anterior view**

*Action* Clavicular portion: Flexion, horizontal adduction, and inward rotation of the glenohumeral joint; abduction when arm is above 90 degrees. Sternal portion: Adduction, horizontal adduction, and inward rotation of the glenohumeral joint: extension to a point just past anatomical position.

When the two portions of the pectoralis major are envisioned in relationship to the shoulder axes, it will be noted that regardless of the height at which the arm is held from the side, the sternal portion crosses the joint inferior to the sagittal axis and will, therefore, function as an adductor. The clavicular portion, however, crosses directly over this axis until the arm is above the horizontal, at which position it is made to cross the joint superior to the axis; the muscle will then act as an abductor.

The flexion ability of the clavicular portion is brought about because of its advantageous attachment on the clavicle. This portion crosses the shoulder joint well in front of the frontal axis to become a powerful flexor. The sternal portion is also located anterior to the frontal axis: however, since its origin is lower than its insertion, it pulls downwardly on the upper humerus to extend the shoulder joint. This extension action ceases when the arm has been moved to a position in which the axis and the two attachments are in a line with each other.

The anterior relationship of both portions to the vertical axis of the glenohumeral joint allows the pectoralis major to be an effective horizontal adductor and inward rotator, regardless of the position of the humerus in the transverse plane. The latter action will be enhanced when the humerus is in a position of outward rotation since the distance over which the muscle pulls against the humerus will be lengthened.

**Coracobrachialis** (coracobrachia'lis) The coracobrachialis (fig. 3.20) is a small muscle located medially on the upper humerus. It may be palpated just medial to the short head of the biceps brachii when the shoulder joint is flexed and resistance is applied at the elbow.

*Origin* Coracoid process of scapula.

*Insertion* Medial and anterior aspect of the humerus opposite the distal attachment of the deltoid.

*Innervation* Musculocutaneous nerve.

*Action* Flexion, horizontal adduction, adduction, and inward rotation of the glenohumeral joint; extension when the arm is overhead.

Figure 3.20. Coracobrachialis, anterior view

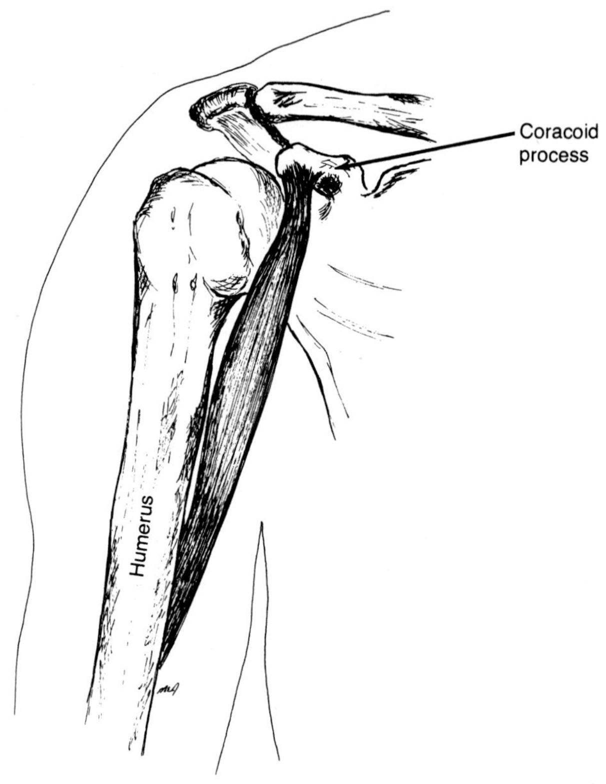


The coracobrachialis, because of its size and the location of its two attachments, is of limited effectiveness in its actions. The muscle crosses the shoulder joint inferior to the sagittal axis for adduction; anterior to the frontal axis for flexion; anterior to the frontal axis if origin is below insertion for extension; and anterior to the vertical axis for horizontal adduction and inward rotation. In all of the actions, the line of pull of the coracobrachialis is quite close to the respective axes. The muscle can act, therefore, in only an assistive manner at best, but is probably most effective as a flexor and an adductor of the shoulder joint.

**Latissimus Dorsi** (latis'simus dor'si) The latissimus dorsi (fig. 3.21), a very broad muscle, is located on the lower back. It is superficial except for a small upper portion which is covered by Part 4 of the trapezius. It can be palpated particularly well at the side of the rib cage during resisted adduction of the glenohumeral joint.

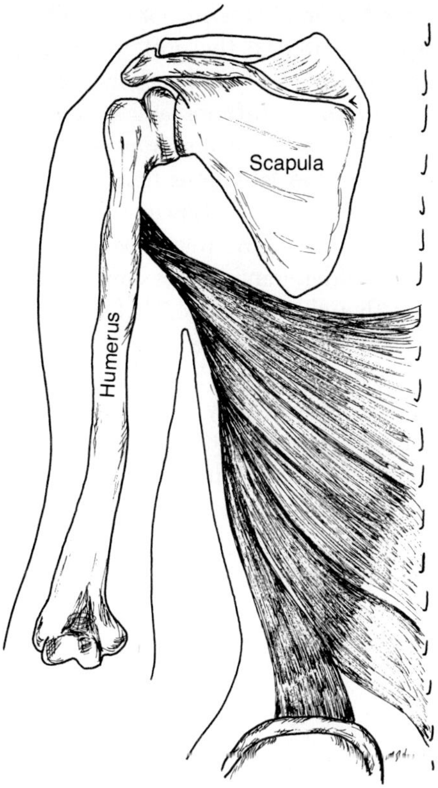

Figure 3.21. Latissimus dorsi, posterior view

*Origin* Spinous processes of lower six thoracic vertebrae and all lumbar vertebrae; posterior surface of sacrum, iliac crest; lower three ribs.

*Insertion* Anterior aspect of the humerus, parallel to the tendon of the pectoralis major.

*Innervation* Thoracodorsal nerve.

*Action* Adduction, extension, hyperextension, horizontal abduction and inward rotation of the glenohumeral joint.

The latissimus dorsi is favorably located with respect to all of the shoulder joint axes. The muscle courses well inferior to the sagittal axis to be a powerful adductor; it is inferior and anterior to the frontal axis of the shoulder regardless of the position of the humerus, and, since its origin is lower than its insertion, is an excellent extensor; it crosses the shoulder joint lateral to the vertical axis when the humerus is in the transverse plane to act as a horizontal abductor; its line of pull is medial to the vertical axis when in anatomical position to function as an inward rotator.

**Teres Major** (te'res ma'jor) The teres major (fig. 3.22) is a thick muscle located at the posterior edge of the axilla just above the latissimus dorsi. The muscle is superficial and may be palpated directly.

*Origin* Inferior angle of the scapula.

*Insertion* Anterior aspect of the humerus, just medial to the tendon of the latissimus dorsi.

*Innervation* Lower subscapular nerve.

*Action* The relationship of the teres major to the three axes of the shoulder joint is the same as that of the latissimus dorsi; it has been thought, therefore, that it performs the same actions as the latissimus dorsi, and is frequently called *the latissimus dorsi's little helper.* This conception has been largely in error, however, because the teres major contracts only when resistance has been applied to the arm, and only when positions are reached and held in the ranges of movement in adduction, inward rotation, and extension. For example, when one performs a chin-up to a bent arm hang, the latissimus dorsi will be strongly active during the lift of the body, but the teres major will be active only during the hang phase.

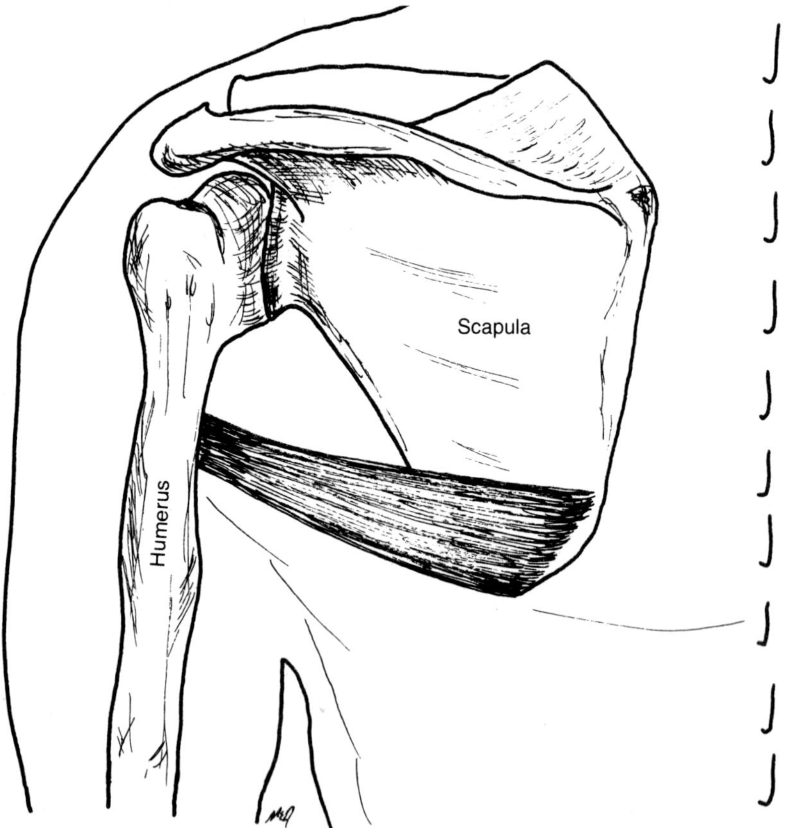


Figure 3.22. Teres major, posterior view

**Infraspinatus—Teres Minor** (infraspina'tus–te'res mi'nor) These two muscles (fig. 3.23) have identical actions and will be discussed together. They lie on the posterior surface of the scapula and are superficial except for a small portion which is covered by the posterior deltoid and the trapezius. They are two of the four rotator cuff muscles.

*Origin* Infraspinatus: Infraspinous fossa. Teres minor: Axillary border of scapula.

*Insertion* Both muscles: Greater tuberosity and adjacent shaft of the humerus.

*Innervation* Infraspinatus: Suprascapular nerve. Teres minor: Axillary nerve.

*Action* Outward rotation, and horizontal abduction of the glenohumeral joint. They also participate in abduction and flexion by pulling downwardly on the greater tuberosity as the deltoid pulls upwardly on the middle of the shaft of the humerus.

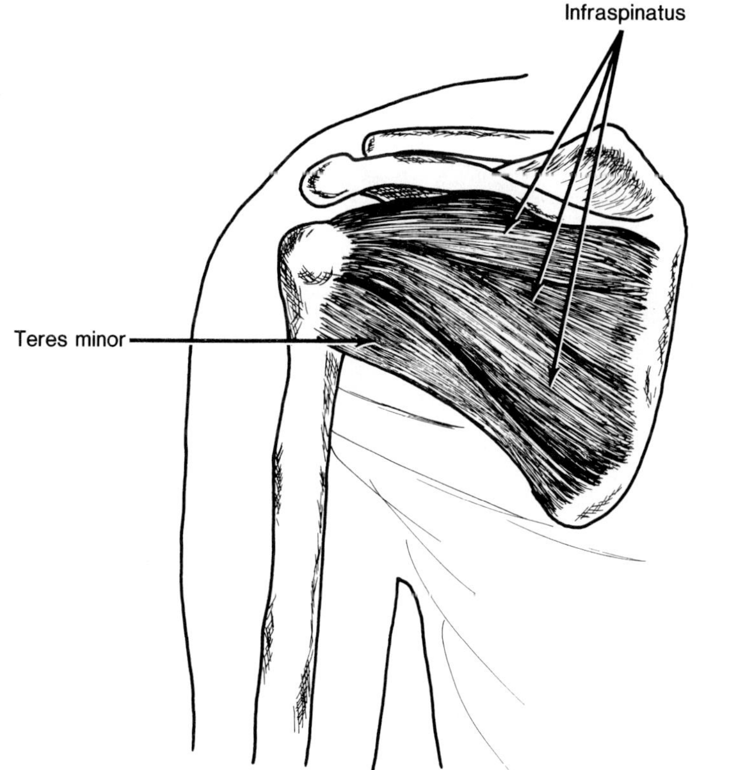


Figure 3.23. Infraspinatus and teres minor, posterior view

The infraspinatus-teres minor pass posterior to the vertical axis of the shoulder joint regardless of the position of the humerus to become outward rotators and horizontal abductors. That they are not also extensors and adductors or abductors is explained by the fact that they pass directly over both the sagittal and frontal axes of the shoulder.

Palpation of these muscles may be accomplished easily on a subject who has inclined the trunk forward and hangs the arms downwardly. The palpating fingers are placed on the axillary border of the scapula below the posterior deltoid. The muscles will be felt to contract as the subject rotates the arms outwardly.

**Subscapularis** (subscapula'ris) The subscapularis (fig. 3.24), one of the rotator cuff muscles, is a triangular muscle located on the scapula and next to the rib cage. It can be palpated on oneself by placing the thumb in the axilla and underneath the scapula as a relaxed toe-touching position is assumed. The weight of the hanging arm pulls the scapula into abduction, making the anterior surface accessible to the thumb. The belly of the muscle can be felt to contract as the arms are inwardly rotated.

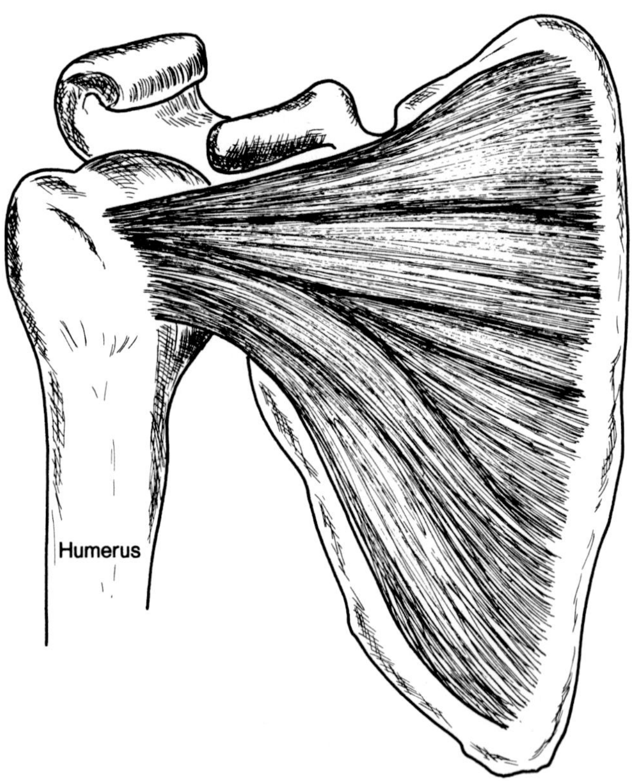


**Figure 3.24. Subscapularis, anterior view**

*Origin* Entire anterior surface of the scapula.

*Insertion* Lesser tuberosity of the humerus.

*Innervation* Subscapular nerve.

*Action* Inward rotation of the glenohumeral joint. The muscle also acts with the infraspinatus-teres minor in participating with the deltoid during abduction and flexion.

The inward rotation function of the subscapularis can be recognized clearly by examining the relationship of the anterior surface of the scapula to the lesser tuberosity of the humerus. As the muscle courses between its two attachments, it crosses medial to the vertical axis and then wraps around the anterior aspect of the upper humerus to give it a very favorable line of pull for rotation.

**Rotator Cuff** The rotator cuff is comprised of the supraspinatus, infraspinatus, teres minor, and subscapularis. These muscles are grouped together both because they all have rotational functions on the humerus, and because their tendons are interwoven into the capsule to form a musculotendinous cuff around the joint. They act together to hold the head of the humerus against the glenoid fossa and thus stabilize the joint against downward dislocation of the humerus. These muscles also perform with the deltoid during abduction and flexion of the shoulder joint. If the deltoid were to contract alone, its line of pull dictates that it would pull the humerus up against the acromion process. If the cuff muscles were to contract alone, they would depress the head of the humerus. Acting together, however, a force couple is produced and abduction or flexion of the joint will occur (fig. 3.25).

**Biceps Brachii** (bi'ceps bra'chii) The biceps brachii (fig. 3.26) lies on the anterior aspect of the upper arm. It is better known as a flexor of the elbow; however, it does cross the shoulder also and has, therefore, some ability to move the humerus. The biceps brachii is superficial, making it easily palpated and observed.

*Origin* Long head: Upper rim of the glenoid fossa. Short head: Coracoid process of the scapula.

*Insertion* Tuberosity of the radius.

*Innervation* Musculocutaneous nerve.

*Action* Long head: Abduction of the glenohumeral joint when the arm is outwardly rotated. Short head: Flexion, adduction, inward rotation, and horizontal adduction of the glenohumeral joint.

The line of pull of the biceps brachii at the shoulder joint is almost identical to that of the coracobrachialis and therefore the actions of the two muscles are similar, but are both of limited effectiveness.

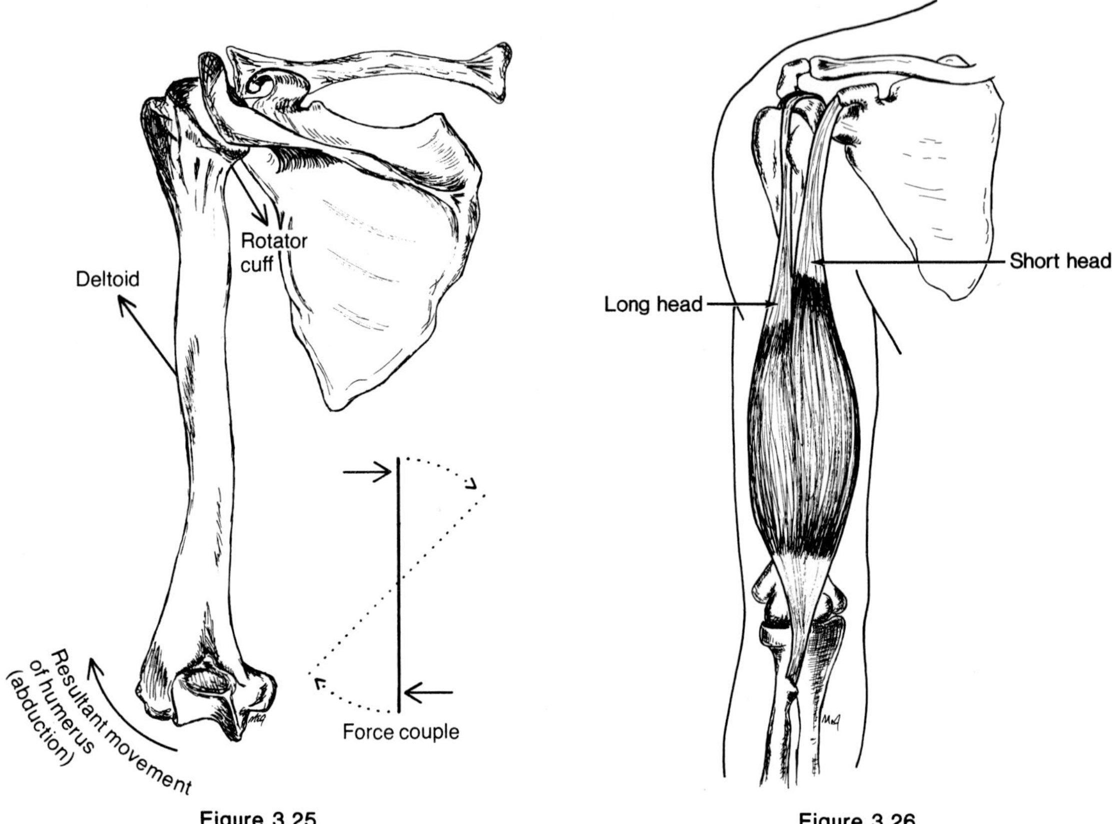

Figure 3.25

Figure 3.26

**Figure 3.25. Mechanics of abduction of the glenohumeral joint**

**Figure 3.26. Biceps brachii, anterior view**

The actions of the biceps at the shoulder joint are enhanced, however, by maintaining the elbow in an extended position, thus putting the muscle slightly on the stretch.

**Triceps Brachii—Long Head** (tri'ceps bra'chii) The triceps brachii (fig. 3.27) is located on the posterior aspect of the upper arm. As its name implies, it has three heads; one of these heads, the long head, crosses the shoulder joint and is, therefore, considered in the musculature of the shoulder joint. The triceps is superficial and is easily palpated and observed.

*Origin* Just inferior to the glenoid fossa.

*Insertion* Olecranon process of the ulna.

*Innervation* Radial nerve.

*Action* Extension and adduction of the glenohumeral joint.

Comparison of the locations of the two attachments of the long head of the triceps indicates that it is ineffectual as a mover of the humerus around the vertical axis because it passes directly over the

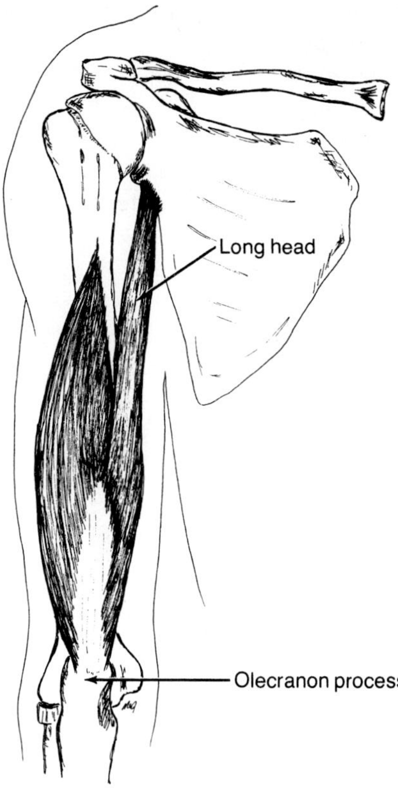

Figure 3.27. Triceps brachii, posterior view

Long head

Olecranon process

axis. The line of pull does pass slightly inferior to the sagittal axis for adduction, and slightly posterior to the frontal axis for extension. In both cases the line of pull produces a strong stabilizing component and a comparatively short angular component. It is to be expected, then, that the triceps is of limited effectiveness as a shoulder joint extensor or adductor. Its effectiveness can be increased, however, by placing the elbow in a flexed position to put the muscle on the stretch.

## Comments

The actions with which the muscles that move the humerus are credited can easily be deduced if their locations relative to the three axes of the shoulder joint are known. The procedure for learning muscle actions can be simplified even further by considering only the aspect of the shoulder on which the muscles are located. For example, the muscles which lie anterior to the frontal axis are generally those which lie on the anterior aspect of the shoulder. The same pattern holds true for the remaining muscles; thus, the four categories of anterior, posterior, superior, and inferior can be used—each category being credited with performing the logical actions on the humerus.

**Anterior Muscles** Flexion, horizontal adduction, inward rotation.

| | |
|---|---|
| *Anterior deltoid* | *Coracobrachialis* |
| *Pectoralis major* | *Latissimus dorsi* (inward rotation only) |
| *Subscapularis* | *Teres major* (inward rotation only) |
| *Biceps brachii* | |

**Posterior Muscles** Extension, hyperextension ,horizontal abduction, outward rotation.

| | |
|---|---|
| *Posterior deltoid* | *Triceps brachii* |
| *Latissimus dorsi* | *Supraspinatus* (outward rotation only) |
| *Teres major* | *Coracobrachialis* (extension only) |
| *Teres minor and Infraspinatus* | |

**Superior Muscles** Abduction.

| | |
|---|---|
| *Middle deltoid* | *Biceps brachii* |
| *Supraspinatus* | |
| *Pectoralis major*—clavicular portion (abduction above 90 degrees) | |

**Inferior Muscles** Adduction.

| | |
|---|---|
| *Latissimus dorsi* | *Coracobrachialis* |
| *Teres major* | *Biceps brachii* |
| *Pectoralis major*—sternal portion | *Triceps brachii* |

## Laboratory Experiences

1. Place the thumb and long finger along the scapular spine of a partner. While palpating, note the movements of the scapula as the arm is moved through the full range of flexion-extension, abduction-adduction, horizontal abduction-adduction, and inward-outward rotation. Which of the actions of the humerus would be limited if each of the following scapular muscles were impaired?

   Pectoralis minor
   Levator scapula
   Part 2 of trapezius
   Serratus anterior

2. Categorize the muscles or muscle portions which move the humerus according to whether they are (1) superior to the sagittal axis, (2) inferior to the sagittal axis, (3) anterior to the frontal axis, (4) posterior to the frontal axis, (5) anterior to the vertical axis, or (6) posterior to the vertical axis. Notice that some muscles or

muscle portions fall in one category only while others may be placed in two or even three categories. What actions will the muscles in the six categories perform?

3. Determine which of the muscles categorized in Experience #2 above are superficial. Palpate these muscles on a partner as the humerus is moved against some resistance through full ranges of motion around the three axes. Does your palpation support your categorizations? For example, the anterior portion of the deltoid will have been categorized as being located anterior to the frontal axis and the vertical axis. As such, it should flex, horizontally adduct, and inwardly rotate the joint. Palpations should confirm these actions.

4. Place a partner in a chair facing the edge of a door so that the two door knobs can be grasped by his right and left hands, respectively. Instruct the subject to extend the elbows and press down on the door knob held by the left hand and lift up on the door knob held by the right hand. Through palpation or observation, determine which portion of the left pectoralis major is active, and which portion of the right pectoralis major is active. Repeat your observations as the subject reverses his actions. Do your observations concur with the actions listed for the pectoralis major?

5. Have a partner lie supine on a table and place electrodes on the belly of the biceps brachii. While monitoring the action potentials, have the partner flex the shoulder joint first with the elbow extended, and then with the elbow fully flexed. Do your results agree with the actions noted for the biceps brachii as a mover of the humerus?

6. Repeat the above procedure on the long head of the triceps brachii of a partner who is lying prone on a table. Compare the action potentials of shoulder extension/elbow straight with those of shoulder extension/elbow flexed. What is your conclusion regarding optimum elbow position for the triceps as a mover of the humerus?

7. With a partner, determine whether the anterior portion of the deltoid acts as an adductor of the humerus. Be careful to eliminate the effects of gravity by having your partner take a supine lying position.

8. Analyze the movements of the humerus during the performance of a pushup. Based upon your analysis, determine which muscles will be involved, and by palpation or observation, confirm your determinations. What actions or exercises would you recommend to stretch these same muscles? Remember that to strengthen a muscle, its attachments must be pulled toward mid-muscle; to stretch a muscle, its attachments must be spread apart from each other.

9. Compare the actions of the humerus during the performance of a chin-up with supinated grip with those during the performance of a chin-up with pronated grip. According to the actions you have determined, list the muscles involved under each type of chin-up. Are the chin-ups alike or different with respect to muscle involvement?

# Elbow

# 4

The elbow is comprised of two joints formed by the articulation of the humerus with both the ulna and the radius. The trochlea of the humerus fits into the trochlear notch of the ulna to form a hinge joint, while the capitulum of the humerus articulates in gliding fashion with the head of the radius. Kinesiologically, the two joints can be thought of as one—a hinge joint which permits rotation about a single axis represented by a line passing through the two epicondyles of the humerus. The only actions which can be performed by the elbow are flexion and extension (fig. 4.1); as a consequence all muscles which cross the elbow will be either flexors or extensors of that joint. Muscles crossing the elbow posterior to the axis will be extensors, while muscles crossing the elbow anterior to the joint axis will be flexors.

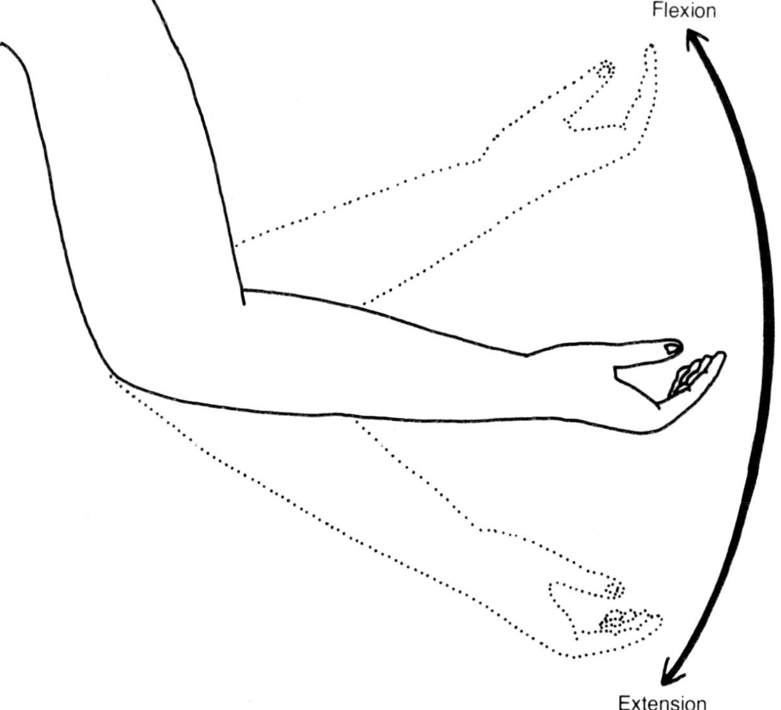


**Figure 4.1. Movements of the elbow joint**

The major ligaments of the elbow joint are the ulnar and radial collaterals (fig. 4.2). The ulnar collateral ligament stabilizes the medial portion of the joint, and runs between the medial epicondyle of the humerus and the olecranon and coronoid processes of the ulna. The radial collateral ligament runs between a depression just below the lateral epicondyle and the annular ligament of the radioulnar joint.

The proximal radioulnar joint, a synovial joint, is formed by the head of the radius and the radial notch of the ulna. The joint is of the pivot variety and allows rotation about a vertical axis which is represented by a line passing through the head of the radius proximally and the head of the ulna distally (fig. 4.3).

The head of the radius is bound firmly to the ulna by the annular ligament which forms a ring within which the radius rotates (fig. 4.2). When the radius is rotated outwardly, the radius and ulna are parallel and the palm of the hand faces forward (supination); when the radius is rotated inwardly, the radius crosses over the ulna and the palm of the hand faces backward (pronation).

The distal radioulnar joint, also of the synovial type, is the articulation between the head of the ulna and the radial notch. The joint is a pivot joint and permits the radius to rotate around the ulna in much the same fashion as is seen in the proximal joint of these two bones. A disc of fibrocartilage is interposed between the head of the ulna and the carpal bones to bind the radius and ulna firmly together.

Since both the proximal and distal radioulnar joints are pivot joints, they can permit only supination (outward rotation of the forearm) and pronation (inward rotation of the forearm). Muscles which cross these two joints are, therefore, supinators or pronators. Supinators cross the joints posterior to the axis of rotation; pronators cross the joints anterior to the axis. When the forearm is midway between supination and pronation, it is said to be in neutral position.

The ligaments of the distal radioulnar joint are the palmar and dorsal radioulnar ligaments. These ligaments run between the radius and ulna on the palmar (anterior) and dorsal (posterior) sides of the joint, and are actually thickenings of the joint capsule.

## Bone Markings

Figure 4.4 notes the various bony landmarks pertinent to the kinesiology of the elbow. The illustration is intended only as review material and should be used with a skeleton for proper perspective.

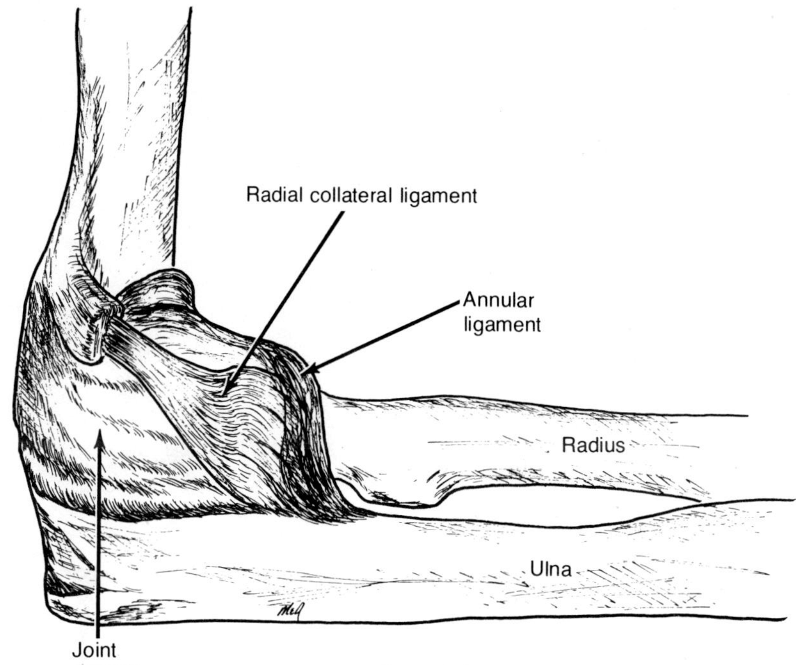


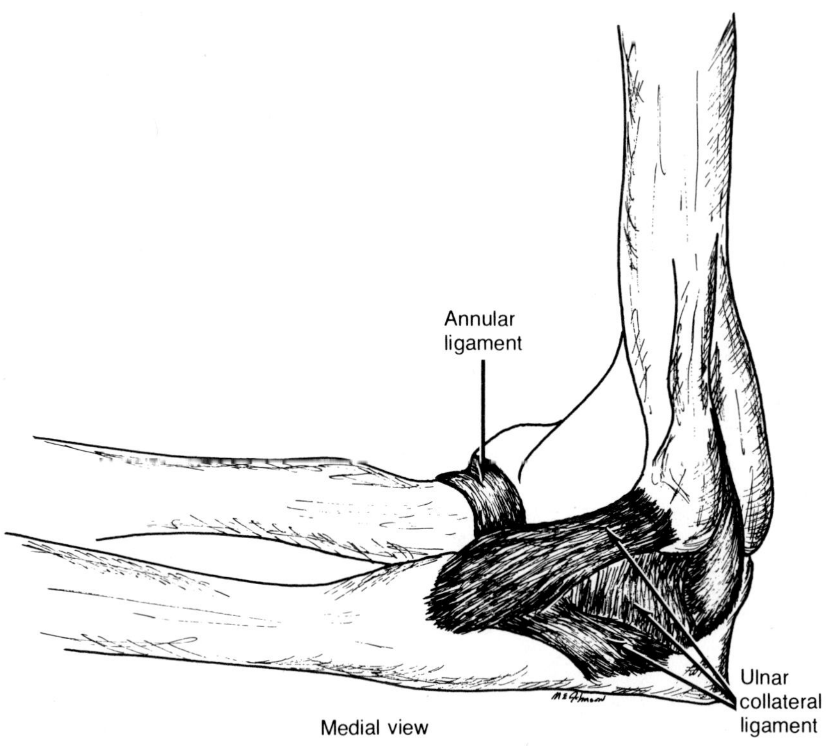


**Figure 4.2. Ligaments of elbow**

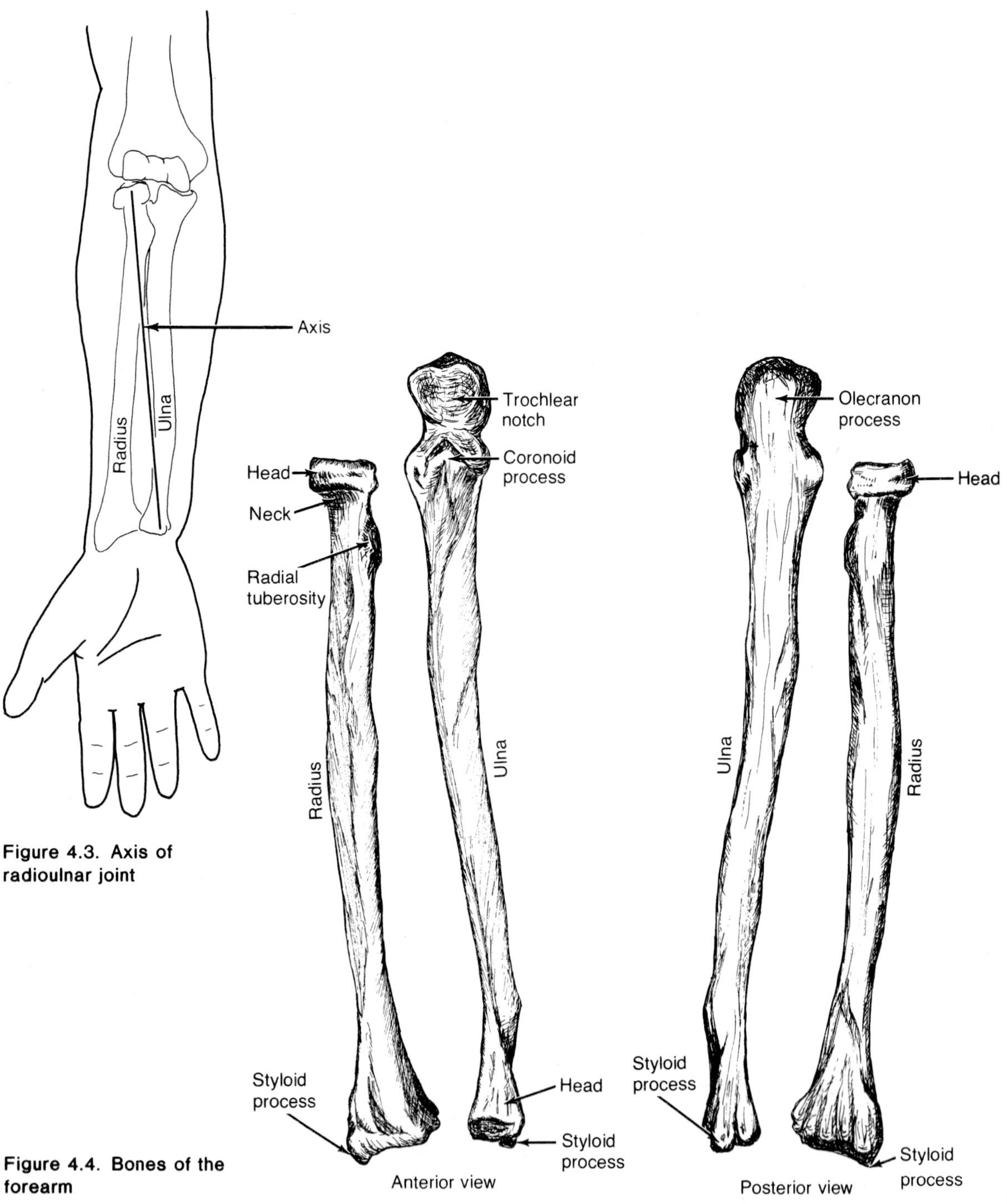


**Figure 4.3. Axis of radioulnar joint**

**Figure 4.4. Bones of the forearm**

## Musculature

**Biceps Brachii** (bi'ceps bra'chii) (See also muscles of shoulder joint, chap. 3)

The biceps brachii (fig. 4.5) is a fusiform muscle located prominently on the front of the upper arm. It is superficial and can be easily palpated and observed.

*Origin* Long head: Upper rim of glenoid fossa. Short head: Coracoid process of scapula.

*Insertion* Tuberosity of the radius.

*Innervation* Musculocutaneous nerve.

*Action* Flexion of the elbow joint and supination of the radioulnar joint.

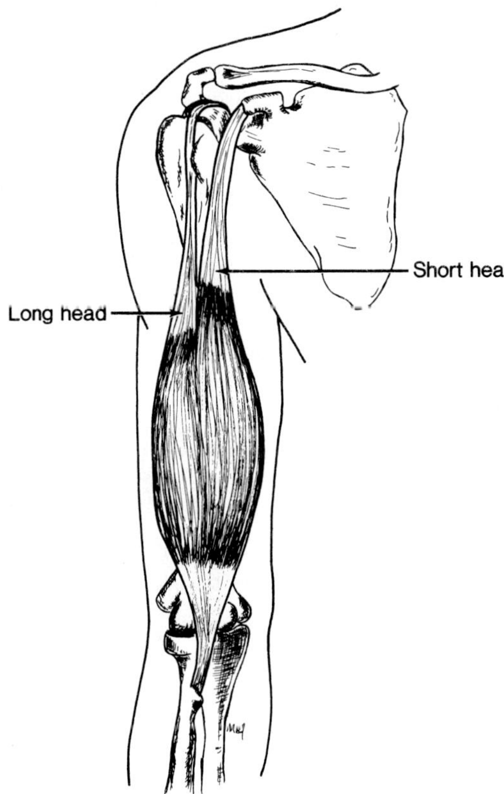


Figure 4.5. Biceps brachii, anterior view

The effectiveness of the biceps as a flexor of the elbow is shown in figure 4.6. The muscle crosses the joint well in front of the axis regardless of the amount of flexion of the elbow. It will be seen, also, that as the forearm is moved through the range from full extension to full flexion, the force components of the pull of the biceps vary in length. At full extension, the contracting biceps is primarily a stabilizer; at full flexion, contraction of the biceps is accompanied by a strong dislocating component. At approximately 90 degrees of elbow flexion, however, the only component provided by the biceps is the angular one. It follows, then, that when strength is desired during elbow flexion, the 90-degree angle of flexion is mechanically best. As the joint angulation changes from 90 degrees as it is either extended farther or flexed farther, the angular component decreases, giving way to the stabilizing or dislocating component, respectively.

It is important to note that the above discussion relates only to the mechanics of contraction and does not reflect any physiological property of the muscle. Because muscle tissue is contractile, extensible, and

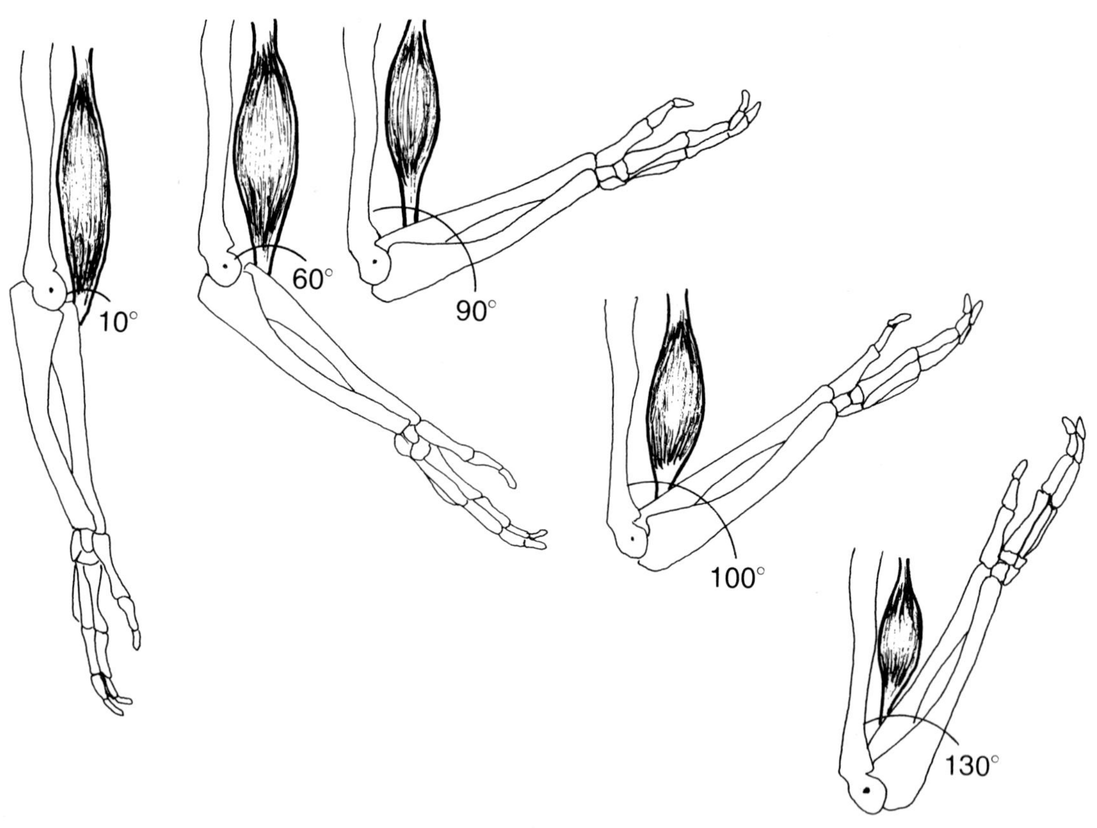


**Figure 4.6. Insertion angles of the biceps brachii at various degrees of elbow flexion**

elastic, it has the ability to adjust itself in length—an ability that materials with which the physicist and engineer work do not have. It is possible to require muscle tissue to so elongate that it cannot contract; it is also possible to shorten muscle tissue to the point at which no further contraction is possible. Hence, as a muscle contracts through its full range of shortening, it begins in a weakened condition, gradually becomes stronger, and then, as it approaches its shortest length, becomes weakened again. It can be seen, then, that if a muscle is required to elongate to accommodate hyperextension of a joint, the muscle contraction will be comparatively weak, both because of the mechanics of its attachments and because of its physiological properties. Similarly, the shortened muscle which accompanies a fully flexed joint is weak both mechanically and physiologically. Somewhere between the ends of the range continuum, peak strength is reached. Mechanically, that point occurs when the muscle inserts at 90 degrees; unfortunately, the physiological point of peak strength does not usually coincide, and is reached sooner, at approximately full extension of the joint. Figure 4.6 is presented to illustrate the difference between the two points of peak strength. The biceps brachii is used as the example; however, the example can be generalized to other muscles, and particularly those which cause angular motion and can, thereby, alter their angles of insertion.

Figure 4.6 indicates that at full extension of the elbow, the biceps inserts at a 10 degree angle; at full flexion, the angle is 130 degrees. Midlength of the biceps will be reached at the approximate insertion angle of 60 degrees

$$\left(\frac{130^\circ - 10^\circ}{2}\right) = 60^\circ$$

At this angle, the muscle is physiologically capable of exerting force, but its angle of insertion is mechanically unsound. At the 90-degree angle demanded by mechanics, however, the muscle is overly shortened and weakened. It is apparent that in order to profit from both concepts, the joint should be positioned half way between the physiological optimum (full extension) and the mechanical optimum (90° flexion).

In summary, when a muscle or muscle group must exhibit maximum strength, position the joint so the angle of insertion is between 90 degrees and the angle of insertion at which the joint is extended. For practical use, the rule can be simplified by first positioning the joint for the 90-degree insertion angle and then adjusting the position of the joint to put the muscle slightly on the stretch.

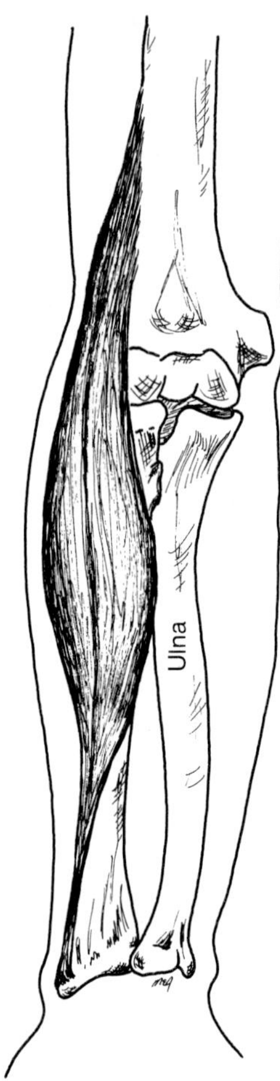

Figure 4.7. Brachioradialis, anterior view

**Brachioradialis** (brachioradia'lis) The brachioradialis (fig. 4.7) is a fusiform muscle located on the radial border of the forearm. It is superficial and may be palpated readily by flexing the elbow and holding the forearm so that the thumb is up. When resistance is applied to the top of the wrist, the brachioradialis is seen to contract just below the elbow.

*Origin* Upper two-thirds of the supracondylar ridge of the lateral epicondyle of the humerus.

*Insertion* Base of the styloid process of radius.

*Innervation* Radial nerve.

*Action* Flexion of the elbow.

The distal attachment of the brachioradialis is considerably farther from the elbow than is the case with the other elbow flexors. The mechanical advantage afforded by this muscle is, therefore, increased. Its proximal attachment is, however, much closer to the elbow than other flexors, and, because of this, the muscle lies very close to the joint axis. During contraction, then, the brachioradialis yields a small angular component at its distal attachment when compared to its large stabilizing component. This angular component can be lengthened slightly by placing the forearm in the neutral position so that the muscle will be made to pass farther anterior to the joint axis. The pull of the brachioradialis will, therefore, be strongest when the forearm is in neutral position.

**Brachialis** (brachia'lis) The brachialis (fig. 4.8), called *the workhorse of the elbow,* is a fusiform muscle located on the anterior aspect of the elbow. It may be palpated just lateral to the biceps when resistance is applied to the wrist.

*Origin* Lower half of anterior surface of the humerus.

*Insertion* Anterior surface of coronoid process of the ulna.

*Innervation* Musculocutaneous nerve.

*Action* Flexion of the elbow.

The brachialis crosses the elbow closer to the axis of flexion/extension than do the biceps or brachioradialis. Per unit of contraction, then, the brachialis is less favorably situated to provide force; however, since its distal attachment is on the ulna rather than the radius, forearm position is inconsequential to the effectiveness of its pull. Regardless of forearm position, degree of elbow flexion or amount of resistance, the brachialis is involved in the flexive action—hence its name, *workhorse of the elbow.*

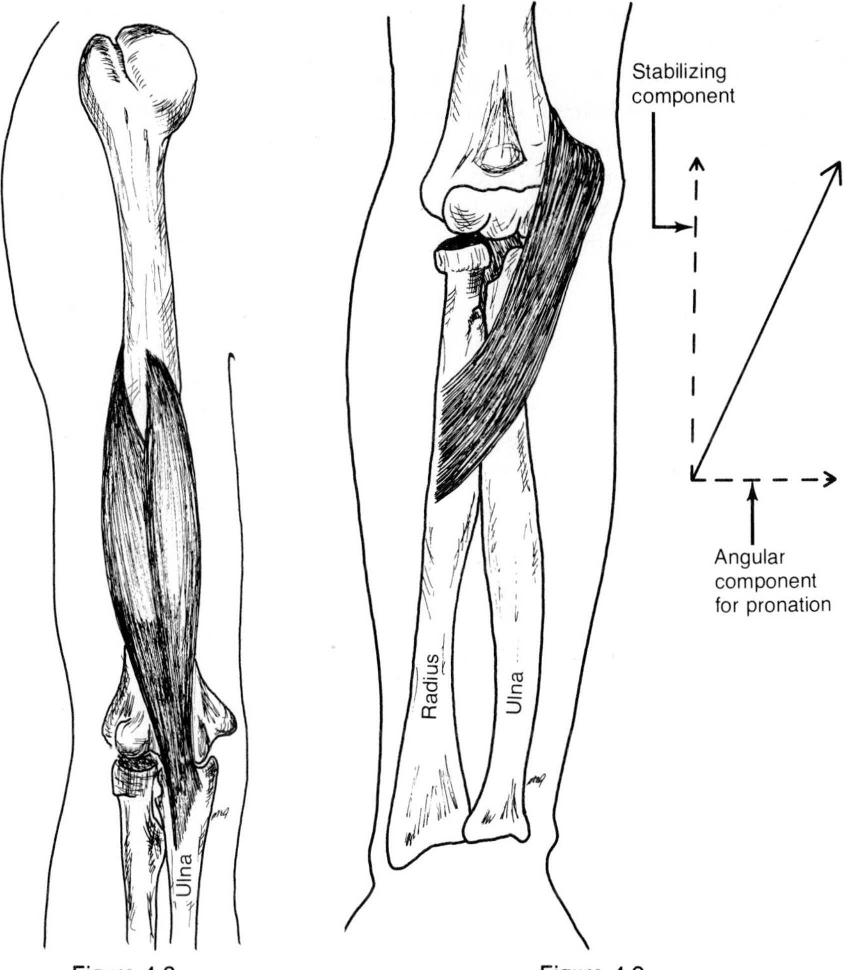


Figure 4.8

Figure 4.9

**Figure 4.8. Brachialis, anterior view**

**Figure 4.9. Pronator teres, anterior view (ulnar head not shown)**

**Pronator Teres** (Prona'tor te'res) The pronator teres (fig. 4.9) is located on the anterior and upper aspect of the forearm. Its distal portion is covered by the brachioradialis; however, the main muscle mass is superficial and may be palpated as the forearm is pronated against resistance with the elbow well-flexed. To help distinguish the pronator teres from surrounding musculature, place the thumb on the medial epicondyle and the long finger on the midpoint of the radius. A ridge of muscle will be seen running obliquely between the thumb and long finger when the forearm is pronated against resistance.

*Origin* By two heads, one (humeral head) from the medial epicondyle of the humerus, and one (ulnar head) from the coronoid process of the ulna. The attachment to the medial epicondyle is by a common tendon which also supports the attachments of the flexor muscles of the forearm.

*Insertion* Lateral surface of the radius near its midpoint.

*Innervation* Median nerve.

*Action* Pronation of the radioulnar joint; flexion of the elbow joint.

The pronator teres is well anterior to the axis of the radioulnar joint. Its approximate angle of insertion on the radius is shown, together with its resolution to the two components, in figure 4.9. The length of the angular component testifies to the high efficiency of the muscle as a pronator whereas the stabilizing vector indicates that contraction of this muscle will be accompanied by a force preventing any tendency of the radius to be dislocated as pronation is performed. Because of its strength and efficiency, the muscle does not participate when pronation is slow or unresisted.

The location of the pronator teres in relationship to the elbow axes can be seen easily through palpation. Regardless of forearm position, the muscle is quite close to the axis throughout the range of flexion, and is, therefore, inefficient as an elbow flexor when compared to the biceps, brachioradialis, and brachialis. As an elbow flexor, the pronator teres would be, at best, an assistant mover. Even then, its contraction may serve to neutralize the supinating tendency of the biceps rather than to contribute to the actual flexion of the joint.

**Pronator Quadratus** (prona'tor quadra'tus) The pronator quadratus (fig. 4.10) is a rhomboidal muscle located at the distal end of the forearm. It is a deep muscle and cannot be palpated.

*Origin* Lower fourth of the palmar surface of the ulna.

*Insertion* Lower fourth of the palmar surface of the radius.

*Innervation* Median nerve.

*Action* Pronation of the radioulnar joint.

The pronator quadratus is the primary mover for pronation. Its size and line of pull allow it to pronate the radioulnar joint without help when the action is performed slowly and without resistance. If speed is required, or if resistance is met, the quadratus will be aided by the pronator teres.

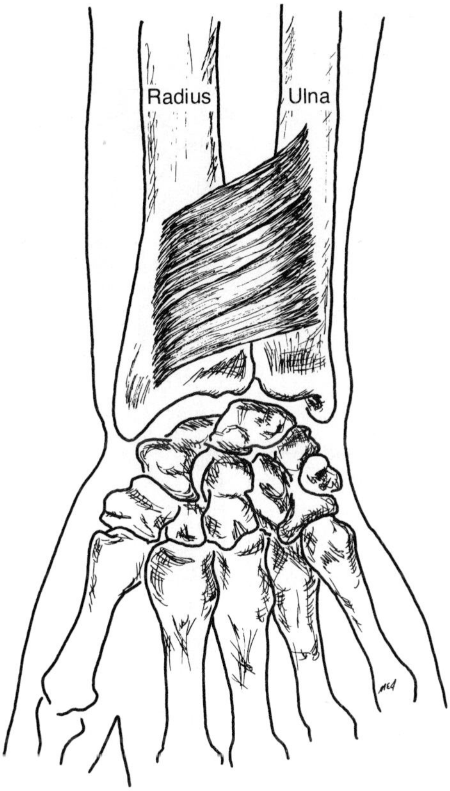

Figure 4.10. Pronator quadratus, anterior view

**Triceps Brachii** (tri'ceps bra'chii) The triceps brachii (fig. 4.11) is a three-headed muscle located superficially on the posterior aspect of the upper arm. Its lateral head may be palpated between the bulge of the deltoid and the lateral epicondyle; its long head may be palpated between the axilla and the olecranon process. The medial head is covered by the other heads and cannot be palpated.

*Origin* Long head: Infraglenoid tuberosity of the scapula. Lateral head: Upper half of posterior surface of the humerus. Medial head: Lower two-thirds of the posterior surface of the humerus.

*Insertion* Olecranon process of the ulna.

*Innervation* Radial nerve.

*Action* Extension of the elbow ioint.

Figure 4.12 illustrates that the triceps, by virtue of its insertion on the olecranon process, applies force for first class leverage. The mechanical advantage is small (approximately .2) to favor speed over power; however, the size of the muscle as well as its angle of attachment on the olecranon give the triceps great power in spite of the poor leverage.

Figure 4.11. Triceps brachii, posterior view

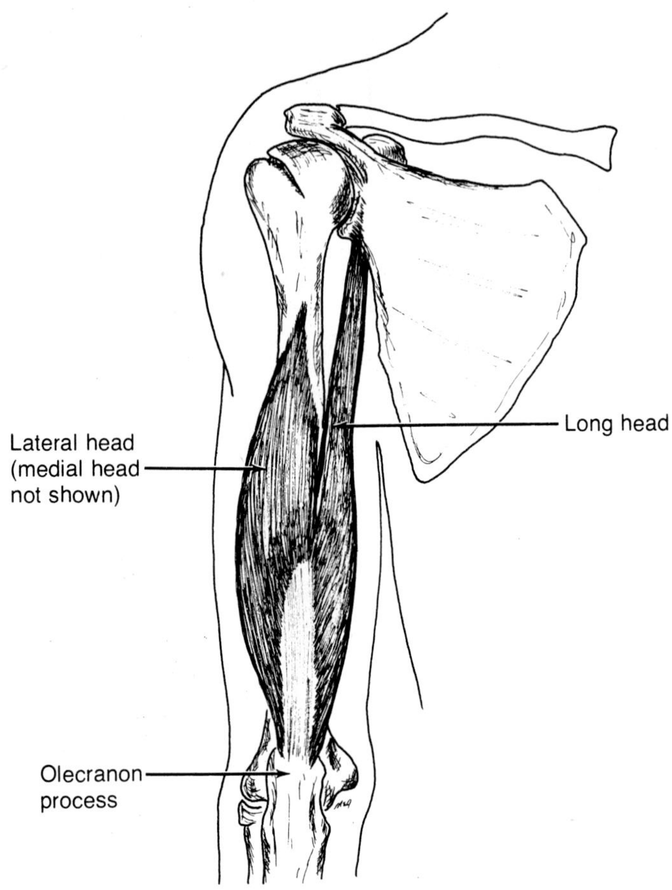


**Anconeus** (ancone'us) The anconeus (fig. 4.13) is a small triangular muscle located on the upper and posterior aspect of the forearm. If the thumb and index finger are placed on the olecranon and lateral epicondyle respectively, they will define the base of an equilateral triangle within which the anconeus may be palpated.

*Origin* Posterior surface of lateral epicondyle of the humerus.

*Insertion* Lateral aspects of the olecranon and posterior surface of upper ulna.

*Innervation* Radial nerve.

*Action* Extension of elbow joint.

As the anconeus courses between its two attachments, it comes very close to the elbow axis. This, in addition to its size, makes the muscle a weak extensor of the joint.

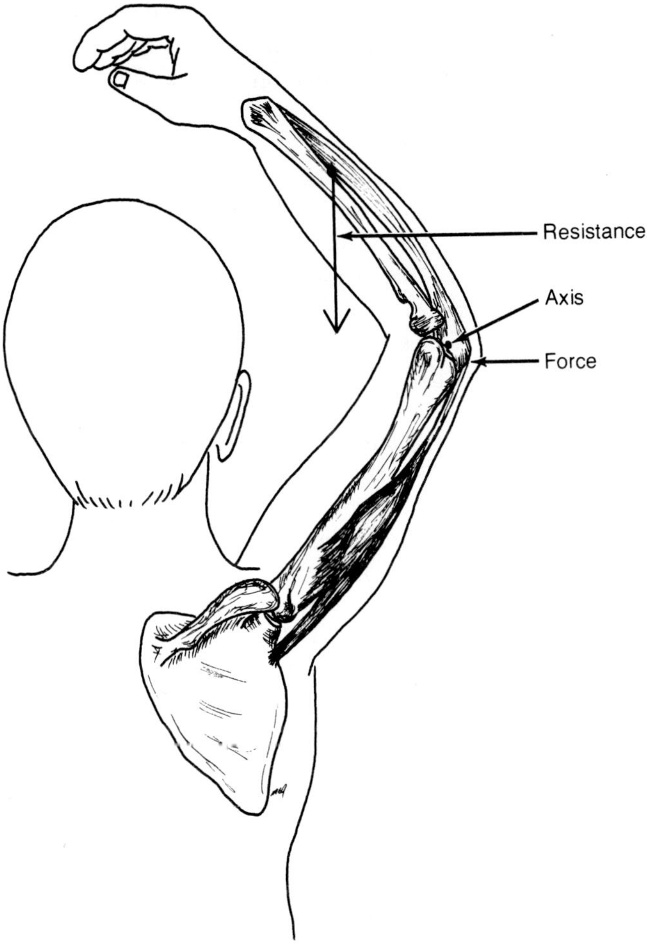

Figure 4.12. First class leverage of the triceps brachii

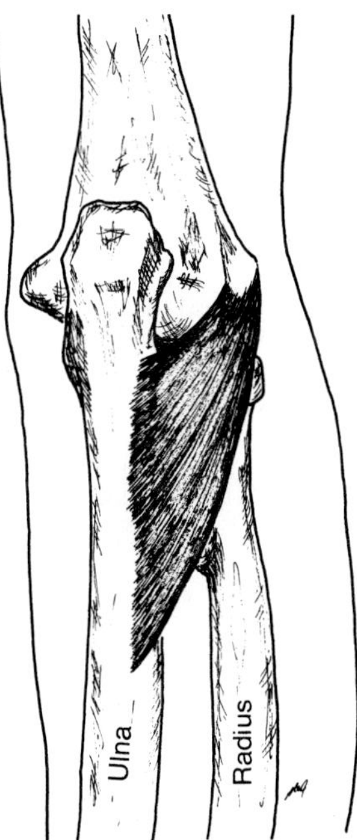


Figure 4.13. Anconeus of the right arm, posterior view

**Supinator** (supina'tor) The supinator (fig. 4.14), a longitudinal muscle of two layers, is located on the dorsum of the forearm. It is covered by the brachioradialis and the wrist extensors, and cannot be palpated.

*Origin* Lateral epicondyle of the humerus; adjacent portion of the ulna; annular and radial collateral ligaments.

*Insertion* Lateral surface of the upper third of the radius.

*Innervation* Radial nerve.

*Action* Supination of radioulnar joint.

The supinator is in its best position to supinate the radioulnar joint when the elbow is extended, thus placing the muscle on the stretch. In this position, it requires assistance from the biceps brachii

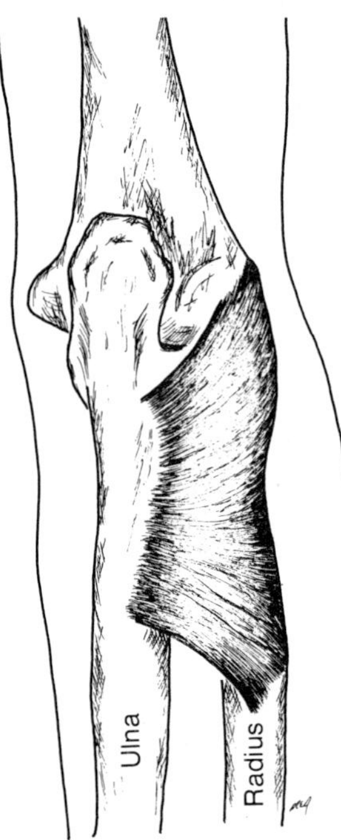

Figure 4.14. Supinator of the right arm, posterior view

only when resistance is met. When the elbow is flexed, however, the supinator is shortened and must have the help of the biceps under all conditions except when supination is performed slowly and without resistance.

**Forearm Muscles** There are eight muscles of the forearm which originate on or just above the epicondyles of the humerus and insert distal to the wrist. The primary actions of these muscles are to move the hand around the wrist joint, or to flex or extend the fingers; however, they do cross the elbow joint, and it is necessary, therefore, to investigate their functions as movers of that joint.

It will be recalled that the axis of flexion-extension of the elbow passes through the two epicondyles of the humerus. Since the eight forearm muscles originate on or adjacent to these bony prominences, there is the possibility that the muscles cross the elbow in line with the axis and will not, therefore, be movers of that joint. Even if some of the muscles should cross the joint either anterior or posterior to the axis, they must, by virtue of their origins, be quite close to the axis, and cannot be powerful movers.

Careful examination of a skeleton will indicate that four of the eight forearm muscles—the extensor carpi radialis longus, extensor carpi radialis brevis, palmaris longus, and flexor carpi radialis—cross the elbow anterior to the axis and are, therefore, in a position to contribute somewhat to elbow flexion. Their contribution is only assistive, and is enhanced when wrist action is required simultaneously with elbow flexion. The origins, insertions, innervations, and additional actions of these muscles are discussed fully in chapter 5.

# Comments

The elbow and radioulnar joints are admirably adapted to the innumerable requirements of sport and dance techniques. The joints are structurally strong, yet allow for satisfactory range of movement. Surrounding musculature is both of the penniform and longitudinal type to meet the demands for strength as well as range of motion, and displays favorable mechanical advantage during both flexion-extension and pronation-supination.

Perhaps the versatility of the elbow region can best be appreciated when one considers the number of sports which involve action of the two joints. Movement patterns comprising activities from archery to waterskiing all require that specific degrees of motion of the elbow be performed with equally specific timing. Even motions which appear to be equivalent involve subtle differences in joint action. The overarm throw is an example. A shortstop and a quarterback both throw overarm but each uses the elbow differently; the javelin thrower exhibits yet a different pattern, as does the volleyball player delivering an overarm serve, and the tennis player executing a smash.

Further respect for the elbow is earned when consideration is given to the size and weight of the objects we throw. Great muscular power is required to accelerate these objects to the point of release, and there is the inevitable stabilizing component which accompanies such forceful contractions. That the joints can withstand so constant a jamming of the articulating bones is, indeed, awesome.

## Laboratory Experiences

1. Place electrodes on the muscle bellies of the biceps brachii and brachioradialis of a partner. Monitor the action potentials as the partner performs arm curls with a two- or three-kilogram weight. Have the partner alternate between the supinated and pronated grips as the arm curls are performed. What conclusions can you make regarding the input of the two muscles relative to the types of arm curls?
2. While monitoring the action potentials of the biceps brachii, supinate the radioulnar joint slowly, and then rapidly. Are there differences in the activity of the muscle? Perform supination against resistance and note differences in the electromyographic record. Do your findings agree with the actions listed for the biceps brachii?
3. Using a cable tensiometer or other device which measures force, determine your maximum strength at 180, 120, 90 and 70 degrees of elbow flexion. At which joint angle are you strongest? Does this agree with the concepts of mechanical and physiological efficiency discussed in this chapter under actions of the biceps brachii?

# 5 The Wrist and Hand

The wrist and hand are comprised of over twenty bones and joints, and twenty-five muscles or muscle groups. That man is able to use so complex a structure with such versatility attests to the perfection of its construction.

The wrist joint (fig. 5.1) is formed by the articulation of the radius and the articular disc with the navicular, lunate, and triquetrum bones. These latter three bones, along with the pisiform, form the proximal row of carpal bones and articulate, in turn, with the distal row—the multangulus major, the multangulus minor, capitate and hamate bones. It is clear that, in actuality, the wrist joint is comprised of

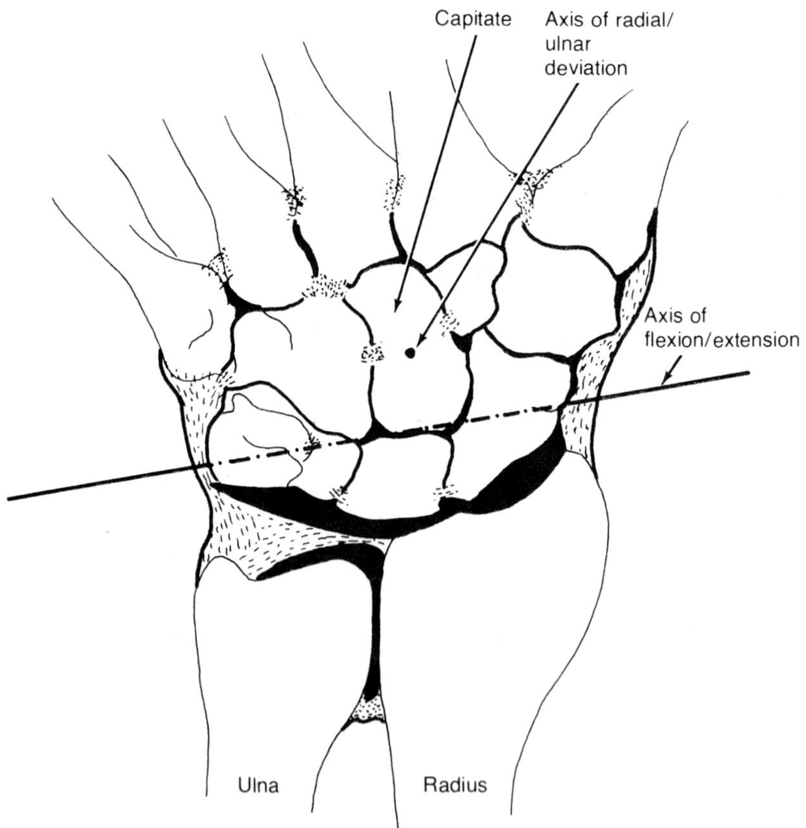


**Figure 5.1. Axes of the wrist joint**

several joints, some between the carpal bones, called *intercarpal joints,* and one between the radius and articular disc and the proximal row of carpals, called the *radiocarpal joint.* It is typical, however, to consider the joints as one and to refer to them collectively as the *wrist joint.*

The distal row of carpals articulate with the five metacarpals via the *carpometacarpal joints.* The metacarpals articulate, in turn, with the proximal phalanges by the *metacarpophalangeal joints,* and between themselves by the *intermetacarpal joints.* The joints between the phalanges are referred to as the *interphalangeal joints.*

## Bone Markings

Figure 5.2 is presented as a review of the bone markings of the wrist and hand which are relevant to the discussion of muscle origins and insertions. A skeleton should be used with the figure for best review.

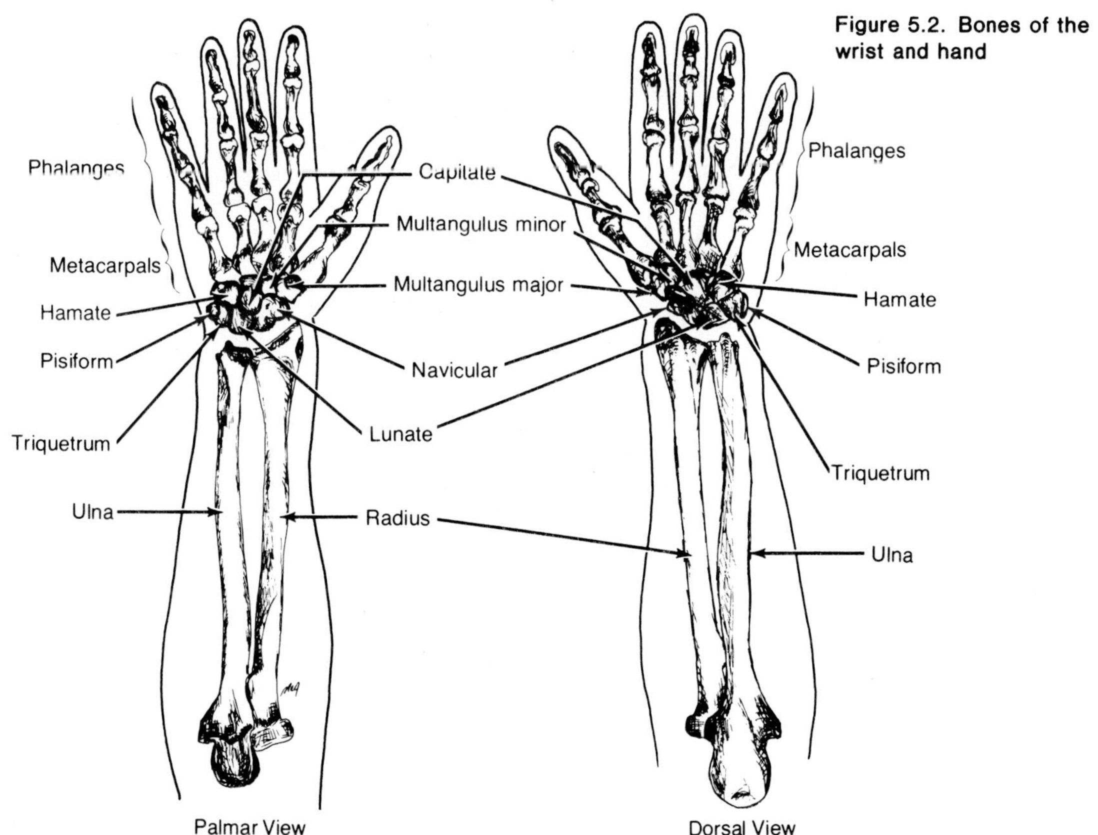


**Figure 5.2. Bones of the wrist and hand**

## Joints of the Wrist and Hand

### Radiocarpal Joint

The radiocarpal joint is a condyloid joint and provides for rotation about two axes. One, the frontal axis, passes through the wrist just distal to the styloid processes of the radius and ulna (fig. 5.1), and is the axis for flexion and extension. The second axis is a sagittal one and passes through the capitate bone at a right angle to the palm (fig. 5.1). Movements of the hand which require rotation around the sagittal axis are radial deviation and ulnar deviation. Sequential combination of movements around the two axes results in circumduction.

The major ligaments of the radiocarpal joint are the volar and dorsal radiocarpal ligaments and the radial and ulnar collateral ligaments. The volar radiocarpal ligament (fig. 5.3) courses between the

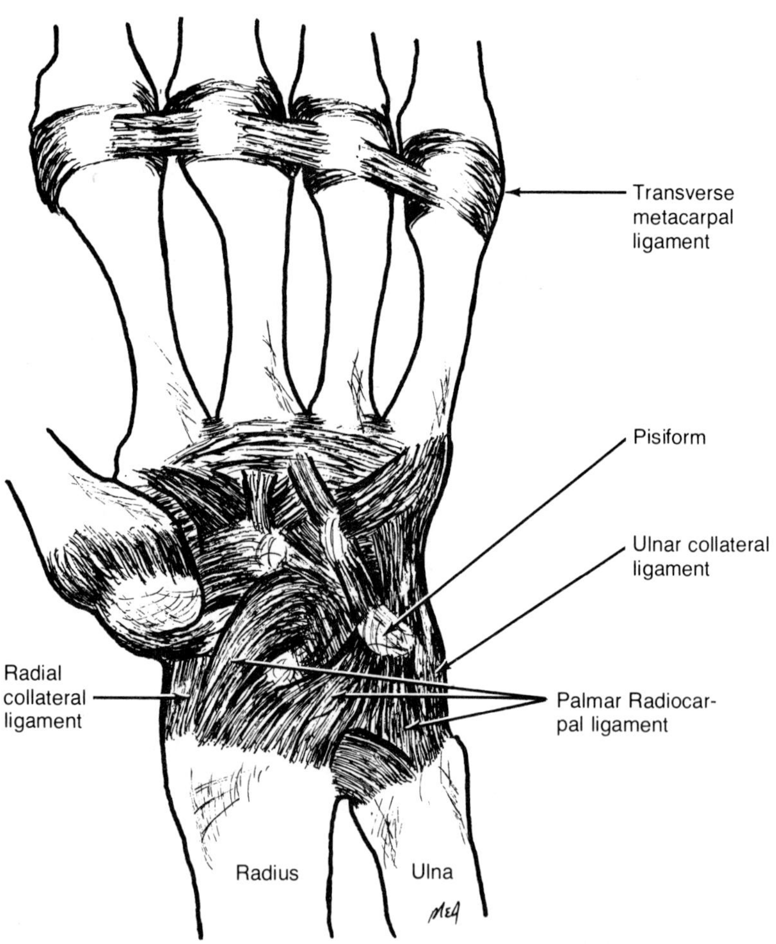


Figure 5.3. Ligaments of the wrist, palmar view

palmar surfaces of the radius and articular disc, and the carpal bones; it also attaches to the volar intercarpal ligament. The dorsal radiocarpal ligament (fig. 5.4) is attached proximally to the posterior surface of the radius and disc, and distally to only the proximal row of carpal bones. The dorsal radiocarpal ligament is thinner and more membranous than its volar counterpart.

The collateral ligaments of the wrist (fig. 5.3) are, as their names imply, on the radial and ulnar sides of the joint. The radial collateral ligament is attached between the styloid process of the radius and the navicular, capitate, and multangulus major. The ulnar collateral ligament attaches to the styloid process of the ulna and the articular disc, and runs distally to the pisiform and the transverse carpal ligament.

The joint capsule is encased by the four ligaments of the wrist joint and thus covers the articular surfaces of the radius and articular disc, and the carpal bones. In order to provide for ease of motion the capsule is quite loose and presents numerous folds, especially when the wrist is flexed.

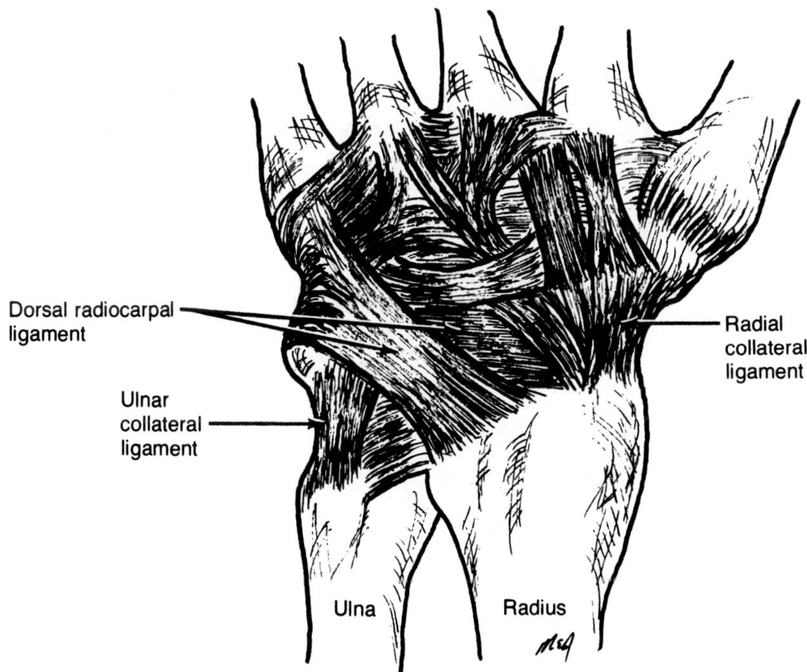


Figure 5.4. Ligaments of the wrist, dorsal view

## Intercarpal Joints

The intercarpal joints are those articulations between the individual bones and between the two rows of bones as well. All of the joints are synovial; however, they are nonaxial and permit only a gliding motion between the bones. Collectively, the several joints contribute to flexion, extension, and radial and ulnar deviation of the radiocarpal joint.

The ligaments of the intercarpal joints are categorized by their location. The palmar and dorsal ligaments run transversely across the hand, connecting several carpal bones. The collateral ligaments are located along the two sides of the hand and are continuous with the radial and ulnar collateral ligaments of the wrist joint. The interosseus ligaments join the articular surfaces of adjacent carpals.

In addition to the ligamentous tissues discussed above, there is a structure of the carpals known as the *flexor retinaculum* (fig. 5.5). It

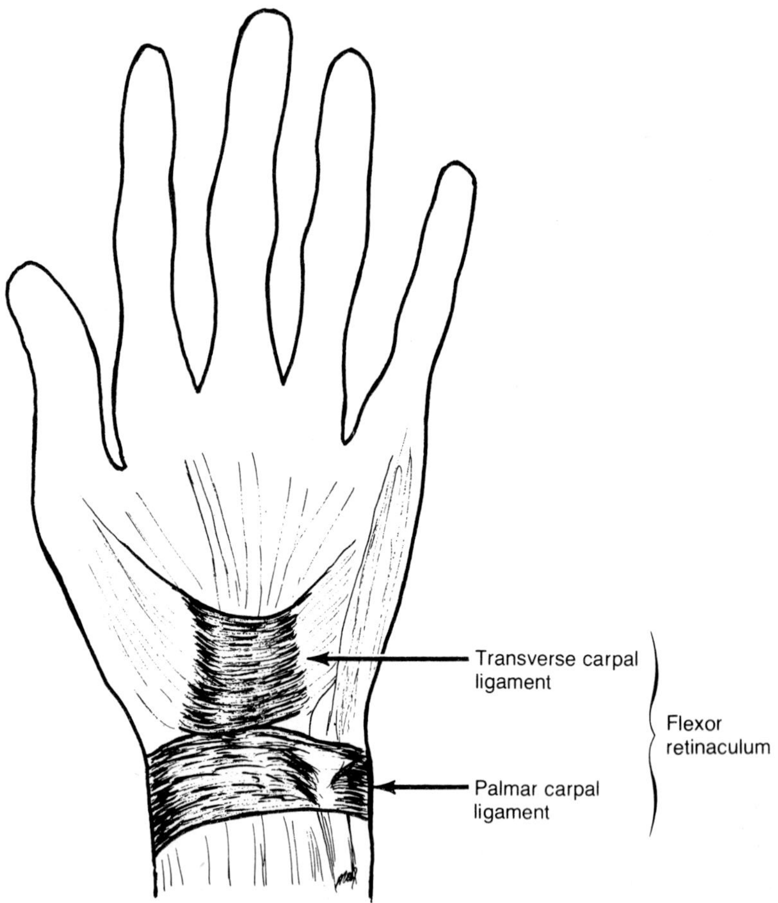


**Figure 5.5. Flexor retinaculum, palmar view**

is comprised of two bands previously known as the *palmar carpal ligament* and the *transverse carpal ligament.* The proximal portion of the flexor retinaculum connects the palmar surfaces of the styloid processes of the ulna and radius. Distally, it is attached between the pisiform and hamate, and the navicular and multangulus major. Under the flexor retinaculum lie the median nerve and the tendons of the flexor digitorum superficialis and the flexor carpi radialis.

The synovial capsule of these joints is extensive and typically allows for communication of the synovial fluid throughout the intercarpal complex. The articulation between the pisiform and triquetrum is an exception, however, and comprises a separate joint capsule.

### Carpometacarpal Joints

The carpometacarpal (referred to as *CMC*) joints are formed by the articulations of the distal row of carpal bones with the base of the five metacarpals. The first CMC joint, that articulation between the multangulus major and the metacarpal of the thumb, is a saddle joint and allows rotation around two axes. One of these axes runs through the base of the first metacarpal and slants toward the base of the ring finger (fig. 5.6). When the metacarpal moves around this axis, the actions of abduction and adduction are performed. These action can easily be repeated by the individual, but care must be taken to restrict action at the knuckle joint of the thumb, and to concentrate attention on the CMC joint. If difficulty is encountered, the actions can be enhanced by placing just the ulnar half of the palm down on a table. Pointing the thumb alternately at the floor and ceiling will produce abduction and adduction at the CMC joint.

The second axis of the first CMC joint also goes through the base of the first metacarpal but is at an approximate right angle to the palm (fig. 5.6). Flexion and extension are performed around this axis.

In addition to flexion/extension and abduction/adduction, the CMC joint of the thumb can allow for actions known as *opposition* and *reposition* (fig. 5.7). These actions are most easily thought of as partial circumductions. If the left hand is held with the palm toward the face, and the thumb circumducted counter-clockwise, the movement described as opposition will be seen to occur as the thumb approaches the palm. Reposition will be performed if the direction of circumduction is reversed. Opposition and reposition are not, therefore, pure actions of the CMC joint of the thumb, but are rather combination actions comprised of flexion and abduction (opposition), and extension and adduction (reposition). The axis of these two actions is, similarly, a combination axis which is aligned between those of flexion/extension and abduction/adduction.

Figure 5.6. Axes of the saddle joint of the thumb

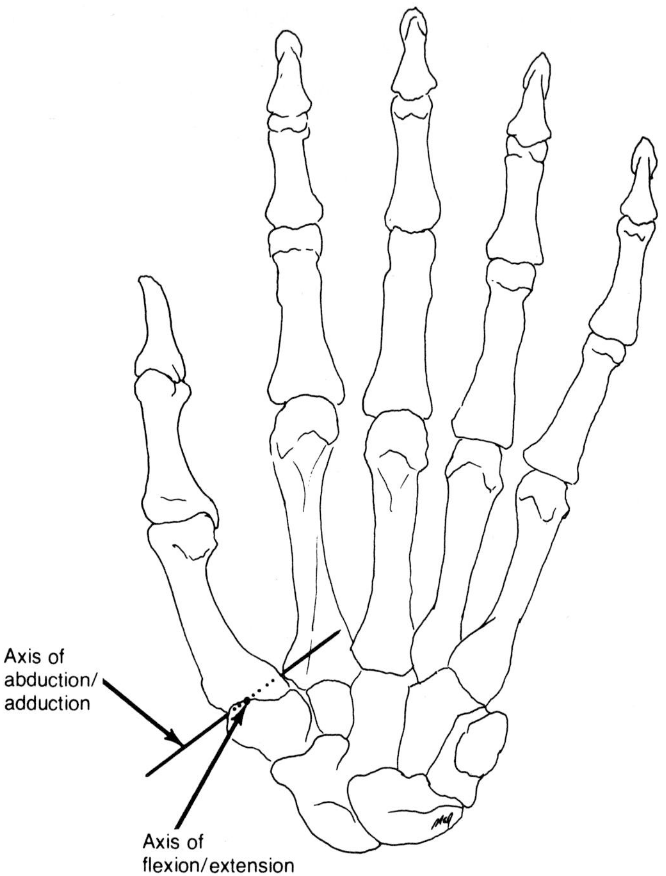


The joint capsule of the first CMC joint is thick but loose. Since there are no ligaments surrounding this joint, the capsule has the responsibility of maintaining joint integrity and therefore must be loose enough to allow for desirable range of motion, yet strong enough to prevent dislocation.

Carpometacarpal joints two through five articulate the metacarpal bones of the four fingers with adjacent carpal bones. These joints are synovial and are classified as modified saddle joints. Movement at these joints is slight, and of a gliding nature, because of the presence of ligaments connecting the bones on their dorsal and palmar surfaces (figs. 5.3, 5.4) as well as between their adjacent surfaces. The ligaments are the dorsal ligaments, palmar ligaments, and interosseus ligaments respectively. The joint capsule, a continuation of the intercarpal capsule, aids in restricting joint movements.

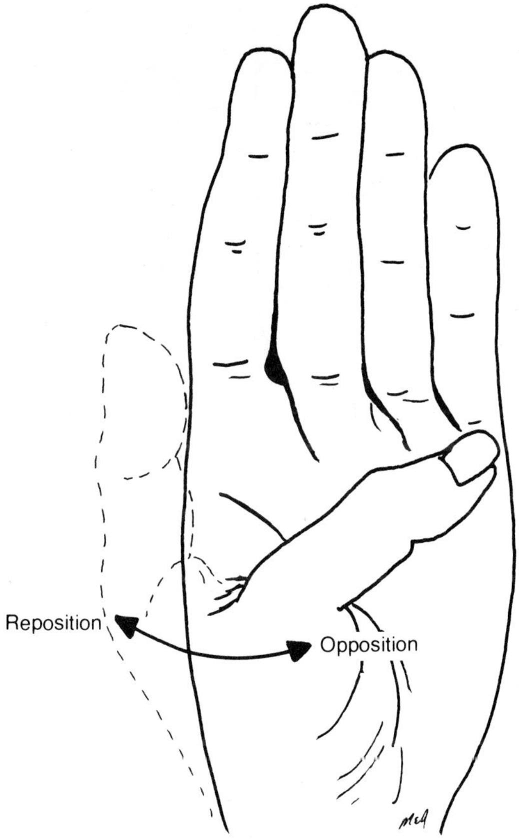

Figure 5.7. Opposition and reposition of the saddle joint of the thumb

Motion at the second through fifth CMC joints is least in joints two and three, and greatest in joint five. Movement contribution of the latter joint may be observed as an attempt is made to touch the base of the thumb to the base of the small finger. The fifth metacarpal will be seen to exhibit limited opposition and reposition (fig. 5.8).

### Intermetacarpal Joints

The intermetacarpal joints are formed by the bases of the second, third, fourth, and fifth metacarpals. The bones are united by dorsal, palmar and interosseus ligaments, and are encased in a joint capsule continuous with that of the intercarpal and carpometacarpal joints. Movements permitted by these joints are slight and are of a gliding nature. Most movement occurs between the fourth and fifth metacarpals during opposition and reposition at the fifth CMC joint.

Figure 5.8. Opposition and reposition of the fifth carpometacarpal joint

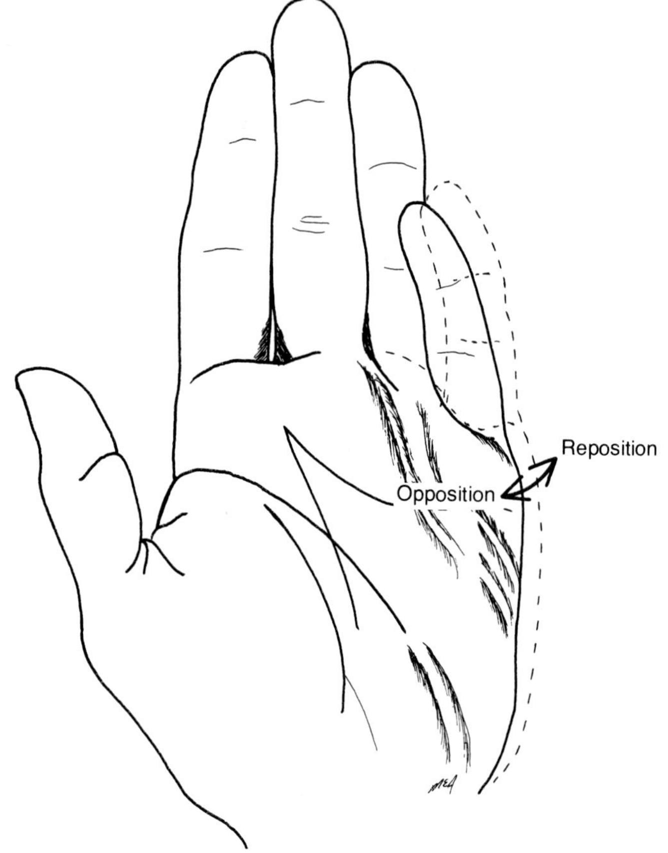


## Metacarpophalangeal Joints

The metacarpophalangeal (abbreviated *MCP*) joints are formed by the heads of the five metacarpal bones, and the proximal phalanx of the thumb and four fingers. The joints are condyloid and allow for flexion/extension around an axis passing from side to side through the joints, and for abduction/adduction around an axis passing from palmar to dorsal surfaces (fig. 5.9). Observation of one's hand will indicate that these movements are much freer in the MCP joints of the hand than they are in the thumb. In fact, it may be necessary to stabilize the first metacarpal to fully observe motion at that MCP joint. Abduction and adduction are particularly difficult to perform, leading one to conclude that the first MCP joint is more of a modified hinge joint than a true condyloid joint.

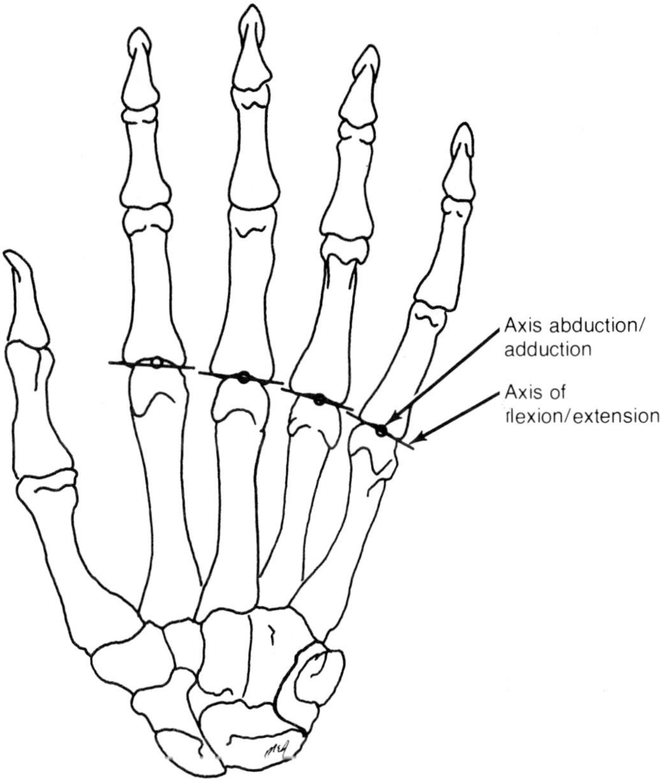

**Figure 5.9. Axes of the metacarpophalangeal joints**

The ligaments of each MCP joint are one palmar ligament and two collateral ligaments. There is also the transverse metacarpal ligament (fig. 5.3) which runs between the heads of the four metacarpals of the hand. This ligament is primarily responsible for limiting sideward spread of the metacarpals; however, since it blends with the palmar ligaments, it has some slight contribution to the integrity of the MCP joints. The capsules of each joint are formed by the deep surfaces of the ligaments.

It has been noted that the movements at the MCP are flexion/extension and abduction/adduction. The movements of abduction and adduction (fig. 5.10) require further explanation in that it is conventional to use the long finger of the hand as the reference position for these actions. When the fingers or thumb are spread away from the long finger, abduction is occurring. When the fingers are closed on the long finger, adduction is occurring. Side to side movements of the long finger are referred to as *radial deviation* (radial flexion) and *ulnar deviation* (ulnar flexion), shown in figure 5.10.

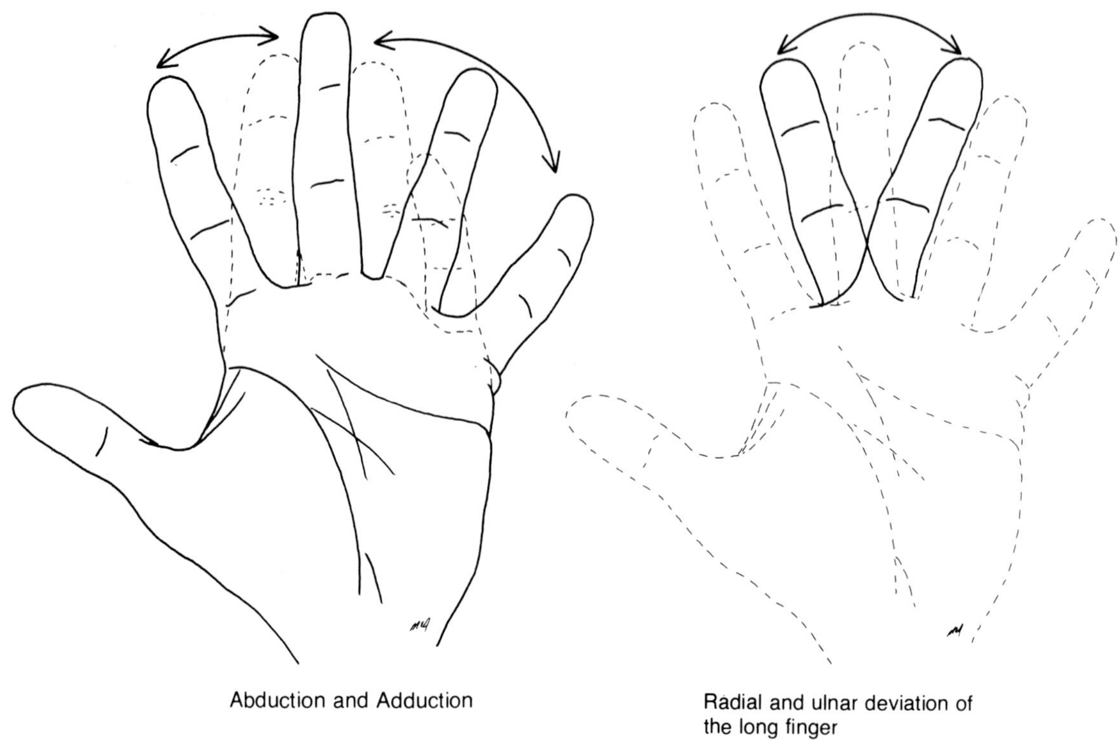


**Figure 5.10. Movements of the fingers in the frontal plane**

## Interphalangeal Joints

The interphalangeal joints are those joints between the phalanges of the fingers and thumb. There are two interphalangeal joints in each finger; the joint between the proximal and middle phalanges is the proximal interphalangeal (abbreviated *PIP*) joint, and the joint between the middle and distal phalanges is the distal interphalangeal *(DIP)* joint. Since there is only one such joint in the thumb, it is referred to simply as the interphalangeal *(IP)* joint of the thumb.

All of the interphalangeal joints are of the hinge type, and permit only flexion and extension around axes which pass from side to side through the joints. The ligaments of the joints are the palmar and collateral ligaments, and are arranged, as are the joint capsules, in similar fashion to those of the MCP joints. The absence of dorsal ligaments at both the MCP and IP joints is noteworthy in that the tendons of the extensor muscles are their substitutes. This arrangement allows for a considerable amount of joint flexion by virtue of the excursion ratio of the extensor muscles, but extension is satisfactorily limited by the palmar and collateral ligaments.

## Muscles of the Wrist and Hand

The twenty-five muscles or muscle groups which are movers of the joints of the wrist and hand have been categorized as forearm muscles, extrinsic muscles, and intrinsic muscles. The forearm muscles are those eight muscles which have origins on or around the epicondyles of the humerus, and insertions distal to the wrist. The four flexor muscles of this group originate, in part at least, from the medial epicondyle of the humerus by the common flexor tendon which also supports the origin of one head of the pronator teres. The four extensors take origin on and around the lateral epicondyle by the common extensor tendon. The muscles of the forearm group are:

| *Flexors* | *Extensors* |
|---|---|
| Palmaris Longus | Extensor Carpi Radialis Longus |
| Flexor Carpi Radialis | Extensor Carpi Radialis Brevis |
| Flexor Carpi Ulnaris | Extensor Carpi Ulnaris |
| Flexor Digitorum Superficialis | Extensor Digitorum |

The extrinsic muscles are those seven muscles which originate between the elbow and wrist and insert distal to the wrist. Four of these muscles move the thumb; one moves the four fingers; the remaining two muscles move the index and small fingers. The extrinsic muscles are:

Extensor Pollicis Longus
Extensor Pollicis Brevis
Flexor Pollicis Longus
Abductor Pollicis Longus
Extensor Indicis
Extensor Digiti Minimi
Flexor Digitorum Profundus

The intrinsic muscles are those ten muscles or muscle groups which originate and insert distal to the wrist. Four of the intrinsics are thumb or thenar muscles and form the palmar muscle mass on the radial side of the hand called the *thenar eminence.* Three intrinsics are movers of the small finger and form the *hypothenar eminence* which is the fleshy part of the palm on the ulnar side of the hand. The remaining intrinsics are muscle groups located between the metacarpals. The intrinsics are:

Flexor Pollicis Brevis
Abductor Pollicis Brevis
Opponens Pollicis
Adductor Pollicis
Abductor Digiti Minimi
Flexor Digiti Minimi Brevis
Opponens Digiti Minimi
Interossei (Palmer and dorsal)
Lumbricales

## Muscles of the Forearm

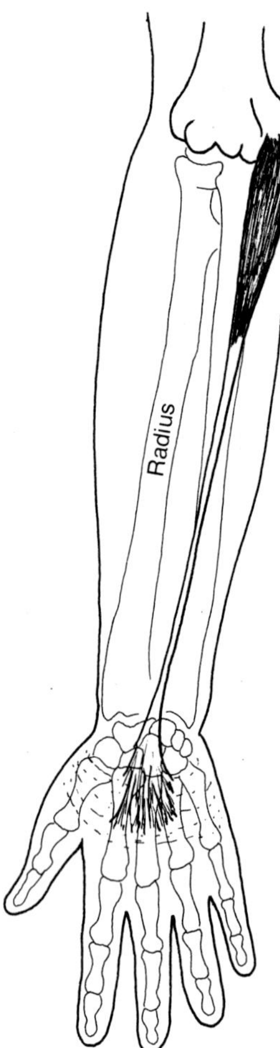


Figure 5.11. Palmaris longus, palmar view

**Palmaris Longus** (palma'ris lon'gus) The palmaris longus (fig. 5.11) is a small fusiform muscle located superficially on the palmar aspect of the forearm. The muscle is absent in 10 to 15 percent of people, but, if it is present, is easily palpated and observed at the wrist when a firm fist is made.

*Origin* Medial epicondyle of the humerus, by the common flexor tendon.

*Insertion* Flexor retinaculum and palmar aponeurosis.

*Innervation* Median nerve.

*Action* Flexion of the wrist joint.

The palmaris longus is in a favorable position to flex the wrist since it crosses the wrist joint farther from the flexion/extension axis than any other flexor. The muscle is so small, however, that, even with its long force arm, it can contribute only weak flexion to the joint.

**Flexor Carpi Radialis** (flex'or car'pi radia'lis) The flexor carpi radialis (fig. 5.12) is a slender muscle on the palmar aspect of the forearm. Its tendon is palpable on the radial side of the tendon of the palmaris longus, and is particularly prominent when one performs resisted radial deviation.

*Origin* Medial epicondyle of the humerus by the common tendon.

*Insertion* Palmar surface of the base of the second metacarpal with a slip to the base of the third metacarpal.

*Innervation* Median nerve.

*Action* Flexion and radial deviation of the wrist joint.

The flexor carpi radialis crosses the wrist joint anterior to the flexion/extension axis and to the radial side of the radial and ulnar deviation axis. The muscle is, therefore, well located to perform its two actions.

Figure 5.12. Flexor carpi radialis, palmar view

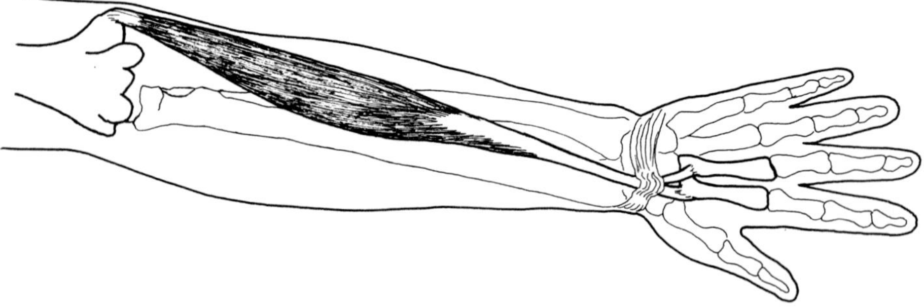

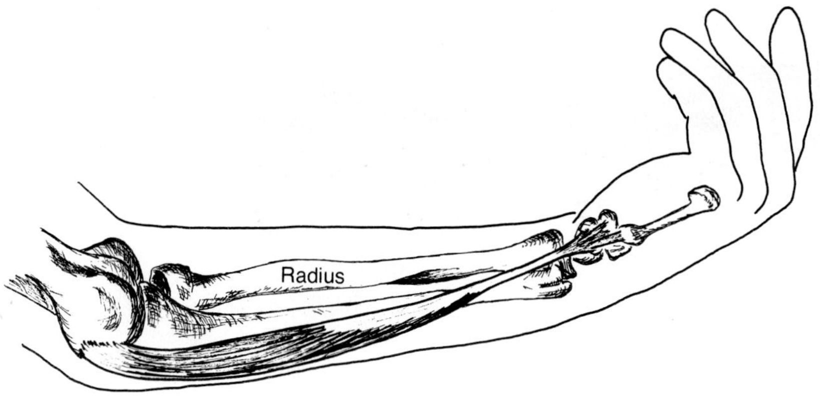

Figure 5.13. Flexor carpi ulnaris, medial view

**Flexor Carpi Ulnaris** (flex'or car'pi ulna'ris) The flexor carpi ulnaris (fig. 5.13) is a superficial muscle located on the palmar aspect of the ulna. Its tendon is palpable just proximal to the pisiform bone when a firm fist is made.

*Origin* By two heads, humeral and ulnar, from the medial epicondyle of the humerus by the common flexor tendon, and the upper two-thirds of the dorsal border of the ulna including the olecranon process.

*Insertion* Pisiform and hamate bones, and the palmar surface of the base of the fifth metacarpal.

*Innervation* Ulnar nerve.

*Action* Flexion and ulnar deviation of the wrist joint.

The flexor carpi ulnaris crosses the wrist joint anterior to the flexion/extension axis and to the ulnar side of the deviation axis, and, therefore, contributes significantly to both flexion and ulnar deviation. In the latter action, it shares responsibility with the extensor carpi ulnaris and, in so doing, neutralizes that muscle's tendency to extend the wrist as it contracts.

**Flexor Digitorum Superficialis** (flex'or digito'rum superficia'lis) The flexor digitorum superficialis (fig. 5.14) is the largest of the flexor muscles of the forearm group. Its tendons can be palpated and observed on the palmar surface of the wrist between the tendons of the flexor carpi radialis and the flexor carpi ulnaris. The tendons may be seen to move within their sheaths as the fingers are flexed to make a fist.

*Origin* By three heads—humeral, ulnar, and radial—from the medial epicondyle of the humerus by the common flexor tendon; the medial aspect of the coronoid process; and the oblique line of the radius.

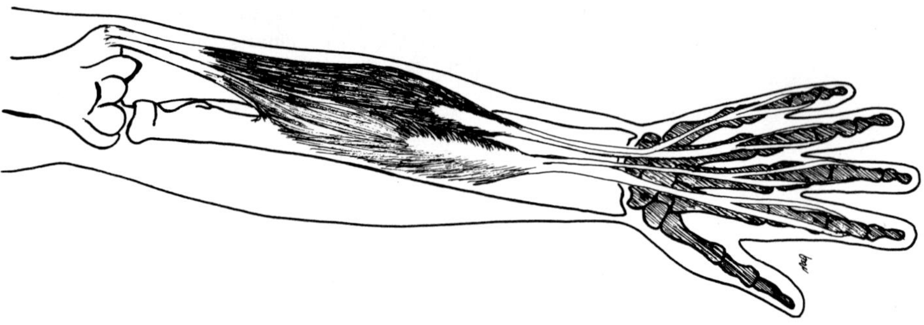

Figure 5.14. Flexor digitorum superficialis, palmar view

*Insertion* By four tendons to the sides of the base of the middle phalanges of the four fingers.

*Innervation* Median nerve.

*Action* Flexion of the metacarpophalangeal and proximal interphalangeal joints of the four fingers; assists in flexion of the wrist.

The flexor digitorum superficialis crosses the wrist, metacarpophalangeal, and proximal interphalangeal joints anterior to the flexion/extension axes of these joints. When these joints are flexed simultaneously, the superficialis has contracted to its shortest length; conversely, when these joints are extended, the muscle is stretched to its fullest.

**Extensor Carpi Radialis Longus** (exten'sor car'pi radia'lis lon'gus) The extensor carpi radialis longus (fig. 5.15) is a partially superficial muscle located on the dorsal surface of the forearm. Its muscular portion may be palpated just above the elbow as the wrist is forcefully extended. Its tendon is prominent also during this action and can be palpated just to the ulnar side of the tendon of the extensor pollicis longus.

*Origin* Distal third of the supracondylar ridge; lateral epicondyle of the humerus by the common extensor tendon.

*Insertion* Dorsal surface of the base of the second metacarpal.

*Innervation* Radial nerve.

*Action* Extension and radial deviation of the wrist joint.

The actions of the extensor carpi radialis longus are logical ones, and follow from the location of the muscle to the wrist axes as it crosses that joint. It is posterior to the flexion/extension axis and to the radial side of the deviation axis.

**Extensor Carpi Radialis Brevis** (exten'sor car'pi radia'lis bre'vis) The muscular portion of the extensor carpi radialis brevis (fig. 5.16) is covered in its proximal part by the extensor carpi radialis longus. It is superficial on the dorsal surface of the middle forearm and may be

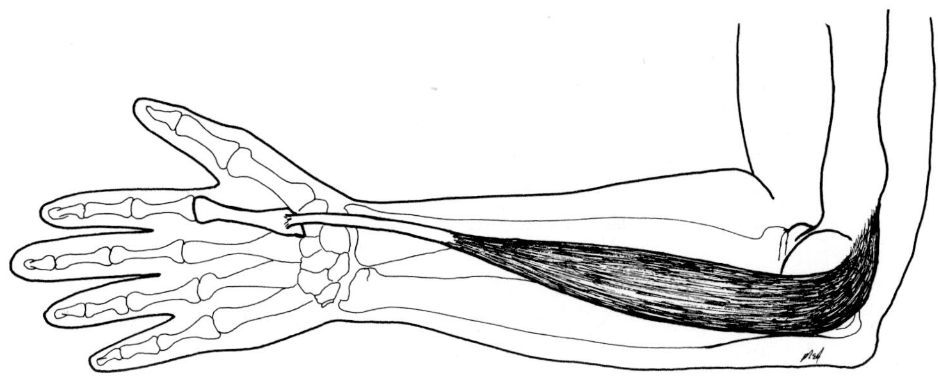

Figure 5.15

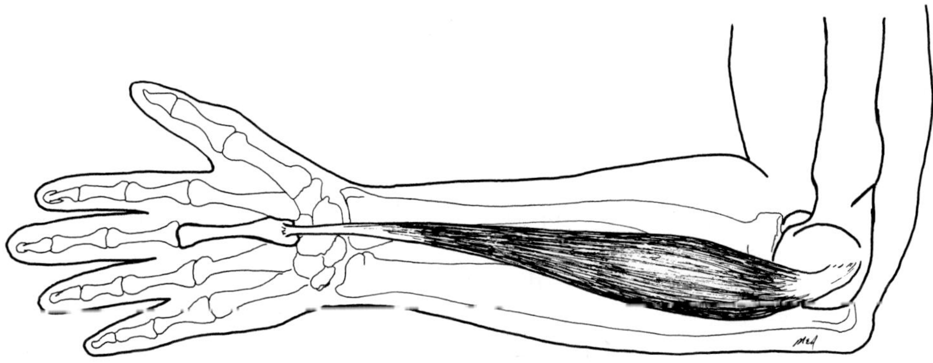

Figure 5.16

Figure 5.15. Extensor carpi radialis longus, dorsal view

Figure 5.16. Extensor carpi radialis brevis, dorsal view

palpated there if care is taken not to confuse it with the extensor digitorum. Its tendon is also difficult to identify because it is crossed by the tendons of the adductor pollicis longus and the extensor pollicis brevis, but it can usually be felt proximal to its insertion if the thumb is placed in the palm of the hand and alternately flexed and relaxed at its interphalangeal joint.

*Origin* Lateral epicondyle of the humerus by the common extensor tendon; and radial collateral ligament.

*Insertion* Dorsal surface of the base of the third metacarpal.

*Innervation* Radial nerve.

*Action* Extension and weak radial deviation of the wrist joint.

The extensor carpi radialis brevis crosses well posterior to the flexion/extension axis of the wrist; however, it courses very close to the deviation axis and thus has scant contribution to radial deviation. The method of palpating the tendon of this muscle attests to its central location in the wrist, because as the thumb is brought toward the palm and then flexed, the palmaris longus contracts to tense the flexor retinaculum. The extensor carpi radialis brevis contracts to prevent the palmaris longus from also flexing the wrist. There is some evidence that "tennis elbow" is caused by microscopic tears of this muscle in the vicinity of its origin. The extensor carpi radialis longus lies over the origin of the brevis and, until recently, has effectively hidden it as one of the causes of "tennis elbow" pain.

**Extensor Carpi Ulnaris** (exten'sor car'pi ulna'ris) The extensor carpi ulnaris (fig. 5.17) is located superficially on the ulnar side of the dorsum of the forearm. Its muscular portion may be palpated next to the anconeus as the wrist is forcefully extended. Its tendon will be prominent just distal to the ulnar styloid process if a fist is made as the wrist is extended.

*Origin* Lateral epicondyle of the humerus by the common extensor tendon; and the middle third of the dorsal border of the ulna.

*Insertion* Ulnar side of the base of the fifth metacarpal.

*Innervation* Deep radial nerve.

*Action* Extension and ulnar deviation of the wrist joint.

Crossing to the posterior and ulnar sides of the two axes of the wrist joint, the extensor carpi ulnaris is well located to perform its actions. Its ability in ulnar deviation is particularly efficient because the wedge-like flare at the base of the fifth metacarpal increases the angle of the muscle's attachment.

**Extensor Digitorum** (exten'sor digito'rum) The extensor digitorum (fig. 5.18) is a fusiform muscle located on the dorsal surface of the forearm. It can be palpated in its entirety except where it is covered proximally by the extensor carpi radialis longus. Its four tendons are

Figure 5.17. Extensor carpi ulnaris, dorsal view

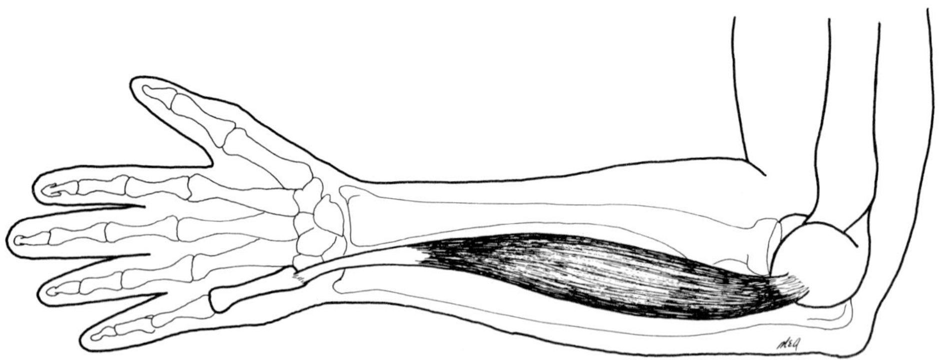

easily observed and palpated as they cross the second, third, fourth, and fifth metacarpophalangeal joints; they are particularly prominent when the metacarpophalangeal joints are fully extended to arch the hand.

*Origin* Lateral epicondyle of the humerus by the common extensor tendon.

*Insertion* By four tendons to the bases of the second and third phalanges of the four fingers.

*Innervation* Deep radial nerve.

*Action* Extension of the metacarpophalangeal joint, and the proximal and distal interphalangeal joints of the four fingers; and if contraction is continued, extension of the wrist joint.

The extensor digitorum crosses more joints than any other muscle of the forearm group. If all of these joints—wrist, metacarpophalangeal, proximal interphalangeal, and distal interphalangeal—are simultaneously extended, the muscle is contracted to its shortest length and is only weakly responsive at the wrist joint. Strength will be quickly restored, however, if the extensor digitorum is lengthened by flexing the PIP and DIP joints of the fingers.

Simultaneous flexion of the wrist, MCP, PIP and DIP joints forces the extensor digitorum to stretch to its fullest; in fact, the extensor digitorum is unable to lengthen sufficiently to allow full flexion at all joints, as can be observed if a firm fist is made followed by an attempt to fully flex the wrist. Full flexion of the wrist can only be performed if the fingers are allowed to uncurl. This principle is used in self-defense to disarm opponents, since by forcing the wrist into flexion, the grip on the weapon is loosened.

**Figure 5.18. Extensor digitorum, dorsal view**

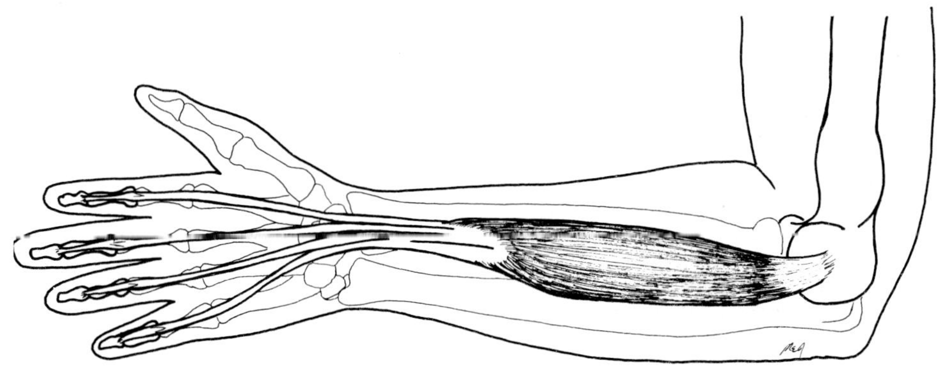

## Extrinsic Muscles

**Extensor Pollicis Longus** (exten'sor pol'licis lon'gus) The extensor pollicis longus (fig. 5.19) is located on the dorsal surface of the forearm. Its muscular portion is difficult to palpate; however, its tendon is clearly prominent when the thumb is fully adducted.

*Origin* Middle third of the ulna on its dorsal surface.

*Insertion* Dorsal surface of base of distal phalanx of the thumb.

*Innervation* Deep radial nerve.

*Action* Extension of metacarpophalangeal and interphalangeal joints of the thumb; reposition, adduction and extension of the carpometacarpal joint; contributes to wrist extension and radial deviation.

The actions of the extensor pollicis longus are several and at first sight may seem difficult to learn. All the actions are straight forward, however, when the respective muscles are viewed with reference to the axes of the joints they cross. At the wrist joint, the tendon of the extensor pollicis longus courses posterior to the flexion/extension axis and to the radial side of the deviation axis to perform the actions of extension and radial deviation. At the CMC joint, the tendon passes to the radial side of that flexion/extension axis to perform extension, and dorsal to the abduction/adduction axis to act as an adductor. The reposition function results from the fact that reposition is a combination movement comprised of adduction and extension. At the metacarpophalangeal and interphalangeal joints, the tendon passes dorsal to the flexion/extension axes to extend the joints.

**Extensor Pollicis Brevis** (exten'sor pol'licis bre'vis) The extensor pollicis brevis (fig. 5.20) lies beneath and to the radial side of the extensor pollicis longus. Its tendon emerges to be superficial as it crosses the

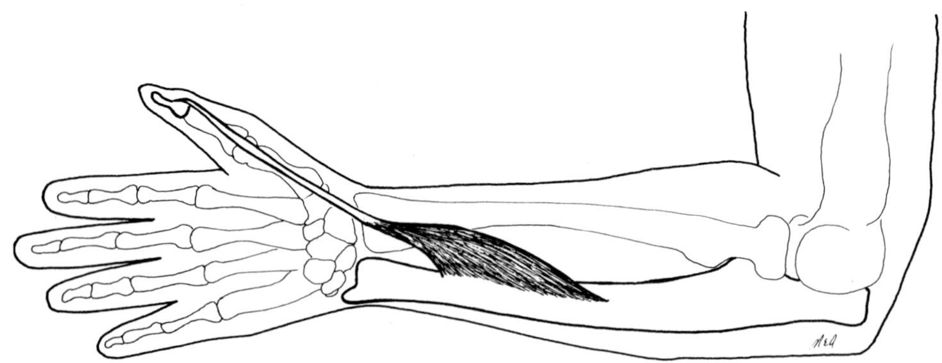

Figure 5.19. Extensor pollicis longus, dorsal view

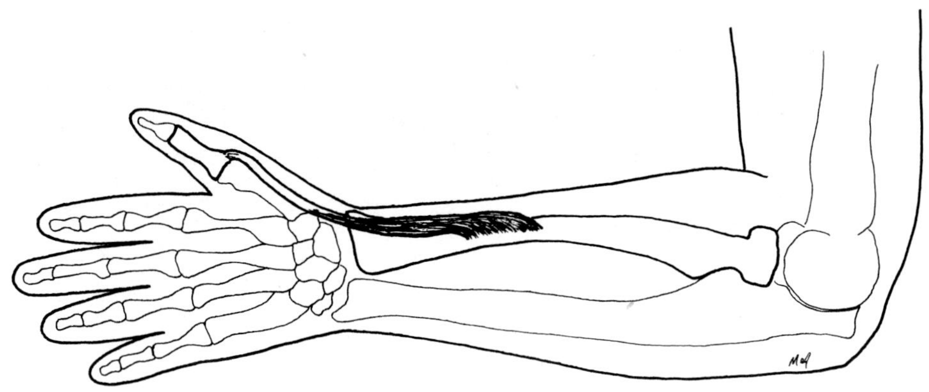

Figure 5.20. Extensor pollicis brevis, dorsal view

wrist joint and may be palpated and observed on the radial side of the extensor pollicis longus during forced extension of the thumb. These two tendons form the "anatomical snuff box" of the hand.

*Origin* Dorsal surface of the radius at its midpoint.

*Insertion* Dorsal surface of the base of the proximal phalanx of the thumb.

*Innervation* Deep radial nerve.

*Action* Extension of the metacarpophalangeal joint of the thumb; extension of that carpometacarpal joint; radial deviation of the wrist.

The actions of the extensor pollicis brevis differ from those of the extensor pollicis longus in three respects: (1) the tendon of the extensor pollicis longus crosses the wrist joint posterior to the axis of flexion/extension to become a wrist extensor; the tendon of the extensor pollicis brevis crosses directly over that axis and is ineffective as an abductor or adductor of that joint; (3) the tendon of the extensor pollicis longus passes dorsal to the axis of abduction/adduction of the carpometacarpal joint to act as an adductor; the tendon of the extensor pollicis brevis crosses directly over the axis and is ineffective as an abductor of adductor of that joint; (3) the tendon of the extensor pollicis brevis does not cross the IP joint of the thumb as does the tendon of the extensor pollicis longus. The brevis has, therefore, no action at that joint.

**Flexor Pollicis Longus** (flex'or pol'licis lon'gus) The flexor pollicis longus (fig. 5.21), a penniform muscle, lies deep on the radial side of the forearm. Its tendon can be palpated on the palmar surface of the thumb between the MCP and IP joints as the IP joint is flexed.

Figure 5.21. Flexor pollicis longus, palmar view

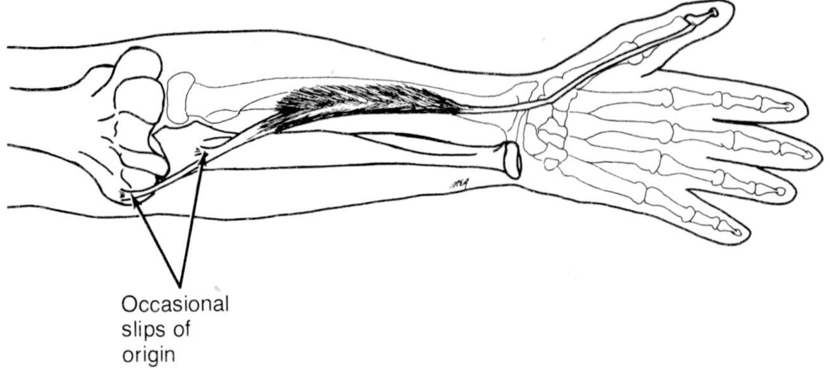


*Origin* Palmar surface of the middle half of the radius.

*Insertion* Palmar surface of the base of the distal phalanx of the thumb.

*Innervation* Palmar interosseous branch of the median nerve.

*Action* Flexes the interphalangeal joint, and by continued contraction, flexes the metacarpophalangeal joint of the thumb; flexes the carpometacarpal joint when resistance is applied.

The tendon of the flexor pollicis longus crosses the IP and MCP joints of the thumb to the palmar side of the flexion/extension axes of those joints to act as a flexor. In addition, the tendon passes to the ulnar side of the CMC axis of flexion/extension to act as a flexor of that joint. The muscle is not credited with wrist joint movement because it lies quite close to both wrist axes and because its contraction powers are largely spent by the time it flexes the three joints of the thumb.

**Abductor Pollicis Longus** (abduc'tor pol'licis lon'gus) The abductor pollicis longus (fig. 5.22) is a deep muscle lying on the dorsal aspect of the forearm just distal to the supinator. Its tendon is superficial as it crosses the wrist joint and may be palpated to the palmar side of the tendon of the extensor pollicis brevis when the thumb is forcefully abducted.

*Origin* Middle third of the dorsal surfaces of the radius and ulna.

*Insertion* Radial side of the base of the first metacarpal.

*Innervation* Deep radial nerve.

*Action* Abduction of the carpometacarpal joint of the thumb and, by continued contraction, radial deviation of the wrist joint.

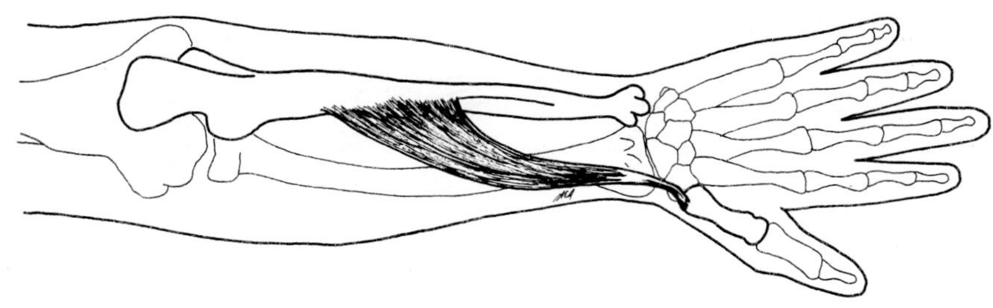

Figure 5.22. Abductor pollicis longus, dorsal view

The abductor pollicis longus crosses only the wrist joint and CMC joint of the thumb. Its tendon is centered directly above the flexion/extension axis of the wrist, but is well to the radial side of the deviation axis of that joint. The tendon is in line, also, with all axes of the CMC joint except that of abduction/adduction. In relation to the latter axis, the tendon is to the radial side. Contraction of the abductor pollicis longus will thus cause abduction of the CMC joint followed by radial deviation of the wrist joint.

**Extensor Indicis** (exten'sor in'dicis) The extensor indicis (fig. 5.23) is a long slender muscle lying deep on the dorsal aspect of the forearm. Its tendon is superficial and can be observed running on the ulnar side of but parallel to the tendon of the extensor digitorum as it approaches the base of the index finger.

*Origin* Dorsal surface of the lower half of the ulna.

*Insertion* Ulnar side of the tendon of the extensor digitorum opposite the second metacarpophalangeal joint.

*Innervation* Deep radial nerve.

*Action* Extension of the second metacarpophalangeal joint with contribution to adduction of that joint. Through the extensor hood, the muscle contributes also to extension of the proximal and distal interphalangeal joints of the index finger. Continued contraction of the muscle assists in wrist extension.

Contraction of the extensor indicis results initially in extension of the MCP joint of the index finger, followed by extension of the PIP and DIP joints and finally extension of the wrist joint. If the MCP joint is held in flexion, however, the muscle's ability to extend the IP joints and then the wrist will be enhanced; if the MCP and IP joints are all held in flexion, the muscle will become an effective wrist extensor.

That the extensor indicis contributes to adduction of the index finger can be observed by forcefully extending the index finger at the MCP and IP joints. As noted above, under palpation procedures, the

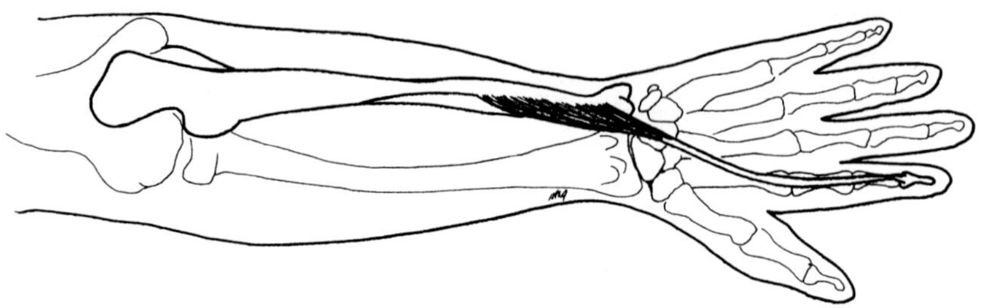
Figure 5.23. Extensor indicis, dorsal view

tendon of the extensor indicis runs parallel to but on the ulnar side of the tendon of the extensor digitorum. The muscle is, thus, just to the ulnar side of the abduction/adduction axis, making it a weak adductor.

**Extensor Digiti Minimi** (exten'sor dig'iti min'imi) The extensor digiti minimi (fig. 5.24) is a long slender muscle located to the ulnar side of the extensor digitorum. The muscle emerges to become superficial slightly proximal to the wrist; its tendon can be palpated and observed on the dorsum of the hand, and especially at the fifth MCP joint when the small finger is extended against resistance.

*Origin* Proximal tendon of the extensor digitorum.

*Insertion* Tendon of the extensor digitorum at a point just distal to the fifth metacarpophalangeal joint.

*Innervation* Deep radial nerve.

*Action* Extension of the fifth metacarpophalangeal joint and, with continued contraction, contributes to wrist extension. The muscle also extends the two interphalangeal joints of the small finger by acting upon the hood of the extensor mechanism.

The actions of the extensor digiti minimi parallel those of the extensor indicis with respect to the order with which the muscle will extend the joints it crosses. The two muscles are similar, also, in that their actions at the wrist joint can be enhanced by holding joints distal to the wrist in flexion; and their extensor abilities at the IP joints can be made more favorable if the respective MCP joint is held flexed.

**Flexor Digitorum Profundus** (flex'or digito'rum profun'dus) The flexor digitorum profundus (fig. 5.25) lies deep on the palmar surface of the forearm. Its tendons are deep also as they cross the wrist and hand and cannot be palpated.

*Origin* Upper three-fourths of the ulna.

*Insertion* By four tendons, to the base of the distal phalanx of each of the four fingers.

*Innervation* Ulnar nerve, and a palmar interosseous branch of the median nerve.

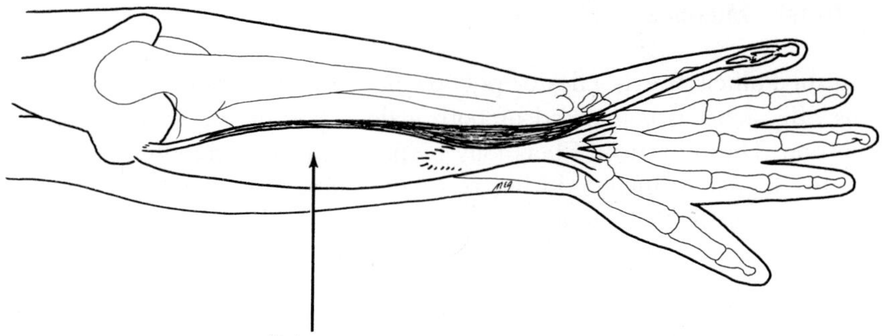

Extensor
digitorum

**Figure 5.24. Extensor digiti minimi, dorsal view**

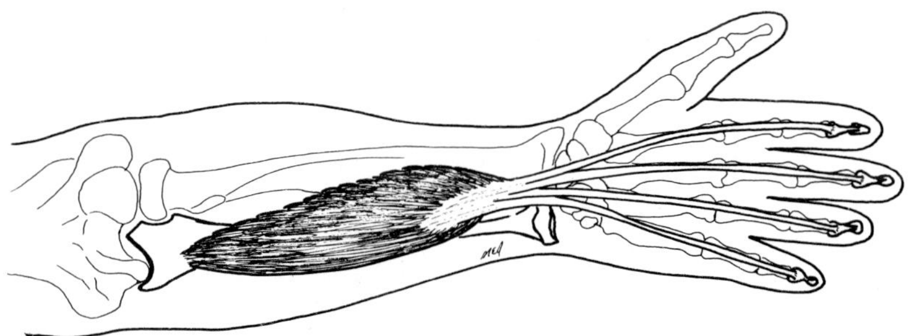

**Figure 5.25. Flexor digitorum profundus, palmar view**

*Action* Flexion of the distal interphalangeal joints of the four fingers and, by continued contraction, flexes the proximal interphalangeal joints, then the metacarpophalangeal joints, and finally the wrist joint.

The flexor digitorum profundus provides a line of pull which is to the palmar side of the flexion/extension axis of each of the joints it crosses. Its only action at these joints is, therefore, flexion which progresses sequentially from the most distal of the joints (the DIP joint) to the most proximal (wrist joint). The strength of its contraction lessens progressively from joint to joint since the muscle must become gradually shorter and, therefore, can contribute only weakly to wrist flexion. Its contribution at the wrist can be enhanced, however, by holding the MCP and IP joints of the fingers in extension to prevent excessive shortening of the fibers.

Unlike the flexor digitorum superficialis, the flexor digitorum profundus has only a single muscle belly, and tends to cause movement in all fingers simultaneously. This can be seen easily as one attempts to flex all joints of the long finger. Invariably, the ring finger moves also, as would the index and small fingers were it not for the neutralizing action of the extensor indicis and extensor digiti minimi.

## Intrinsic Muscles

**Flexor Pollicis Brevis** (flex'or pol'licis bre'vis) The flexor pollicis brevis (fig. 5.26) is comprised of both a deep portion and a superficial portion. The superficial fibers may be palpated along the ulnar border of the thenar eminence during resisted flexion of the metacarpophalangeal joint of the thumb.

*Origin* Deep head: Ulnar surface of first metacarpal. Superficial head: Multangulus major and adjacent portion of flexor retinaculum.

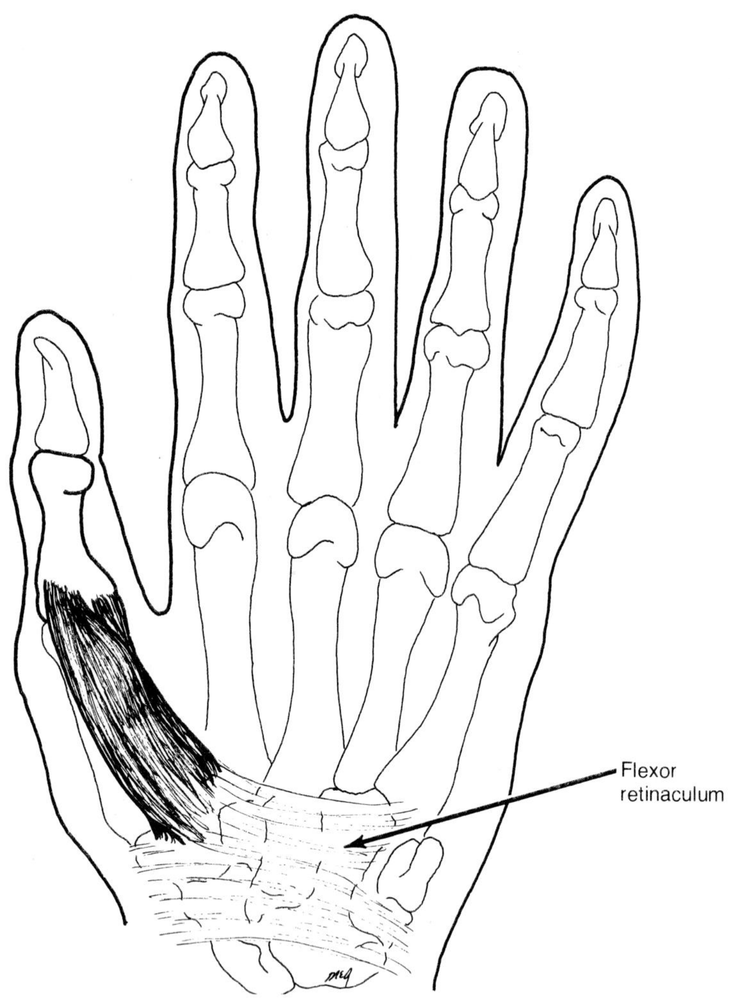


Figure 5.26. Flexor pollicis brevis, palmar view

*Insertion* Deep head: Ulnar side of the palmar surface of the base of the proximal phalanx of the thumb. Superficial head: Radial side of the palmar surface of the proximal phalanx of the thumb.

*Innervation* Deep head: Deep ulnar nerve. Superficial head: Median nerve.

*Action* Both heads: Flexion of the metacarpophalangeal joint of the thumb. Deep head: Adduction of the metacarpophalangeal joint of the thumb. Superficial head: Flexion of the carpometacarpal joint.

The two heads of the flexor pollicis brevis, with their insertions on the palmar surface of the proximal phalanx, cross the flexion/extension axis of the MCP joint well to the palmar side to become effective flexors of that joint. The deep head of the muscle, as it courses between its two attachments, crosses only the MCP joint, and is located to the ulnar side of the abduction/adduction axis of the MCP joint to be additionally active as an adductor of that joint. The superficial head crosses both the MCP and CMC joints of the thumb. At the latter joint, the muscle lies to the palmar side of the flexion/extension axis, and slightly medial to the opposition/reposition axis, to function as both a flexor and a weak opposer. Being inserted on the radial side of the proximal phalanx, the muscle would appear to be capable of abducting the metacarpal joint; however, study of a skeleton will confirm that the muscle runs directly across that axis and cannot contribute significantly to any side-to-side movement at that joint.

**Abductor Pollicis Brevis** (abduc'tor pol'licis bre'vis) The abductor pollicis brevis (fig. 5.27) is the most superficial muscle of the thenar eminence. It may be palpated in the center of the eminence during resisted abduction of the carpometacarpal joint of the thumb.

*Origin* Multangulus major and navicular bones, and adjacent portion of flexor retinaculum.

*Insertion* Radial side of the base of the first phalanx of the thumb.

*Innervation* Median nerve.

*Action* Abduction of the carpometacarpal joint of the thumb; flexion and abduction of the metacarpophalangeal joint of the thumb.

The abductor pollicis brevis and the superficial head of the flexor pollicis brevis have similar lines of pull; however, the origin of the abductor pollicis brevis is somewhat more to the radial side of the hand than the flexor pollicis brevis. By this slight lateral displacement, the abductor pollicis brevis is made to be ineffectual as a mover around all but the abduction/adduction axis of the CMC joint; and,

Figure 5.27. Abductor pollicis brevis, palmar view

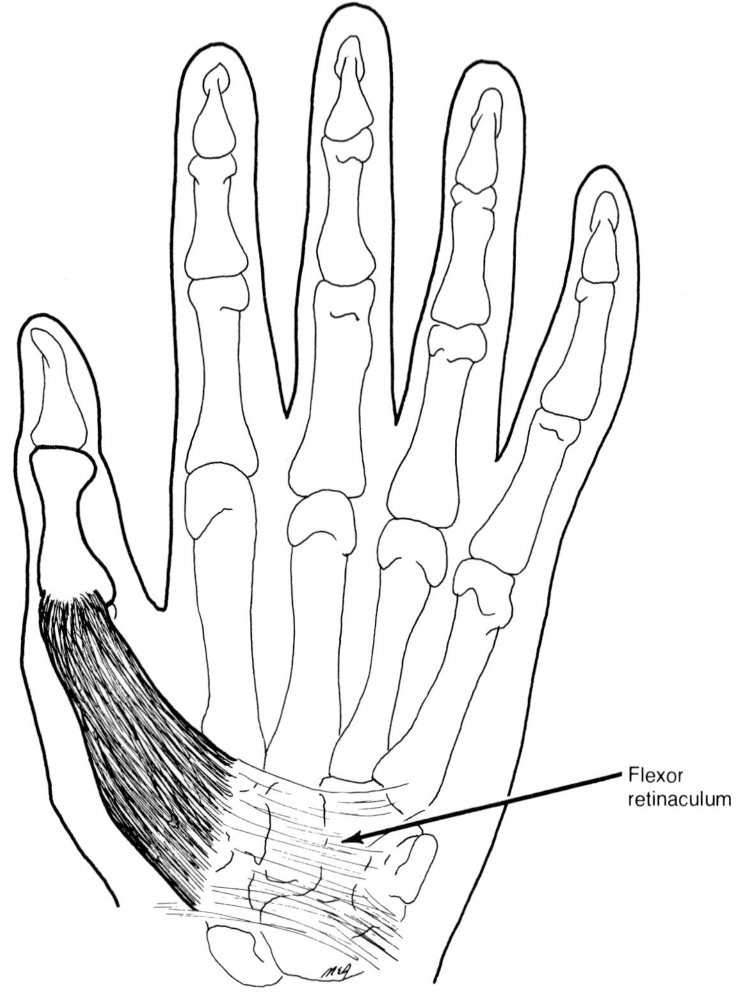


being well to the palmar side of this axis, it is a strong abductor. At the MCP joint, the muscle crosses both to palmar side of the flexion/extension axis and to the radial side of the abduction/adduction axis. Since the muscle must share its strength between both axes, it is only an assistive mover in either of the actions of flexion or abduction.

**Opponens Pollicis** (oppo'nens pol'licis) The opponens pollicis (fig. 5.28) is located beneath the abductor pollicis brevis. It is superficial along the radial border of the thenar eminence next to the first metacarpal and can be palpated when the thumb is pressed firmly against the tip of the long finger.

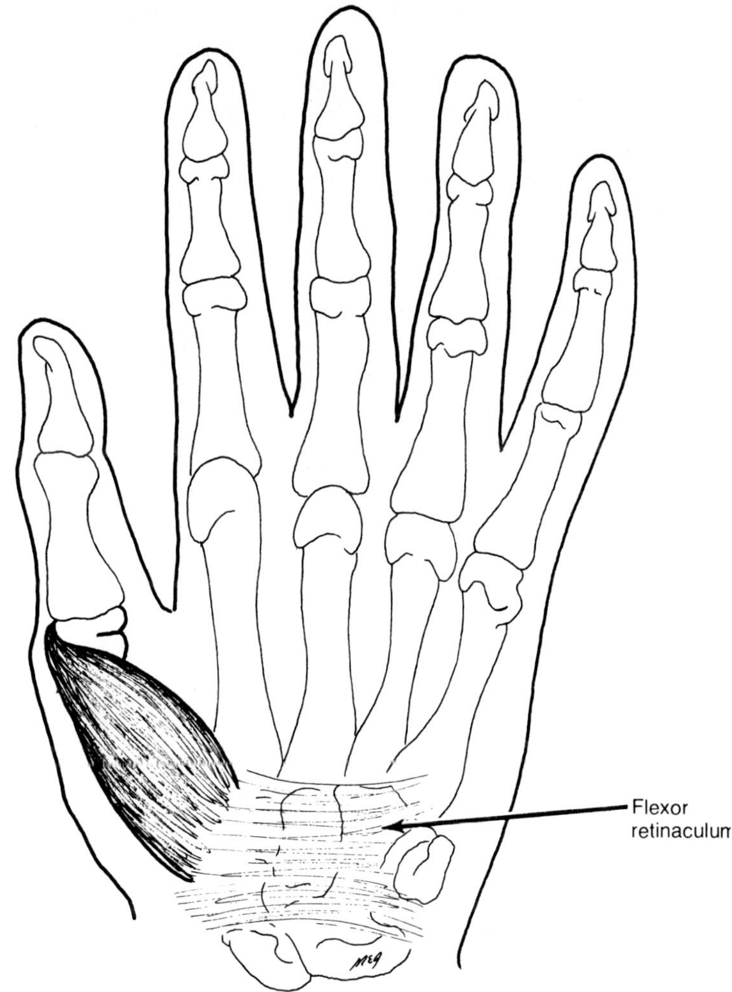


Figure 5.28. Opponens pollicis, palmar view

*Origin* Multangulus major and adjacent portion of flexor retinaculum.

*Insertion* Radial surface of entire length of the first metacarpal.

*Innervation* Medial nerve.

*Action* Opposition of the carpometacarpal joint of the thumb; contributes to abduction and flexion of that joint.

The opponens pollicis is triangular in shape and located so that its uppermost fibers are in a favorable position to cause flexion of the CMC joint, while its lowermost fibers are situated to cause abduction. When the muscle contracts, it performs both actions, and opposition results.

**Adductor Pollicis** (adduc'tor pol'licis) The adductor pollicis (fig. 5.29) lies deep in the palm of the hand but emerges to be superficial just before its insertion. It can be palpated between the first and second metacarpals as the thumb is pressed firmly against the tip of the index finger.

*Origin* By the oblique and transverse heads, from the capitate and bases of the second and third metacarpals, and the distal two-thirds of the third metacarpal.

*Insertion* Both heads converge to insert on the ulnar side of the proximal phalanx of the thumb.

*Innervation* Deep palmar branch of the ulnar nerve.

*Action* Adduction and flexion of the carpometacarpal joint of the thumb.

Figure 5.29. Adductor pollicis, palmar view

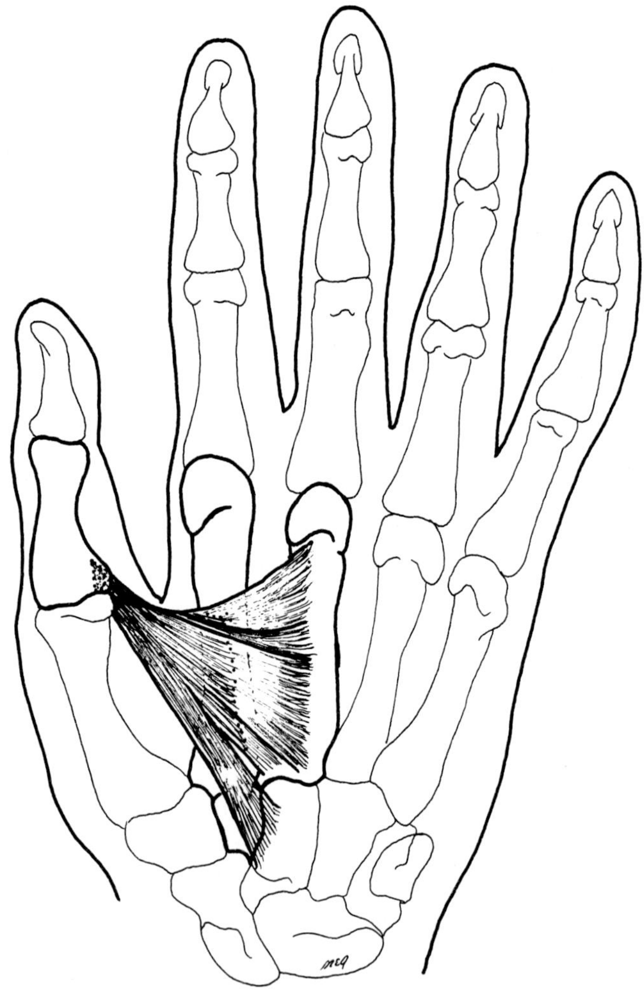

The adductor pollicis is favorably located to flex the first CMC joint regardless of the position of the thumb. Its ability to adduct the CMC joint is greatest when the joint is fully abducted and diminishes gradually as the muscle pulls the metacarpal closer and closer to the palm. When the thumb is positioned even with the palm, the adductor pollicis is no longer effective since its two attachments are then aligned with the abduction axis.

**Abductor Digiti Minimi** (abduc'tor dig'iti min'imi) The abductor digiti minimi (fig. 5.30) is superficial on the ulnar border of the hypothenar eminence. It may be palpated next to the fifth metacarpal during resisted abduction of the small finger.

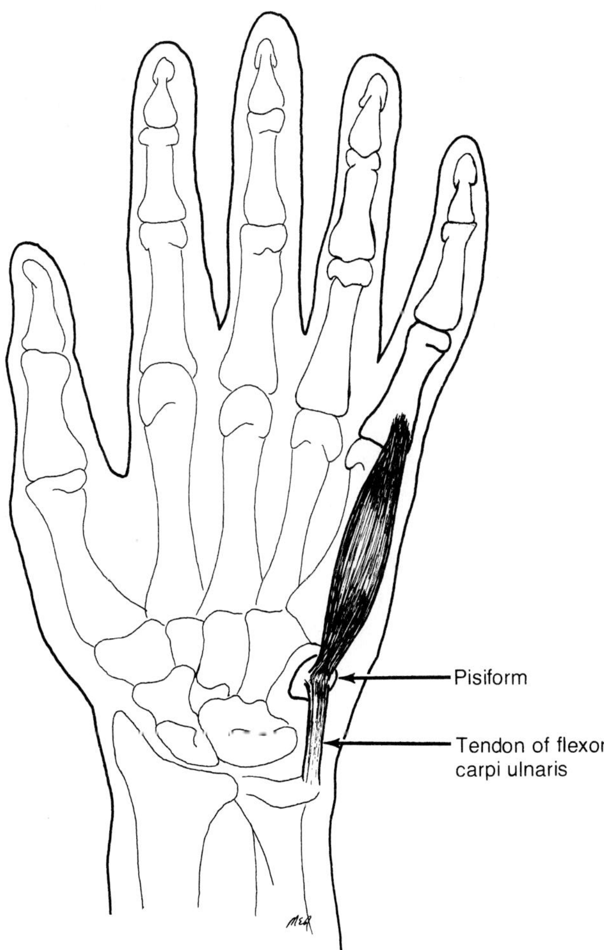


**Figure 5.30. Abductor digiti minimi**

*Origin* Pisiform bone and tendon of the flexor carpi ulnaris.

*Insertion* By two tendinous slips, to the ulnar side of the base of the proximal phalanx of the small finger, and the ulnar surface of the aponeurosis of the extensor digiti minimi.

*Innervation* Ulnar nerve.

*Action* Abduction and flexion of the metacarpophalangeal joint of the small finger.

The line of pull of the abductor digiti minimi is much more favorable for abduction than it is for flexion since the muscle is farther from the abduction/adduction axis than it is from the flexion/extension axis of the joint. The muscle's primary function is, therefore, to abduct; it is only assistive as a flexor.

**Flexor Digiti Minimi Brevis** (flex'or dig'iti min'imi bre'vis) The flexor digiti minimi brevis (fig. 5.31) runs parallel to and on the radial side of the abductor digiti minimi. It is superficial, but palpation is difficult because it is easily confused with the abductor digiti minimi.

*Orgin* Hook of the hamate and adjacent portion of the flexor retinaculum.

*Insertion* Ulnar surface of the base of the proximal phalanx of the small finger.

*Innervation* Ulnar nerve.

*Action* Flexion of the metacarpophalangeal joint of the small finger.

The flexor digiti minimi brevis crosses to the palmar side of the axis of flexion/extension of the fifth MCP joint to be a flexor of that joint; however, its oblique direction across the hypothenar eminence aligns it with the abduction/adduction axis to permit no side-to-side action.

**Opponens Digiti Minimi** (oppo'nens dig'iti min'imi) The opponens digiti minimi (fig. 5.32) lies beneath the abductor digiti minimi and the flexor digiti minimi brevis in the hypothenar eminence. It is not palpable.

*Origin* Hook of the hamate and adjacent portion of the flexor retinaculum.

*Insertion* Ulnar border of the entire length of the fifth metacarpal.

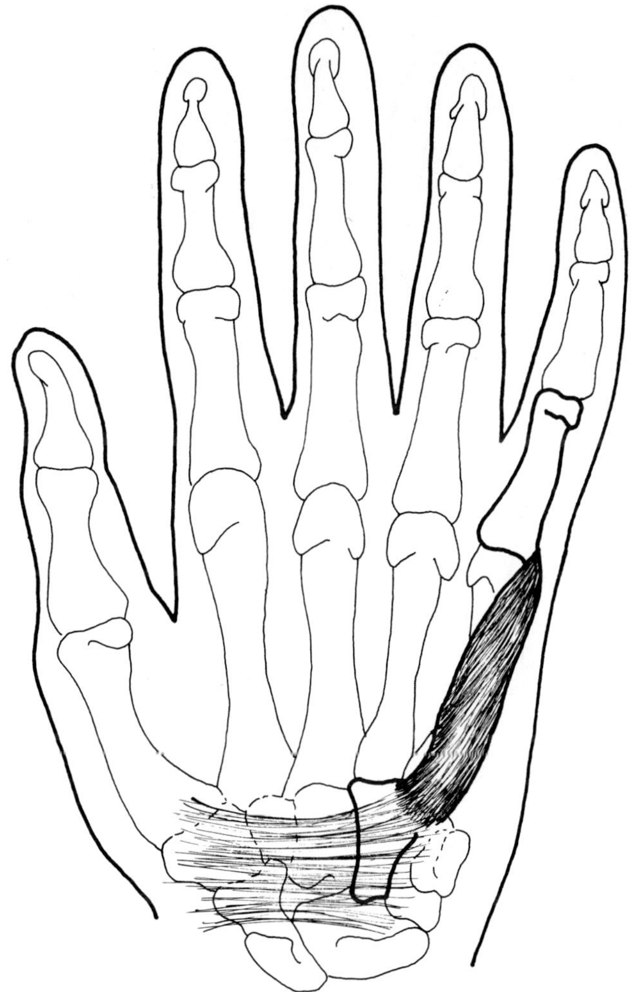

Figure 5.31. Flexor digiti minimi brevis, palmar view

*Innervation* Ulnar nerve.

*Action* Opposition of the carpometacarpal joint of the small finger.

The proximal fibers of the opponens digiti minimi are well situated to flex the fifth CMC joint while the distal fibers are more favorably placed to adduct that joint. Contraction of the muscle thus causes the metacarpal to move in both directions simultaneously, and opposition results.

Figure 5.32. Opponens digiti minimi, palmar view

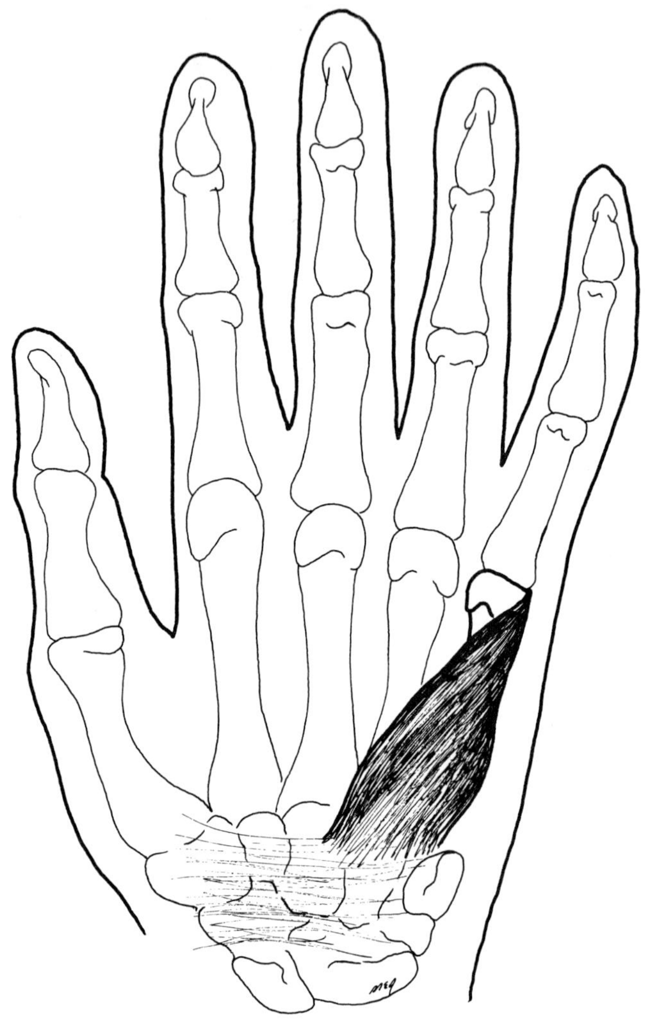

**Dorsal Interossei** (dor'sal interos'sei) The dorsal interossei (fig. 5.33) are four muscles located superficially on the dorsum of the hand. As their name implies, they lie between the metacarpals and, except for the first dorsal interosseous, are difficult to palpate. Dorsal interosseus 1 lies between the thumb and the hand and can be observed as a firm fist is made.

*Origin* Each of the four muscles arises by two heads from adjacent sides of the metacarpals.

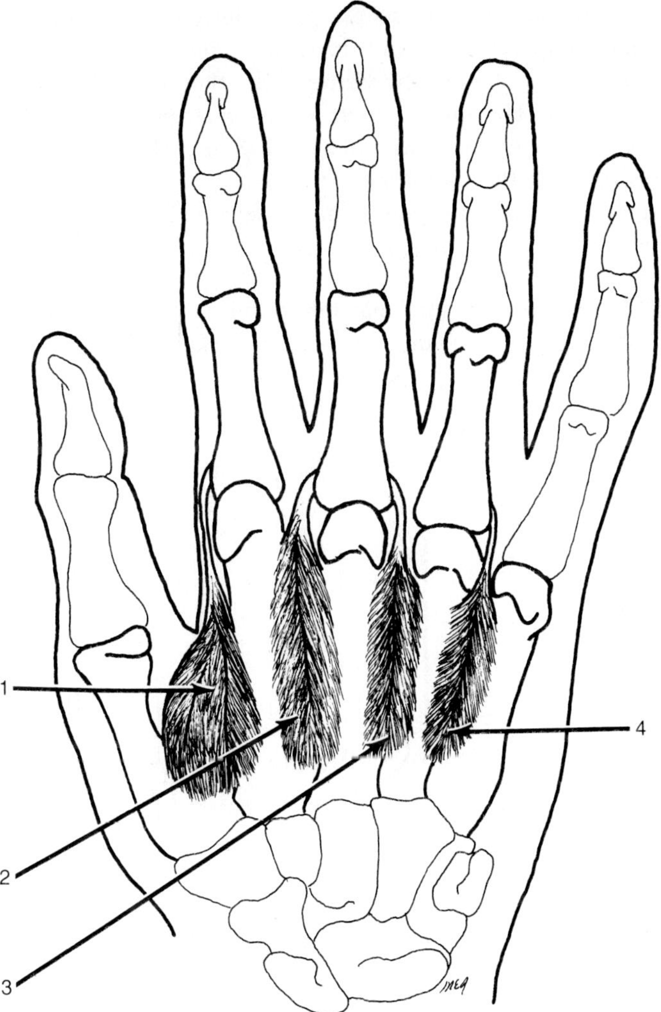


Figure 5.33. Dorsal interossei, palmar view

*Insertion* Base of the proximal phalanx and aponeurosis of the tendons of the extensor digitorum on the radial aspect of the index finger, the radial and ulnar sides of the long finger, and the ulnar side of the ring finger.

*Innervation* Deep palmar branch of the ulnar nerve.

*Action* Abduction of the second and fourth metacarpophalangeal joints; radial and ulnar deviation of the third metacarpophalangeal joint; flexion of the second, third and fourth metacarpophalangeal joints; extension (through the extensor hood) of the interphalangeal joints of the index, long, and ring fingers.

The dorsal interossei are particularly well-located to perform their abduction/adduction and deviation actions, since they display a relatively long force arm by virtue of the flair at the bases of the proximal phalanges. The muscles perform their strongest flexion actions at the MCP joints with extension of the PIP and DIP joints during the pinch grasp when the thumb and fingers are used to pick up a small object such as a pin or a coin. The muscles are also very active during a power grip.

**Palmar Interossei** (pal'mar interos'sei) The palmar interossei (fig. 5.34) are three in number and are located beneath the dorsal interossei. They are not palpable.

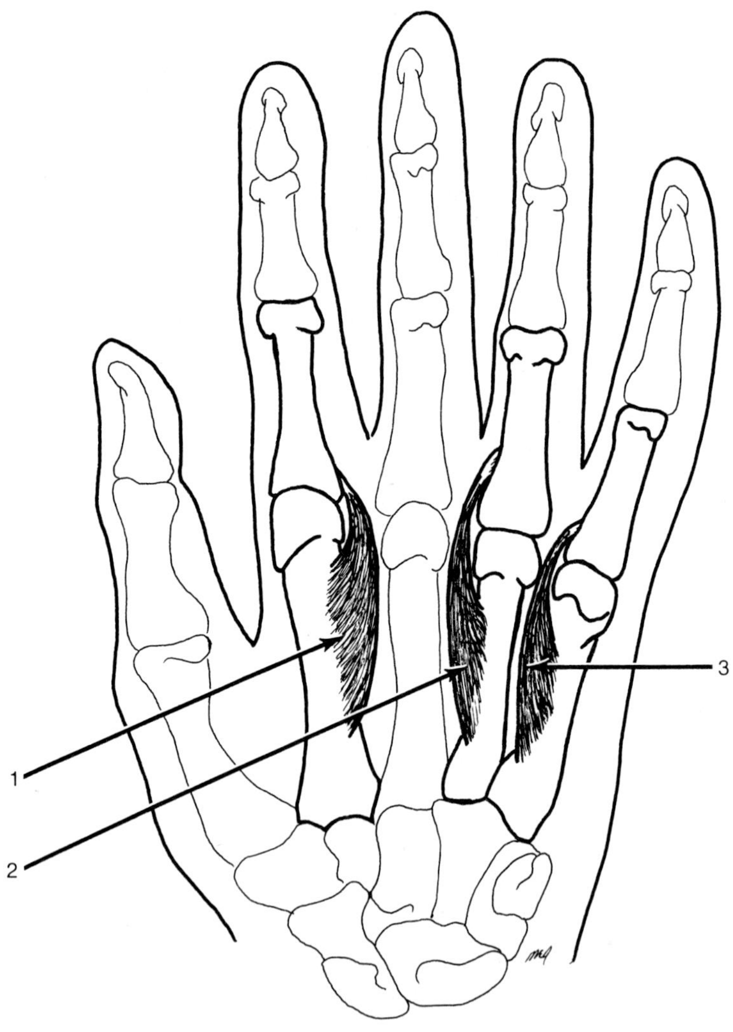


**Figure 5.34. Palmar interossei, palmar view**

*Origin* First palmar interosseus: Ulnar surface of the second metacarpal. Second palmar interosseus: Radial surface of the fourth metacarpal. Third palmar interosseus: Radial surface of the fifth metacarpal.

*Insertion* Base of the proximal phalanx and the aponeurosis of the tendons of the extensor digitorum on the ulnar side of the index finger; the radial side of the ring finger; and the radial side of the small finger.

*Innervation* Deep palmar branch of the ulnar nerve.

*Action* Adduction and flexion of the metacarpophalangeal joints of the index, ring, and small fingers; extension (through the extensor hood) of the interphalangeal joints of those fingers.

The flexion and extension functions of the palmar interossei and the dorsal interossei are similar; however, the palmar interossei are somewhat farther from the flexion/extension axis of those joints than are the dorsal interossei. The palmar muscles have, therefore, greater efficiency as flexors. The adduction action of the palmar set follows from their medial locations with respect to those axes.

**Lumbricales** (lumbrica'les) The lumbricales (fig. 5.35) comprise four muscles located around the tendons of the flexor digitorum profundus. They are deep in the palm and cannot be palpated.

*Origin* From the four tendons of the flexor digitorum profundus.

*Insertion* Aponeuroses of the tendons of the extensor digitorum. After passing to the radial sides of the metacarpals, the points of insertion are opposite the metacarpophalangeal joints.

*Innervation* Lumbricales one and two: Median nerve. Lumbricales three and four: Deep palmar branch of ulnar nerve.

*Action* Flexion of the second through fifth metacarpophalangeal joints; extension through the extensor hood of the interphalangeal joints of the four fingers.

The lumbricales are primarily involved in extending the IP joints of the fingers since their contractions pull the extensor hood proximally to tighten the entire expansion. A secondary result of their contractions is to produce slack in the profundus tendons so that extension of the IP joints will be allowed.

The lumbricales pass to the palmar side of the flexion/extension axis of the MCP joints as they course between their two attachments, and can be expected to make some contribution in the flexing of those joints. Their effectiveness is limited, however, since they do not have a firm origin on the profundus tendons, and is displayed more as neutralizing action against the extensor digitorum rather than as observable flexion of the joints.

Figure 5.35. Lumbricales, palmar view

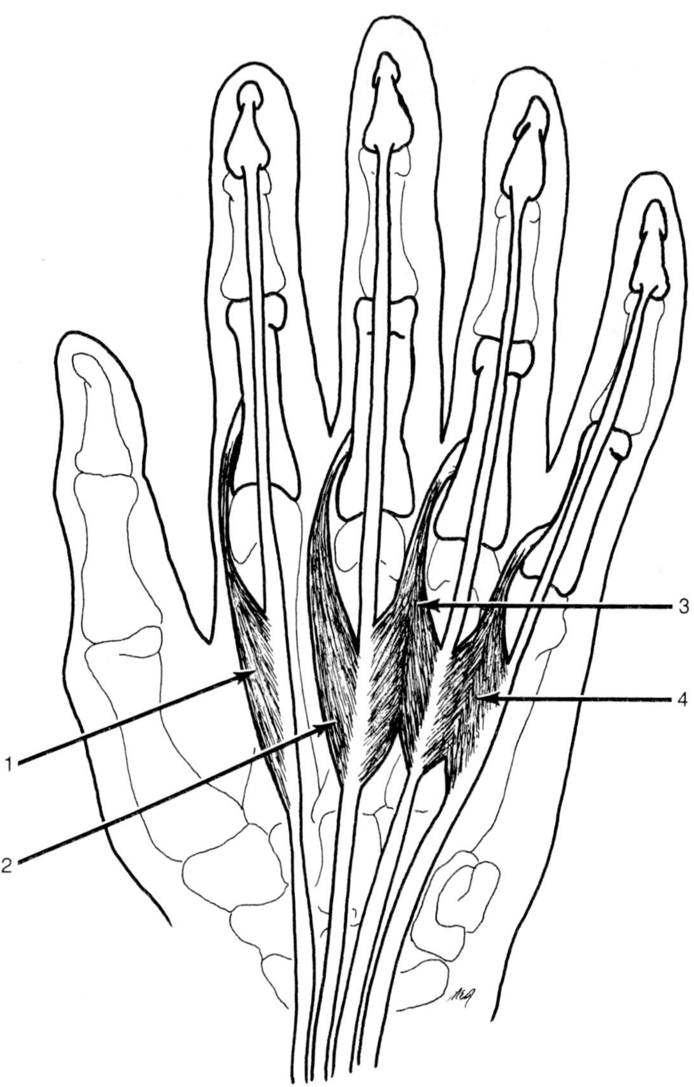


## Comments

Of the muscles of the wrist and hand, the larger ones originate above the wrist. When rackets and similar sports implements are gripped over long periods of time, the forearm muscles of the preferred arm hypertrophy and are often responsible for a considerable difference in the girth of the two arms. Hand size may differ, also, because of hypertrophy of the intrinsic muscles. The degree of hypertrophy is related to the weight of the racket used and, therefore, to the size of the racket grip. Rackets used in tennis, squash racquets, and badminton all vary in both weight and grip size. A comparison of these three rackets will suffice to illustrate the mechanics involved in executing the power grip with the hand.

The tennis racket is the heaviest of the three rackets and has the largest grip. When the hand grasps the grip, both the flexors and the extensors contract forcefully. This may seem unusual since the flexors are the gripping muscles; however, it must be remembered that when the flexors contract they tend to cause wrist flexion as well as flexion of the joints of the hand. Neutralization must be provided by the extensors in order to maintain a straight wrist. The more forceful the grip, the more neutralization is required of the extensors.

The appropriate grip size of a tennis racket is one which allows the thumb to overlap the distal interphalangeal joint of the long finger. With this grip size, the metacarpophalangeal joints are flexed to an approximate 90-degree angle, allowing the interossei, prime power grip muscles, to insert at an optimum angle for strength. Since the racket is comparatively heavy, strength is important to the maintenance of hand contact through the swing, contact, and follow-through. If the size of the handle is too large for the player, strength of grip will be sacrificed, and the racket will twist or even be dislodged from the hand. Grip size of a racket must match its weight as well as the hand size of the player.

The badminton racket is the lightest of the three rackets and has the smallest grip. It must be pointed out that the badminton racket of this discussion is of the type that would be used by a tournament player; it should not be confused with the less expensive, heavier version built for its lasting qualities rather than for its high performance. The grip of a tournament racket is quite small—small enough to allow the entire distal phalanx of the thumb to overlap that phalanx of the long finger. The metacarpophalangeal joints, as well as the interphalangeal joints, are required to flex to acute angles in order to grip the racket, and there is an accompanying loss of strength of the flexor muscles. Since the racket is so light, however, the loss is not critical. Far more important than the strength loss is the fact that the extensor digitorum is near its maximum length when the joints of the hand are flexed to such an extent. When wrist flexion is required to execute a stroke, the small amount of extensibility remaining to the muscle is limiting to the range of motion. To offset this disadvantage, the badminton player grips the racket with only the first two or three fingers. By allowing the remaining finger or fingers to be free, the extensor digitorum is given some slack, and wrist flexion will be enhanced.

The squash racket occupies the middle position of the three rackets mentioned. The mechanics of gripping this racket are a compromise between those enumerated for the tennis racket and those for the badminton racket, and indicate that the grip, being smaller than that of the tennis racket but larger than that of the badminton racket, is well-matched to its intermediate weight.

Even though the above application of grip mechanics has been specific to the racket sports, the concepts can be generalized to other situations in which objects must be held or swung. When power is the most important requirement, the size of the object to be gripped should allow for an approximate 90-degree angle at the metacarpophalangeal joints. If the object is small in circumference, wrist flexion will be limited unless one or two fingers can be relieved of their gripping responsibilities and are allowed to curl passively. Large objects such as footballs and softballs cannot be gripped securely, but they can be thrown with a great deal of wrist "snap." As a side comment, it is noted that the baseball pitcher is faced with a serious problem of grip mechanics. A baseball is small enough to permit the hand to close around it to the extent that wrist flexion will be limited. To compensate, the pitcher grips the ball with the fingers and thumb in such a way that the metacarpophalangeal joints are extended. The responsibility of gripping the ball is, thus, relegated to the digits in order to afford the extensor digitorum some slack which can be used subsequently to permit the wrist "snap" at the time of ball release.

## Laboratory Experiences

1. Determine, through the use of a goniometer, your range of motion in flexion and extension of the wrist joint while maintaining a firm fist. Repeat your observations while maintaining the metacarpal and interphalangeal joints in extension. How should the hand be held for greatest wrist flexion? for greatest wrist extension?
2. Abduct the index finger against resistance while palpating dorsal interossei 1. You should notice tension in the muscle. Continue to palpate as you make a firm fist, and again tension should be noted. Explain the activity of this muscle as it is involved in these two dissimilar movements.
3. Grasp the handle of a tennis racket, bat, or other such implement, and have a partner pull it from your grip in the direction of your thumb. Notice the comparative weakness of your grip against the pull. Generalize this to the releases taught in lifesaving classes.

4. Use a grip dynomometer to determine your grip strength while holding the wrist in full extension. Repeat the observation while holding the wrist in line with the forearm, and while maintaining full wrist flexion. Generalize your findings to explain the various forehand grips used in tennis and racketball.
5. The intrinsic muscles of the hand are difficult to study electromyographically because they are small and are frequently not superficial. The muscles comprising the superficial layer of the thenar and hypothenar eminences can be monitored, however, through the use of small electrodes. If appropriate electrodes are available, attach them to the midpoints of the two eminences and investigate the involvement of the various muscles during opposition, reposition, abduction, and flexion of the thumb and small finger.

# 6 The Spine and Pelvic Girdle

## The Spine

The spine is formed by thirty-three bones called vertebrae. The vertebrae are categorized, according to their locations, as cervical, thoracic, lumbar, sacral, and coccygeal. There are seven cervical, twelve thoracic, five lumbar, five sacral, and four coccygeal vertebrae (fig. 6.1).

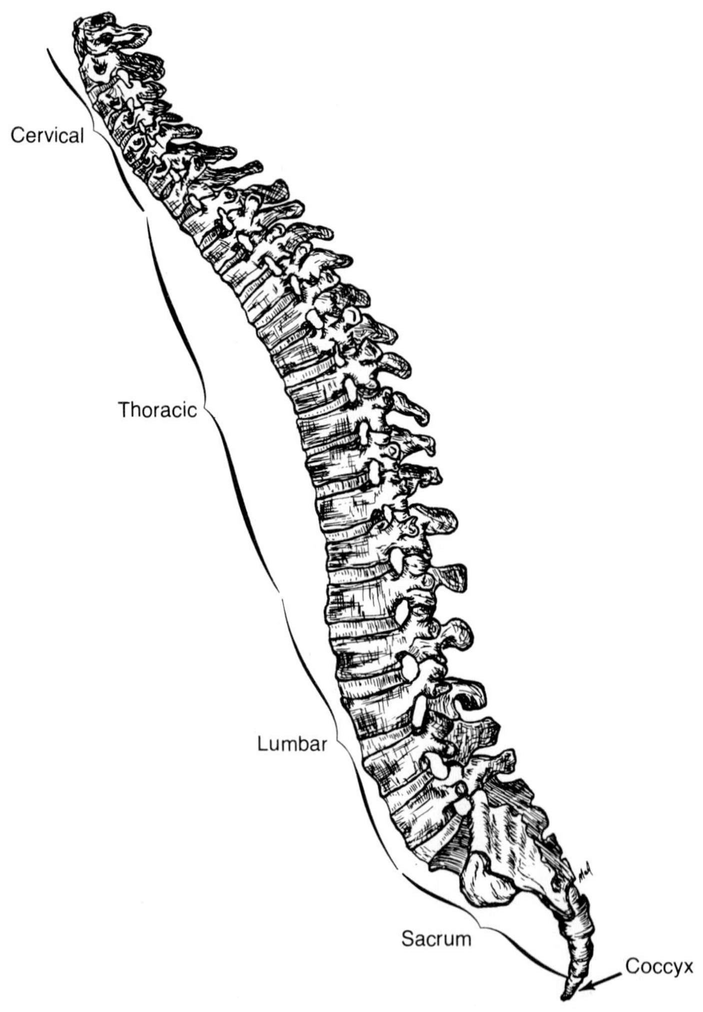


Figure 6.1. The spinal column, lateral view

### The Vertebrae

A vertebra is characterized generally by several parts (fig. 6.2). The body is the largest of the parts and is cylindrical in shape. Intervertebral discs of fibrocartilage are attached to its superior and inferior surfaces through which each vertebra articulates with its neighbors.

Extending posteriorly from the body are the pedicles, and then to complete the vertebral foramen are the laminae. A spinous process extends posteriorly from the laminae and two transverse processes extend from the junctions between the laminae and pedicles. Two superior and two inferior articular processes extend upwardly and downwardly in the frontal plane (fig. 6.3); just anterior to the inferior articulating processes and below the pedicles are the intervertebral notches through which nerves leave the spinal column. The pedicles and laminae, together with the processes they support, are referred to collectively as the vertebral arch.

**Cervical Vertebrae** In the cervical area, three of the vertebrae, the first, second and seventh, exhibit certain peculiarities. The first cervical vertebra (fig. 6.4), called the *atlas* because it supports the cranium, has no body but rather resembles a bony ring. Its spinous process is shortened but the transverse processes are long. On its superior surface are two large concavities which articulate with the occipital condyles of the skull to allow for flexion and extension around the frontal axis.

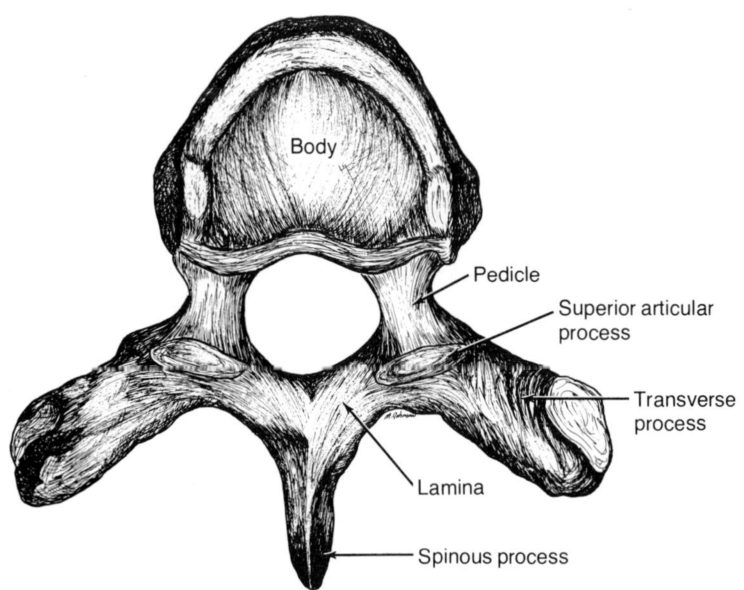


Figure 6.2. A typical vertebra, superior view

Figure 6.3. A lumbar vertebra, cross section

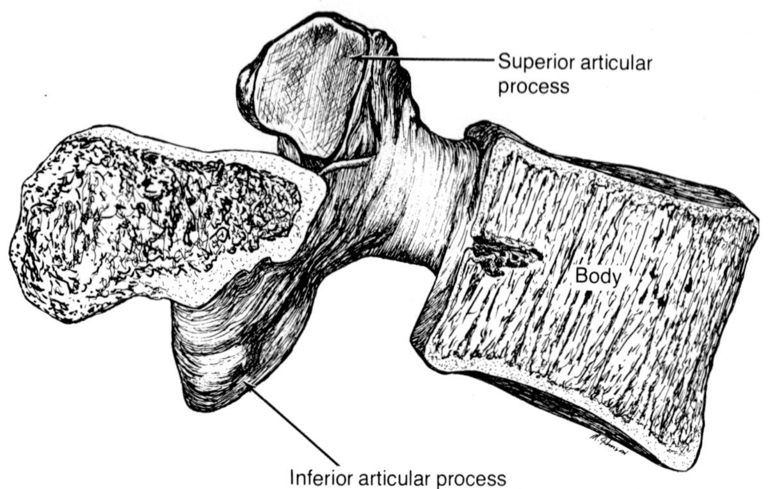


Figure 6.4. The first cervical vertebra (*atlas*), superior view

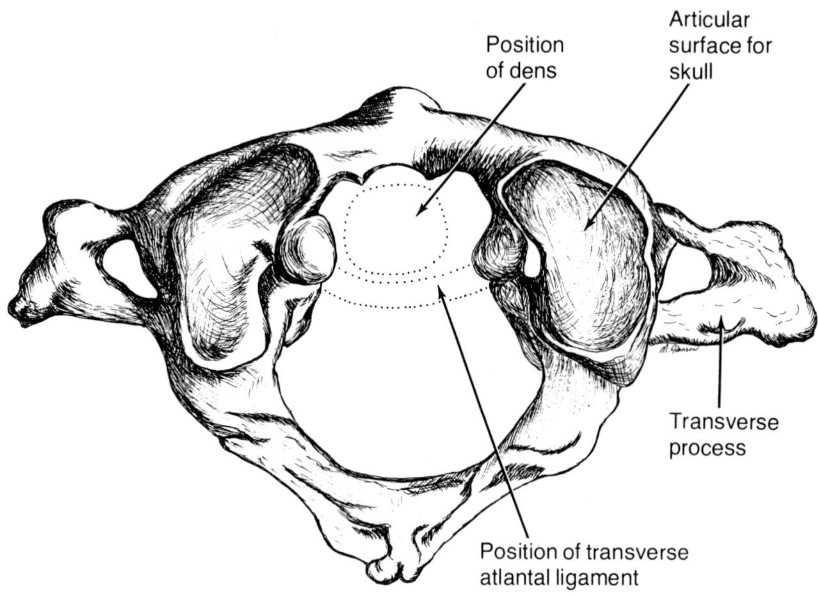


The second cervical vertebra (fig. 6.5) is called the axis because it is characterized by a short peg, the dens, which is the pivot around which the first vertebra, carrying the head, rotates. The dens extends into the vertebral foramen of the first vertebra where it is separated from the spinal cord by the large transverse atlantae ligament. This arrangement permits extensive range of movement around the vertical axis; as, for example, turning the head to look from side to side.

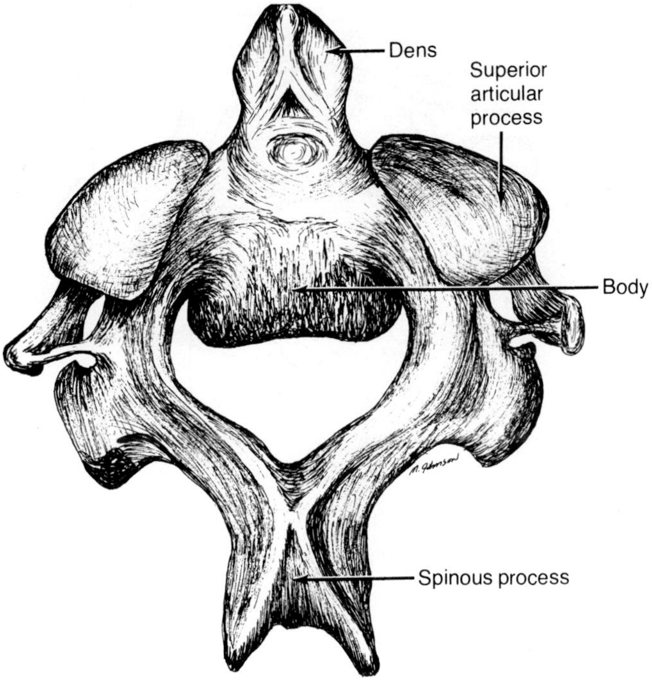

Figure 6.5. The second cervical vertebra (axis), superior view

The seventh cervical vertebra (fig. 6.6) is distinguished by its unusually long spinous process. It is easily palpated on the posterior base of the neck and provides a convenient point of separation between the cervical and thoracic regions of the spine.

**Thoracic Vertebrae** Of the thoracic vertebrae, all exhibit four articular facets which are not to be found on other vertebrae (fig. 6.7). These facets form the articulations with the twelve ribs, to place an effective anatomical splint on the thoracic area. Resulting ranges of motion in flexion and lateral flexion are limited to the ability of the ribs to spread and close. An additional peculiarity of the thoracic vertebrae is that the spinous processes are projected downwardly, particularly in the second through the tenth vertebrae—a characteristic which limits the ability of the thoracic spine to hyperextend.

**Lumbar Vertebrae** The lumbar vertebrae (fig. 6.8), being the largest of the movable vertebrae, must support the weight of the body above them. Their articular processes are more defined than in other vertebrae and provide more of an interlocking articulation which limits

**Figure 6.6. The seventh cervical vertebra, superior view**

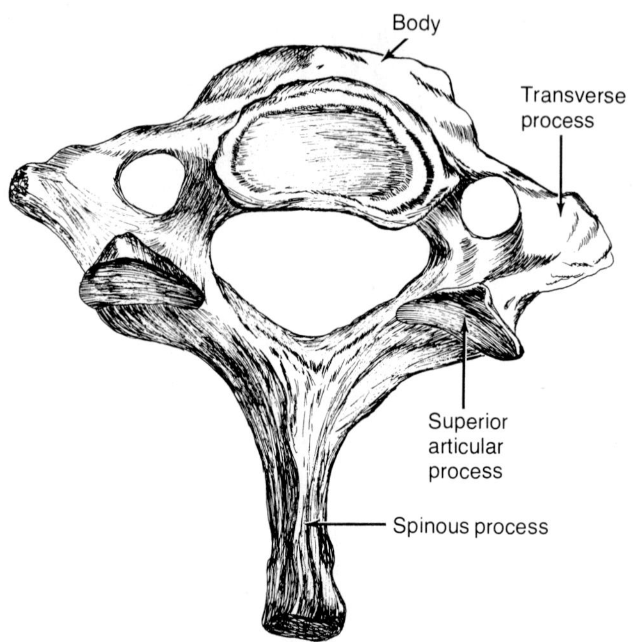


**Figure 6.7. A thoracic vertebra, lateral view**

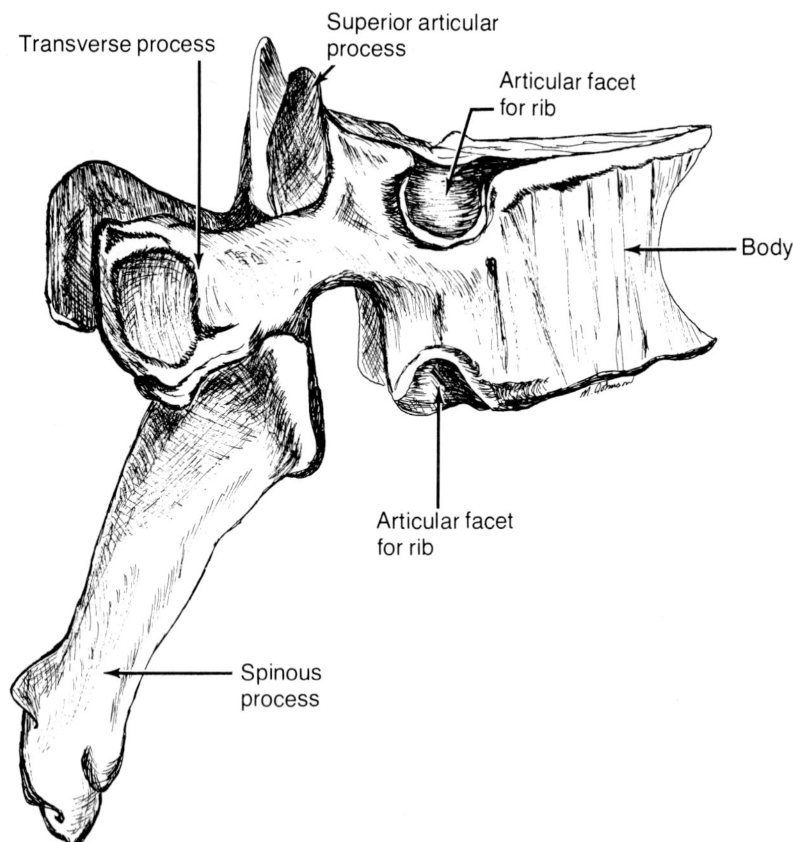

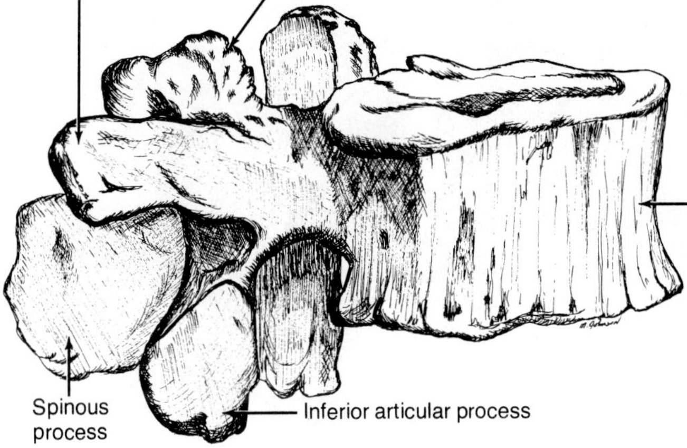

Figure 6.8. A lumbar vertebra, lateral view

movement around the vertical axis. The fifth lumbar vertebra deserves special comment in that it articulates distally with the sacrum through the lumbrosacral junction. The range of movement is greater in this junction than elsewhere in the lumbar spine.

**Sacral Vertebrae** The sacrum (fig. 6.9) represents the fusion of five sacral vertebrae to form a large triangular bone located like a wedge between the two hip bones. It articulates proximally with the last lumbar vertebra and distally with the coccyx. No movement is possible in this area of the spine.

**Coccygeal Vertebrae** The coccyx (fig. 6.10) is formed of four rudimentary vertebrae, the last one of which is only a nodule of bone. Like the sacrum, no movement is possible.

Viewed laterally, the spinal column is seen to comprise four curves. Two of these, the curves of the thoracic and sacrococcygeal regions, are convex posteriorly whereas the remaining two curves, those of the cervical and lumbar regions are convex anteriorly. Since the former two curves existed before birth, they are referred to as *primary curves*. The cervical and lumbar curves develop during infancy and early childhood, and are called *secondary curves*.

## Ligaments of the Spine

Seven ligaments of the spine will be discussed briefly. Two of these are ligaments of the vertebral bodies, and five are associated with the pedicles, laminae, and vertebral processes (the vertebral arches). The

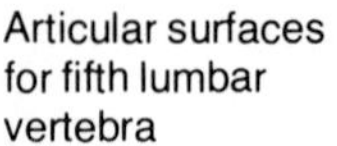


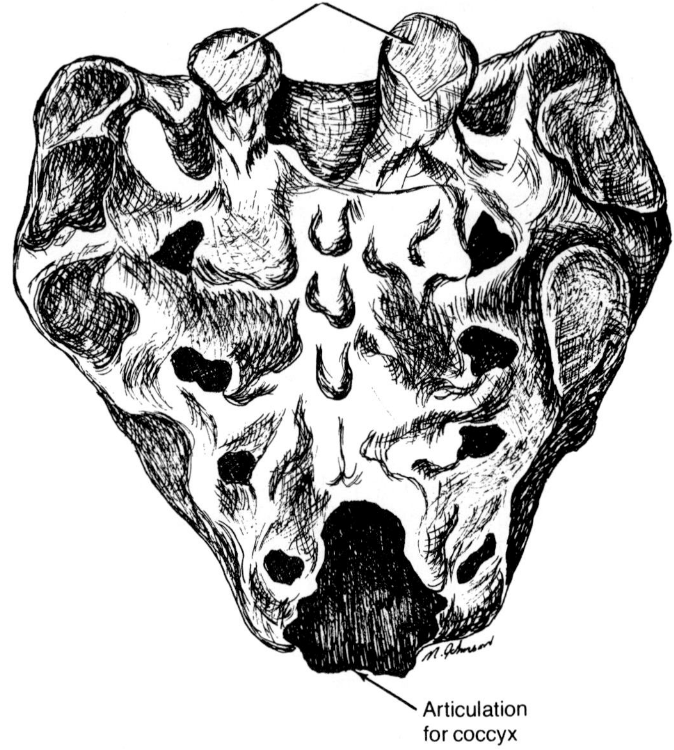


Figure 6.9. The sacrum, posterior view

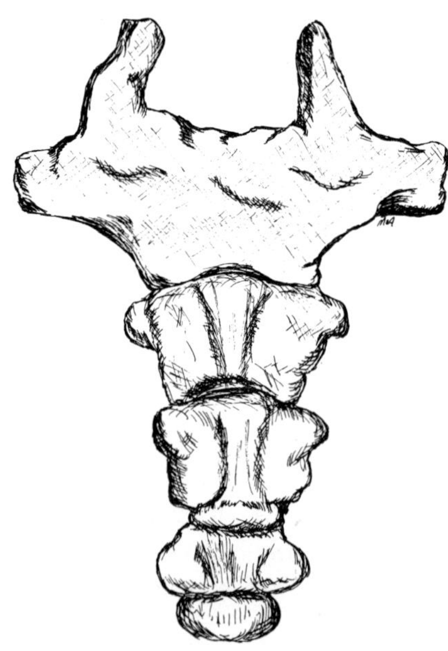

Figure 6.10. The coccyx, posterior view

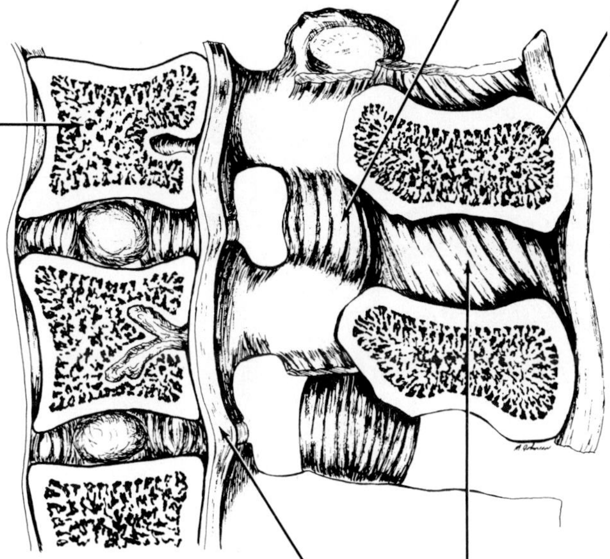

**Figure 6.11. Ligaments of the spine, cross section**

anterior longitudinal ligament (fig. 6.11) extends from the inner surface of the occipital bone down the anterior surface of the vertebral bodies to the sacrum. It is thickest in the thoracic area. The posterior longitudinal ligament (fig. 6.11) extends from the occipital bone down the posterior surface of the vertebral bodies to the coccyx. It is thickest in the thoracic area. The ligamenta flava (fig. 6.11) connect the laminae of adjacent vertebrae. They are thickest in the lumbar region. The interspinous ligaments (fig. 6.11) connect neighboring borders of the spinous processes. They are thin ligaments but are best developed in the lumbar region. The supraspinal ligament (fig. 6.11) connects the posterior tips of the spinous processes. It extends from the seventh cervical vertebra to the sacrum and is thicker in the lumbar than in the thoracic region. The ligamentum nuchae (fig. 6.12), or ligament of the neck, is an extension of the supraspinal ligament upwards from the seventh cervical vertebra to the occipital bone. It forms a division between the muscles on either side of the neck. The intertransversii ligaments are poorly developed ligaments which course between the transverse processes of adjacent vertebrae. They are best developed in the thoracic region.

Figure 6.12. Ligamentum nuchae, lateral view

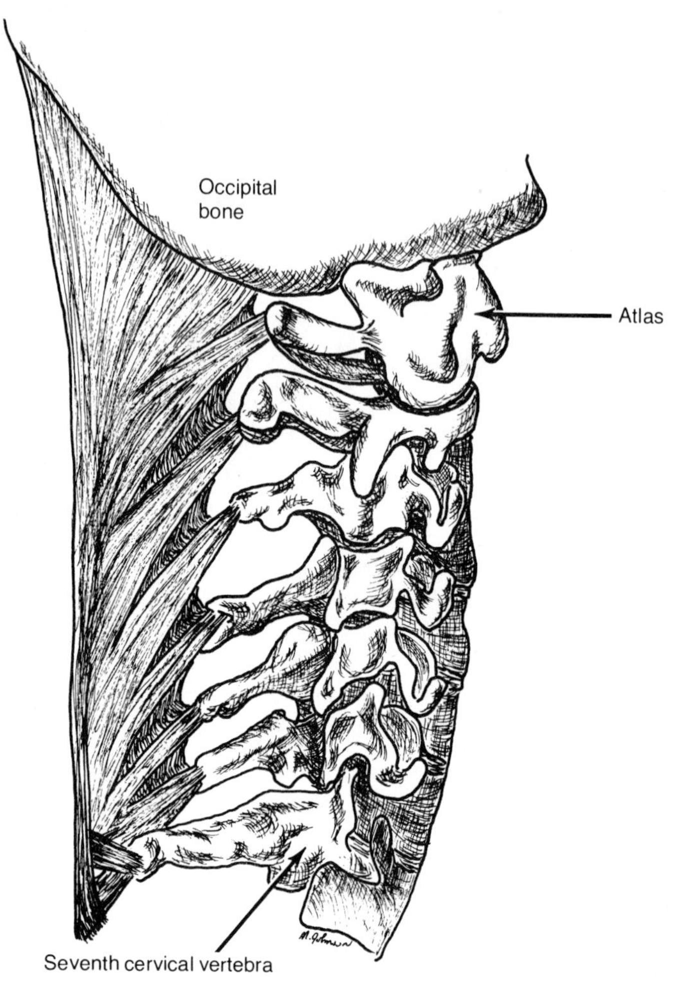


## Movements of the Spine

The movements of the spine are made possible by two types of articulations; those between the vertebral bodies, and those between the vertebral arches. With the exception of the joint between the first and second cervical vertebrae, the joints between the bodies are classified as cartilaginous because of the discs of fibrocartilage which occupy the intervertebral spaces. Each disc consists of an outer rim, the annulus fibrosis, and a pulpy nucleus, the nucleus pulposus (fig. 6.13). The nucleus pulposus is firmly compacted material with elastic properties to permit compression in any direction around it.

Whereas no single disc can provide for more than slight compression, a cumulation of the compressive movement over several discs

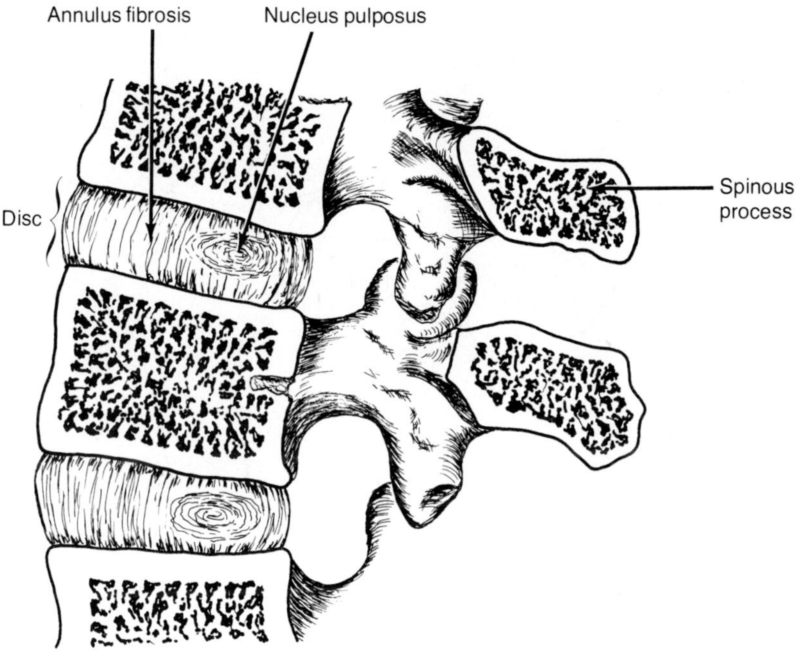

Figure 6.13. Intervertebral discs of lumbar spine, cross section

yields impressive ranges of motion not unlike those of a triaxial ball and socket joint (fig. 6.14). Flexion, extension and hyperextension of the spine occur in the sagittal plane around multiple axes, each one passing from side to side through the nucleus pulposus of the compressing discs. Lateral flexion occurs in the frontal plane around sagittal axes passing, again, through the nucleus pulposus. Rotation of the spine, described as being either right or left, occurs in the horizontal plane around a vertical axis passing downward from the top of the head through the discs to the sacral region. Circumduction combines the actions in the sagittal and frontal planes.

The muscles acting on the spine can be categorized generally as anterior or posterior muscles. Anterior muscles function mainly to flex the spine; posterior muscles extend and hyperextend it. Lateral flexion is caused by either anterior or posterior muscles when only one side of each pair is contracted; rotation is caused by these muscles, also, but only if they do not lie parallel to the vertical axis.

It should be noted that the action of spinal rotation is always accompanied by a certain amount of lateral flexion to that side. Lateral flexion is, similarly, always accompanied by some rotation to the same side. This phenomenon explains the tendency of most individuals to exhibit a slight pelvic rotation when standing erect, or perhaps an asymmetrical projection of an upper rib. Because use of the preferred

Figure 6.14. Movements of the spine

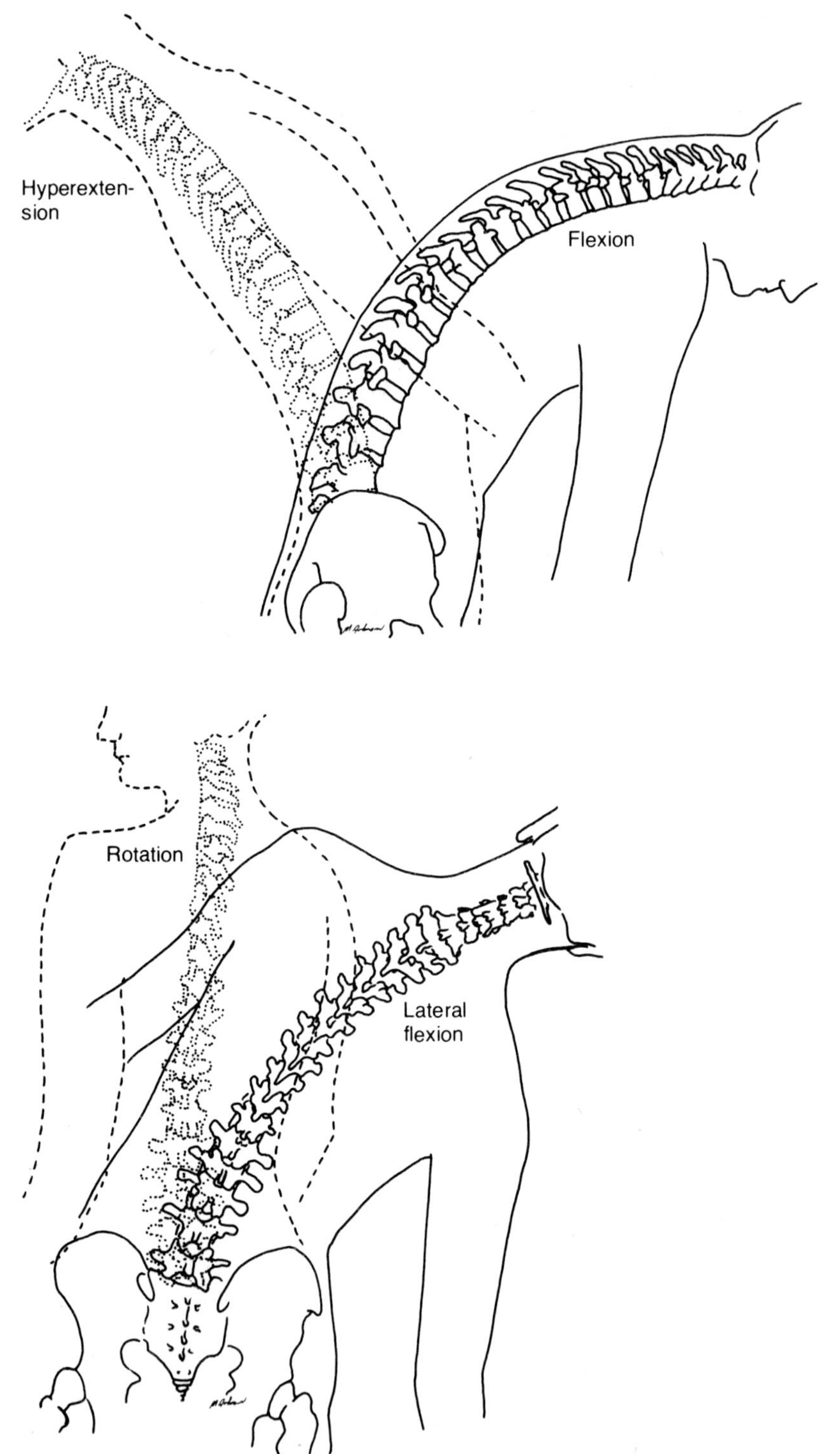

arm is so much greater than that of the nonpreferred arm, the musculature on the preferred side of the body is usually better developed, and pulls the spine into slight lateral flexion. The accompanying rotation can manifest itself in the thoracic region causing malalignment of the ribs, or in the lumbar area causing a right or left facing of the hips.

The articulation between the first and second cervical vertebrae, the atlantoaxial joint, has been discussed previously as being a pivot joint allowing only for rotation around the vertical axis. It should be remembered also that the occipitoatlantal articulation contributes to the overall flexion-extension-hyperextension movement of the spine.

The joints between the vertebral arches are nonaxial synovial joints which allow for a limited amount of gliding between the articulating surfaces. Such an arrangement permits the spinal column to change its shape in response to the temporary distortions of the intervertebral discs.

Figure 6.15 is presented to summarize the movements of the various regions of the spine. The spinal column is depicted in extension as it would be in upright posture, with notations regarding the type and extent of movements of which the several regions are capable. These notations are rather consistent regardless of whether the initial position of the spine is flexed, extended, or hyperextended, with this generalized exception: lateral flexion and rotation occur higher than usual when the starting position involves the flexed spine, and lower than usual when the spine is hyperextended.

## The Pelvic Girdle

The pelvic girdle (figs. 6.16, 6.17) is comprised of two hip bones, each of which is formed by the fusion of the pubis, ilium, and ischium. The two hip bones themselves are joined around the sacrum, and then tied together at the symphysis to form a single unit.

The sacroiliac articulation defies precise categorization. It presents characteristics of a nonaxial synovial joint in that a joint space containing synovial fluid is present in a portion of the articulation. Movement is extremely limited, however, and is never voluntary. The articulation also presents characteristics of a cartilaginous joint. There is an intervening plate of cartilage between the two bones which, together with the anterior and posterior sacroiliac ligaments and the interosseus ligament, is responsible for the near immobility of the joint.

The symphysis is a cartilaginous joint which joins the two pubes. The joint is only slightly movable, being reinforced heavily by the superior pubic and arcuate pubic ligaments.

Figure 6.15. Locations of spinal movements

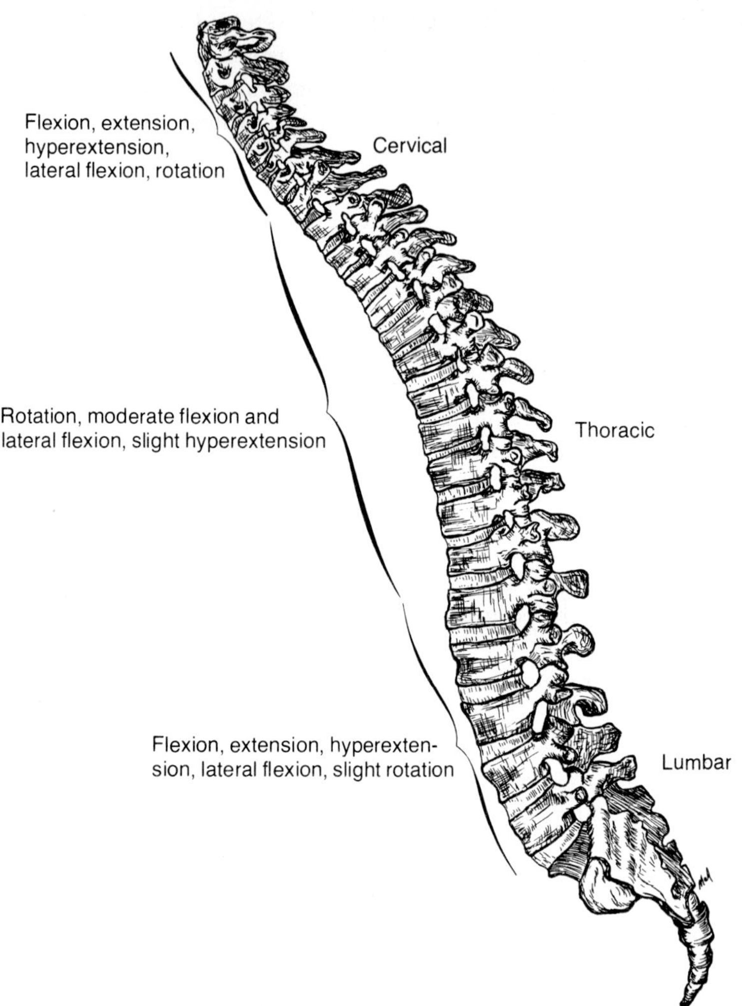


The lumbrosacral joint, discussed previously in this chapter, is the most important articulation to pelvic movement. All movements of the pelvic girdle occur around this joint and are classified as follows:

*Forward Tilt* Hyperextension of the lumbrosacral joint resulting in a dowward and backward movement of the symphysis.

*Backward Tilt* Reduction of hyperextension of the lumbrosacral joint resulting in an upward and forward movement of the symphysis.

*Lateral Tilt* Lateral flexion of the lumbrosacral joint resulting in the raising or lowering of one iliac crest.

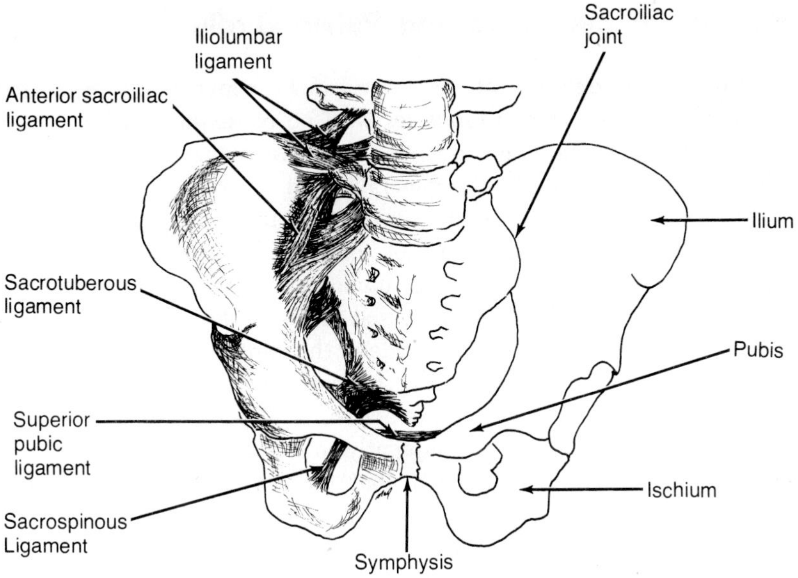

**Figure 6.16. The pelvis, anterior view**

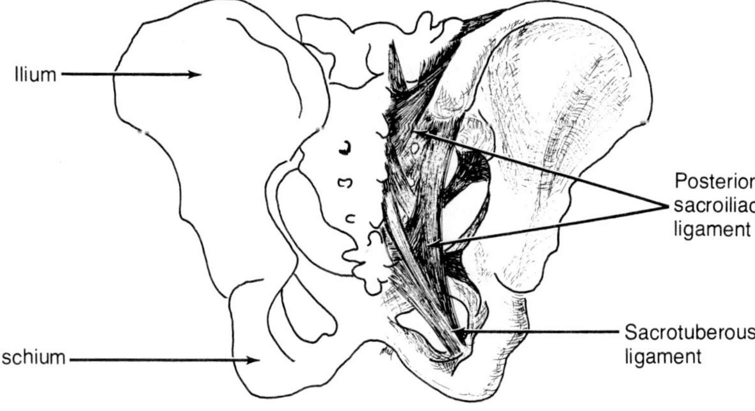


**Figure 6.17. The pelvis, posterior view**

*Rotation* Rotation to the right or left at the lumbrosacral joint resulting in a pivotal movement of the hips around the vertical axis.

The muscles acting on the lumbrosacral joint are those which move the spine and will be discussed in the following section. In general, muscles which cause forward and backward tilt will be those located on the posterior and anterior aspects of the spine, respectively. Lateral tilt and rotation will be caused by the contraction of only one side of paired muscles; rotation results specifically from contraction of those muscles which are not parallel to the vertical axis.

## Muscles of the Spine and Pelvic Girdle

Most of the musculature of the spine can be conveniently organized into groups of two or more muscles with no consequential loss to the learning of the underlying concepts. It must be realized, however, that this approach necessitates the generalization of origins, insertions, innervations, and actions. Frequent referral to the illustrations and to a skeleton should clarify any confusion, but if more precision is required, one of the several classical texts of human anatomy may be consulted.

All of the muscle groups discussed in this section are paired, with one of each pair located on either side of the vertical axis. Their actions are, therefore, described according to whether both sides of the pair are contracting or only one side is active.

Reference will be made frequently to the axes around which the muscles act. It was noted earlier that there is no single sagittal or frontal or vertical axis of the spine. Rather, there are multiple axes passing through the discs between the compressing vertebrae. For practical purposes, however, it will suffice to refer to the three axes in the singular when describing the actions of the muscle groups.

**Prevertebral Muscles** The prevertebral muscles (fig. 6.18) are the rectus capitis anterior, rectus capitis lateralis, longus capitis, and longus colli (rec'tus cap'itis ante'rior, rec'tus cap'itis latera'lis, lon'gus cap'itis, and lon'gus col'li). They are deep muscles and cannot be palpated.

*Origin* Anterior surfaces of all cervical and the first three thoracic vertebrae.

*Insertion* Anterior aspect of the occipital bone and the cervical vertebrae.

*Innervation* Cervical nerves.

*Action* Both sides: Flexion of atlantooccipital joint and the cervical spine. One side: Lateral flexion of cervical spine.

The muscles of the prevertebral group are located anterior to the spine; however, with their attachments on the spine itself, they have short force arms. This, together with their small size, enables them to be only assistive in their actions.

**The Scaleni** The scaleni (fig. 6.19) are the scalenus anterior, scalenus posterior, and scalenus medius (scale'nus ante'rior, scale'nus poste'rior, and scale'nus medius). They are located on the side of the neck between the sternocleidomastoid and Part 1 of the trapezius and are easily confused with those muscles during palpation.

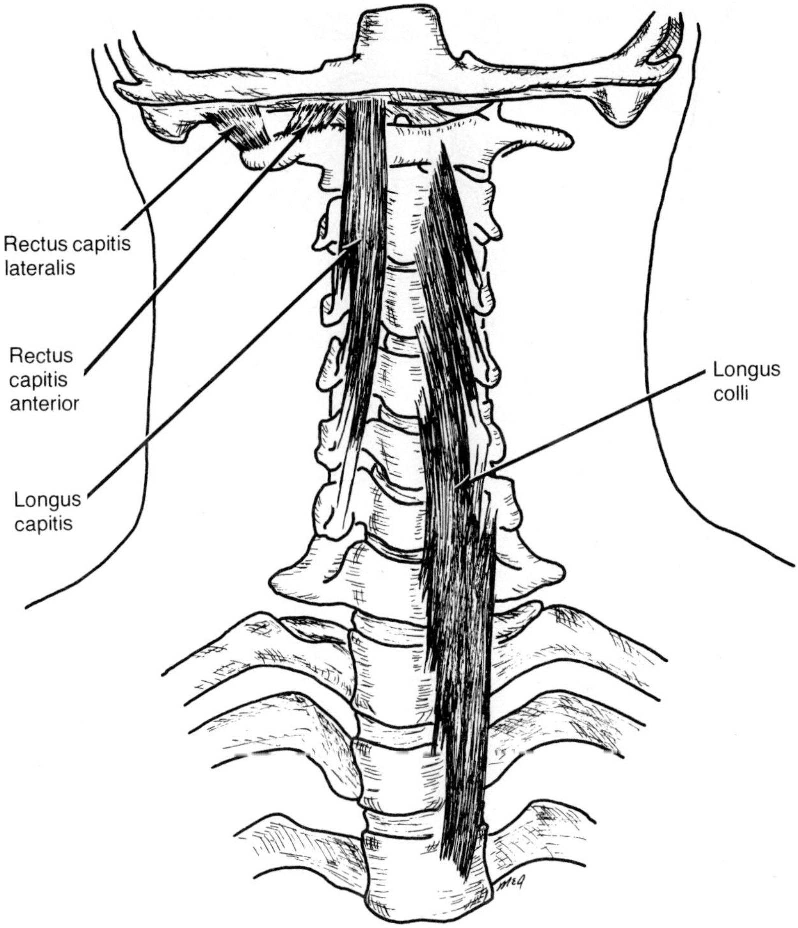

**Figure 6.18. Prevertebral muscles, anterior view**

*Origin* Upper two ribs.

*Insertion* Transverse processes of the cervical vertebrae.

*Innervation* Second to seventh cervical nerves.

*Action* Both sides: Flexion of cervical spine. One side: Lateral flexion of cervical spine.

The attachments of the scaleni locate the muscles only slightly anterior to the spine; hence, they are not capable of more than a weak contribution to flexion of the cervical spine. They are, however, well located for lateral flexion in that their attachments on the ribs serve to extend their force arms from the sagittal axis.

Figure 6.19. The scaleni muscles, anterior view

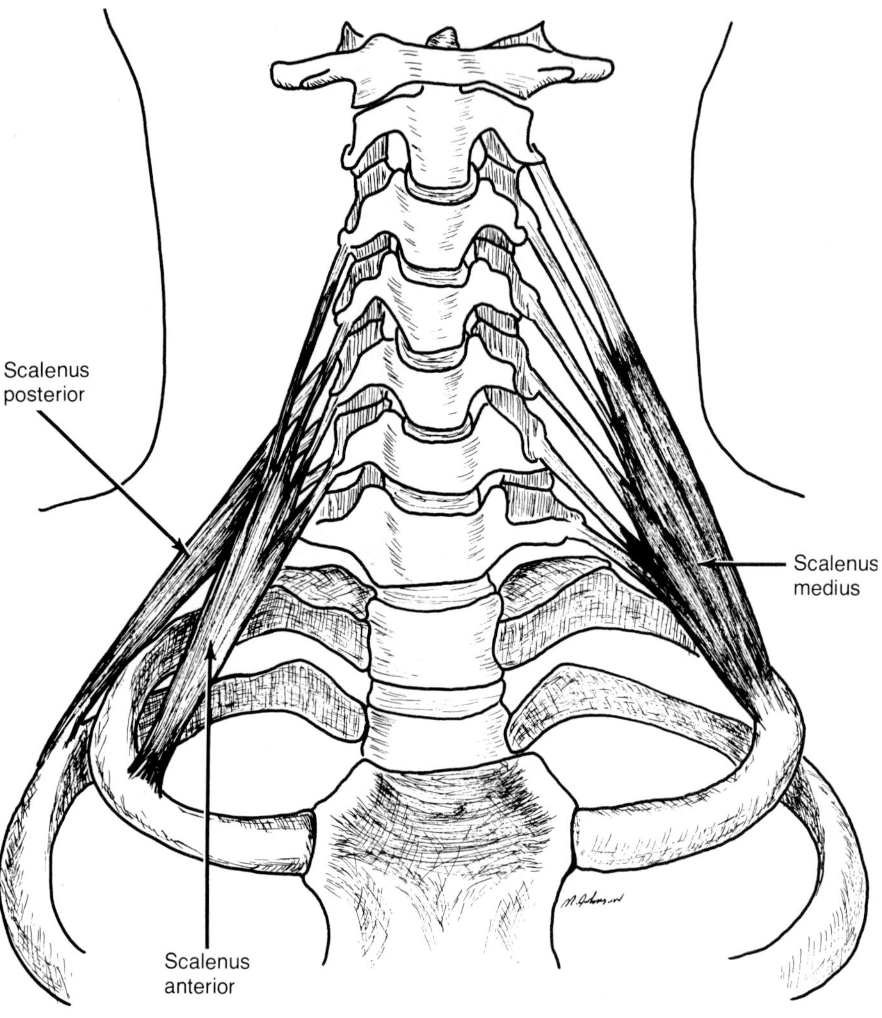


**Sternocleidomastoid** (ster'no cleid'o mas'toid) The sternocleidomastoid (fig. 6.20) is the large cord-like muscle located on each side of the neck. It may be palpated easily as the head is rotated to the opposite side.

*Origin* By two heads, from the superior aspect of the sternum and the inner third of the clavicle.

*Insertion* Mastoid process of the temporal bone.

*Innervation* Spinal assessory and second and third cervical nerves.

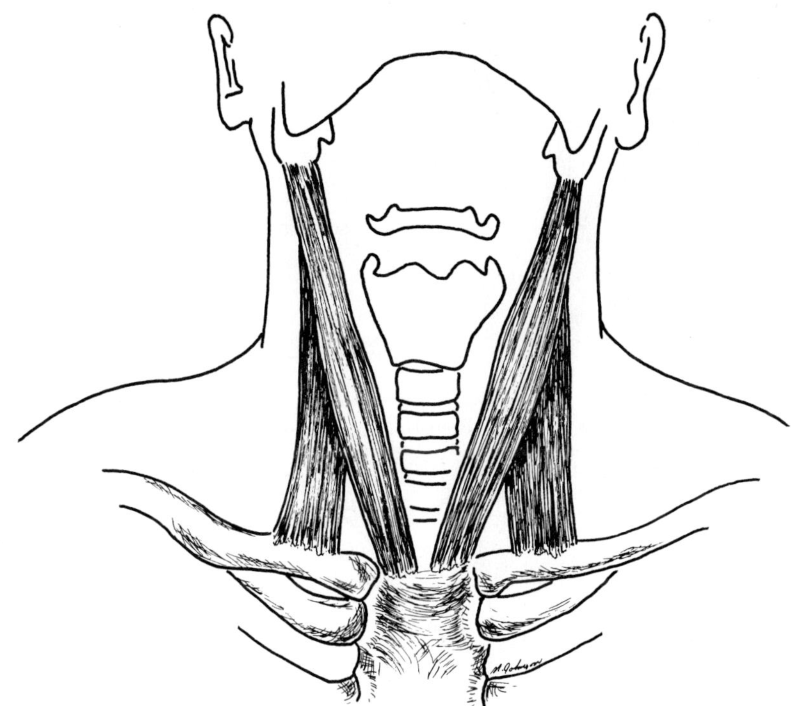

Figure 6.20. Sternocleidomastoid of both sides of neck, anterior view.

*Action* Both sides: Flexion of atlantooccipital joint and by continued action, flexion of the cervical spine. One side: Lateral flexion of cervical spine; rotation to opposite side of atlantoaxial joint and cervical spine.

The sternocleidomastoid is the largest of the anterior muscles acting on the head and neck. Its relatively long moment arm to all three axes enables the muscle to exert a great deal of force in all of its actions.

**Levator Scapulae** (leva'tor scap'ulae) The levator scapulae (fig. 6.21) is located on the lateral and posterior aspect of the neck. It lies beneath Part 1 of the trapezius and cannot be palpated except through that muscle portion.

*Origin* Vertebral border of the scapula, between the superior angle and the root of the scapular spine.

*Insertion* Transverse processes of the first four cervical vertebrae.

*Innervation* Dorsal scapular and third and fourth cervical nerves.

*Action* Both sides: Stabilization of the cervical spine. One side: Lateral flexion of the cervical spine.

Figure 6.21. Levator scapulae, posterior view

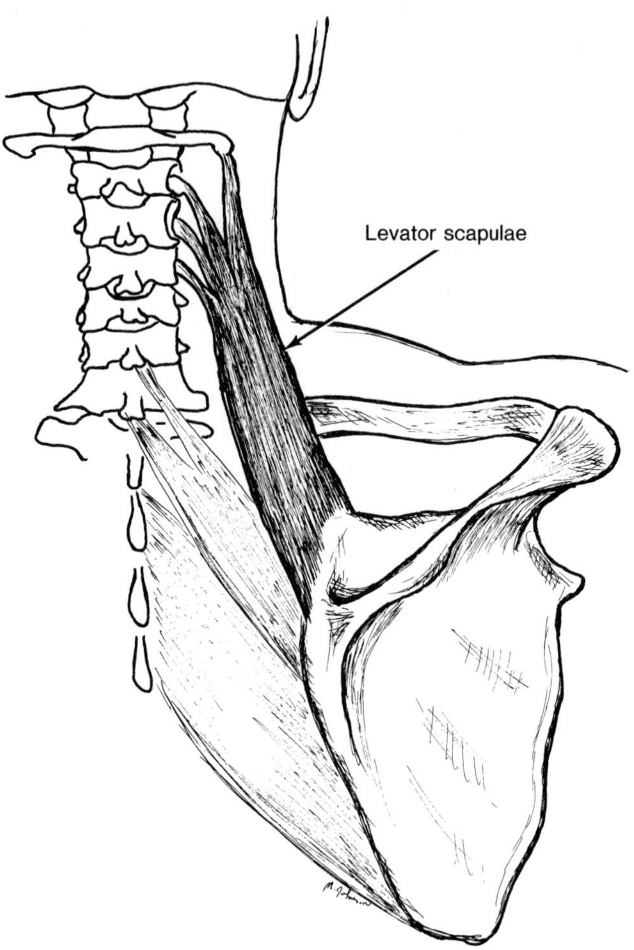


The primary function of the levator scapulae is to elevate the scapula; however, when the scapula is stabilized to provide an origin, the muscle, if only one side is contracted, will pull the cervical spine into lateral flexion. If both muscles are contracted, they neutralize each other's tendency to laterally flex, and cervical stability results.

**Splenius Muscles** The splenius muscles (fig. 6.22) are the splenius capitis and splenius cervicis (sple'nius cap'itis and sple'nius cer'vicis). The capitis is superficial between the sternocleidomastoid and trapezius, just below the skull.

*Origin* Inferior half of ligamentum nuchae; spinous processes of last cervical and upper six thoracic vertebrae.

*Insertion* Mastoid process of temporal bone; transverse processes of first three cervical vertebrae.

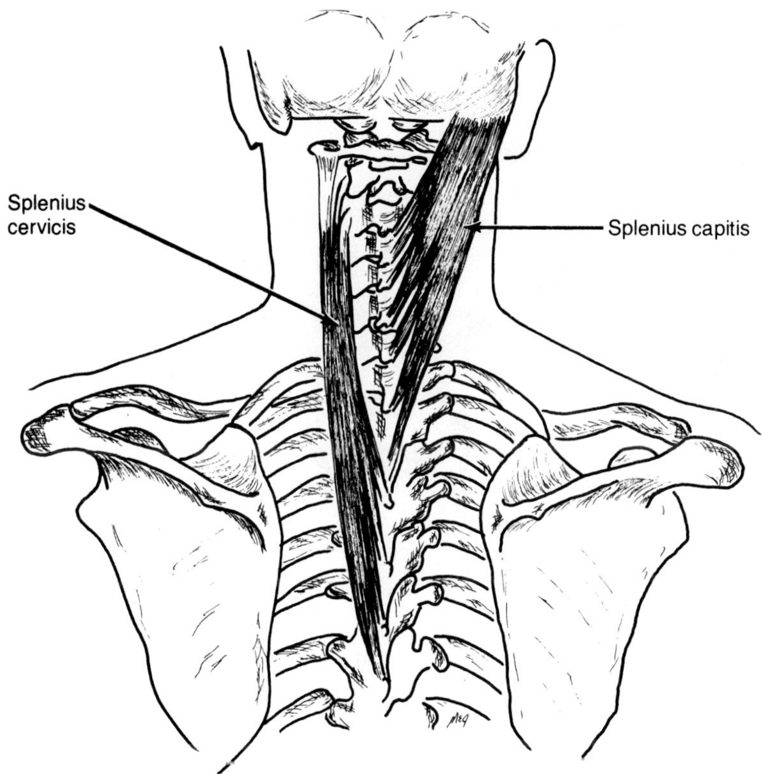


**Figure 6.22. Splenius muscles, posterior view**

*Innervation* Branches of the middle and lower cervical nerves.

*Action* Both sides: Extension and hyperextension of atlanto-occipital joint and cervical spine. One side: Lateral flexion and rotation to the same side of the cervical spine.

The splenius muscles are located posterior to the frontal axis, lateral to the sagittal axis, and by virtue of the attachment of the capitis on the mastoid process, are diagonal to the vertical axis. If both sides are contracted simultaneously, they neutralize their tendencies to rotate and laterally flex; the resultant action is a backward movement of the head and neck in the sagittal plane. If only one side is contracted, the muscles spend their action in lateral flexion and/or rotation.

**The suboccipitals** The suboccipitals (fig. 6.23) are the obliquus capitis superior, obliquus capitis inferior, rectus capitis posterior major, and rectus capitis posterior minor (obli'quus cap'itis supe'rior, obli'quus cap'itis infe'rior, rec'tus cap'itis poste'rior ma'jor, and rec'tus cap'itis poste'rior mi'nor). They lie deep below the skull and cannot be palpated.

Figure 6.23. The suboccipital muscles, posterior view

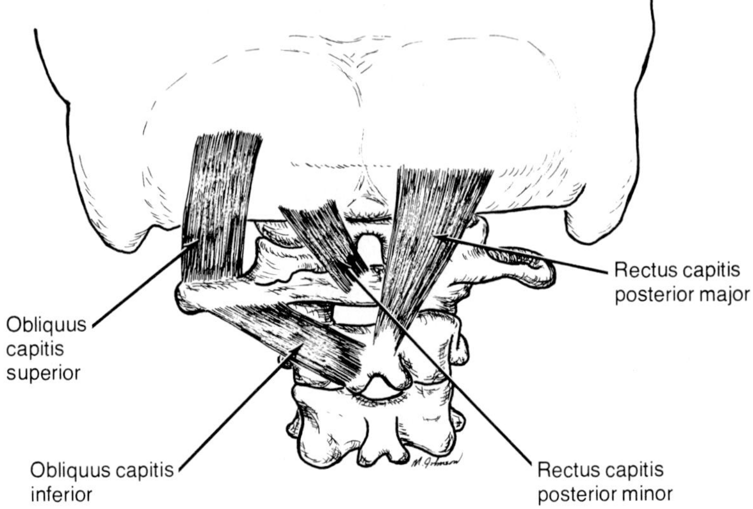


*Origin* Posterior surfaces of the first two cervical vertebrae (atlas and axis).

*Insertion* Occipital bone and transverse process of the first cervical vertebra (atlas).

*Innervation* Suboccipital nerve.

*Action* Both sides: Extension and hyperextension of the atlantooccipital joint. One side: Lateral flexion of the cervical spine and rotation to the same side.

The vertical line of pull of the two rectus muscles favors the extension/hyperextension function of the suboccipitals, whereas the two oblique muscles, with their diagonal lines of pull, favor rotation. None of the muscles is sufficiently large, however, to contribute more than assistively to any action.

**Erector Spinae** (erec'tor spi'nae) The erector spinae (fig. 6.24) is a massive muscle of the back consisting of the iliocostalis, longissimus, and spinalis (iliocosta'lis, longis'simus, and spina'lis) branches. Each branch is further subdivided according to its location as follows:

*Illiocostalis:* Cervicis, thoracis, lumborum.

*Longissimus:* Capitus, cervicis, thoracis.

*Spinalis:* Cervicis, thoracis.

*Origin* Lower portion of ligamentum nuchae; posterior aspects of cervical, thoracic, and lumbar spine; angles of the lower nine ribs; iliac crest; posterior sacrum.

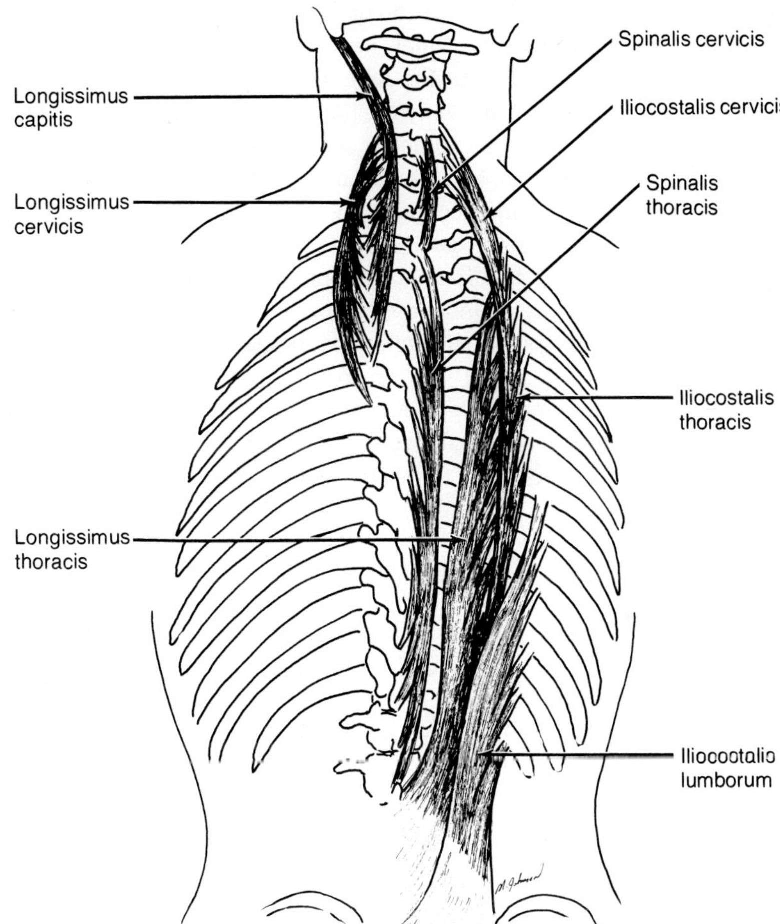


**Figure 6.24. The erector spinae, posterior view**

*Insertion* Mastoid process of temporal bone; posterior aspects of cervical, thoracic, and lumbar vertebrae; angles and adjacent portions of the twelve ribs.

*Innervation* Posterior branches of spinal nerves.

*Action* Both sides: Extension and hyperextension of atlanto-occipital joint and entire spine. One side: Lateral flexion of entire spine and rotation to the same side.

The erector spinae is recruited completely during almost all movements of the spine; however, certain portions of the muscle will predominate according to whether the movement is in the sagittal, frontal, or transverse plane. In general, it might be said that the portions of the muscle closer to the spine favor extension and hyperextension, and those farther from the spine favor lateral flexion. Rotation is accomplished by those portions which have a diagonal rather than vertical line of pull with respect to the long axis of the spine.

The erector spinae is not only an important mover of the spine, it functions also to stabilize the spine by contracting eccentrically to control flexion and lateral flexion. For example, when the trunk is flexed from the anatomical reference position, the erector spinae becomes active in order to control the torso against the effects of gravity. Activity gradually ceases as full flexion is approached. At full flexion, the muscle is quiet, and the support of the trunk becomes the responsibility of the fasciae and posterior ligaments. Similarly, when the trunk is lifted through extension, the erector spinae does not resume activity until after the initial phase of the movement has been accomplished. The frequent warning, "lift with your legs, not your back," would appear to have validity if one is to avoid the dangers of overstressing the vertebral ligaments.

**Semispinalis Muscles** (semispina'lis) The semispinalis muscles (fig. 6.25) are the semispinalis capitis, semispinalis cervicis, and semispinalis thoracis (semispina'lis cap'itis, semispina'lis cer'vicis, semispina'lis thora'cis). The muscles lie in the neck and upper back; they cannot be palpated.

*Origin* Articular processes of the fourth through sixth cervical vertebrae; transverse processes of seventh cervical through tenth thoracic vertebrae.

*Insertion* Occipital bone; spinous processes of second cervical through fourth thoracic vertebrae.

*Innervation* Posterior branches of cervical and thoracic nerves.

*Action* Both sides: Extension and hyperextension of atlanto-occipital joints and joints of cervical and thoracic spine. One side: Lateral flexion of cervical and thoracic spine; rotation of thoracic spine to opposite side.

The line of pull of the capitis portion of the semispinalis group is vertical, and whereas it is well-situated for extension, hyperextension and lateral flexion, it cannot contribute to rotation. The cervical and thoracic portions have a slightly diagonal direction and, in addition to moving the spine backwardly and laterally, can rotate it by pulling the spinous processes toward the transverse and articulating processes of the vertebrae below them. When the spinous processes are pulled in one direction, the resulting spinal rotation is in the opposite direction.

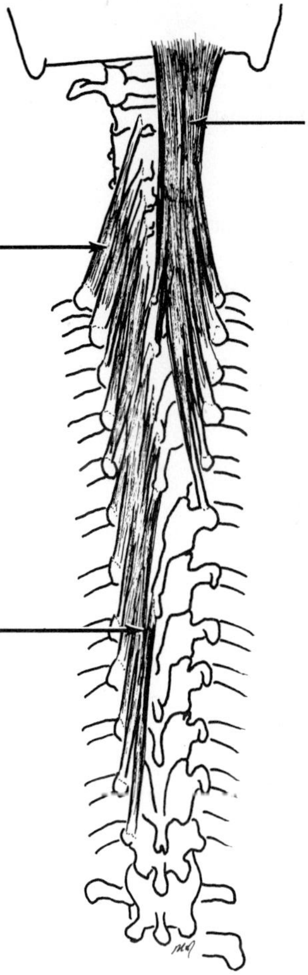

Semispinalis capitis
Semispinalis cervicis
Semispinalis thoracis

**Figure 6.25. The semispinalis muscles, posterior view**

**Deep Posterior Muscles** The deep posterior muscles of the spine (fig. 6.26) are the rotatores, multifidus, interspinalis, intertransversii, and the levatores costarum (rotato'res, multif'idus, interspina'lis, intertransversa'rii, levato'res costa'rum). None of these muscles can be palpated.

*Origin* Posterior processes of all vertebrae; posterior surface of sacrum.

*Insertion* Spinous and transverse processes, and laminae of vertebrae above those on which the muscle portions originate.

*Innervation* Spinal and intercostal nerves, and eighth cervical nerve.

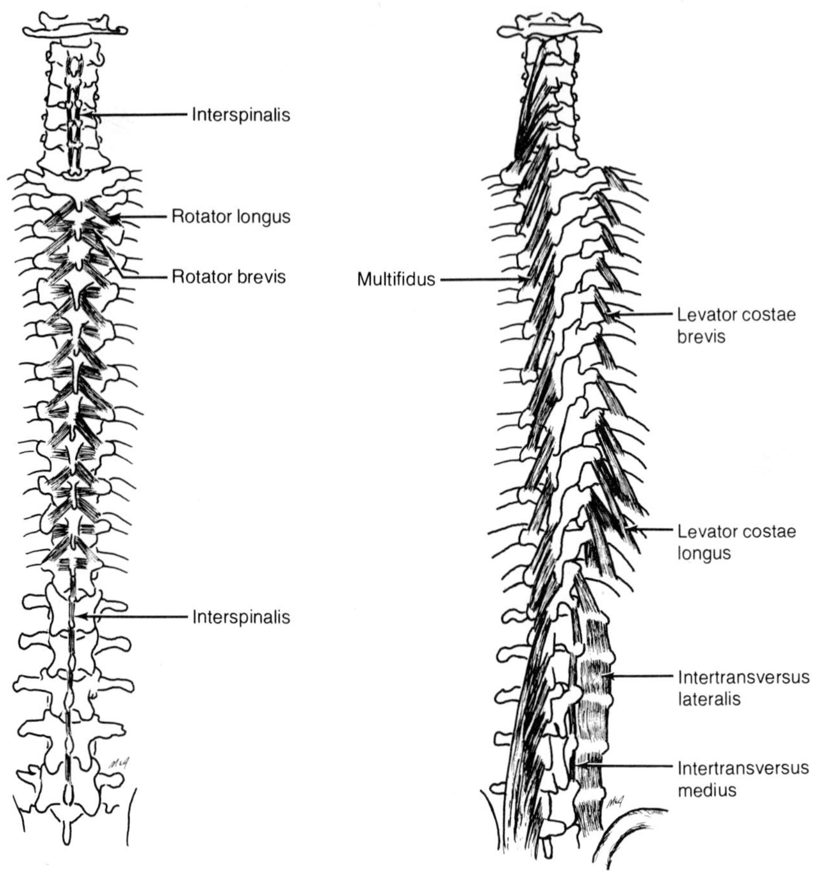


Figure 6.26. Deep posterior muscles, posterior view

*Action* Both sides: Extension and hyperextension of entire spine. One side: Lateral flexion of spine; rotation to opposite side.

These muscles are quite small, consisting of short slips which seldom span more than one vertebra from origin to insertion. The interspinalis and intertransversii lie parallel to the vertical axis and hence favor extension, hyperextension, and lateral flexion. The other portions lie diagonally to the vertical axis and thus are able to contribute the additional actions of rotation.

**Quadratus Lumborum** (quadra'tus lumbo'rum) The quadratus lumborum (fig. 6.27) is located on either side of the spine in the lumbar area. It is difficult to palpate because of the fatty tissue in the area.

*Origin* Iliolumbar ligament and adjacent portion of iliac crest.

*Insertion* Last rib; transverse processes of first four lumbar vertebrae.

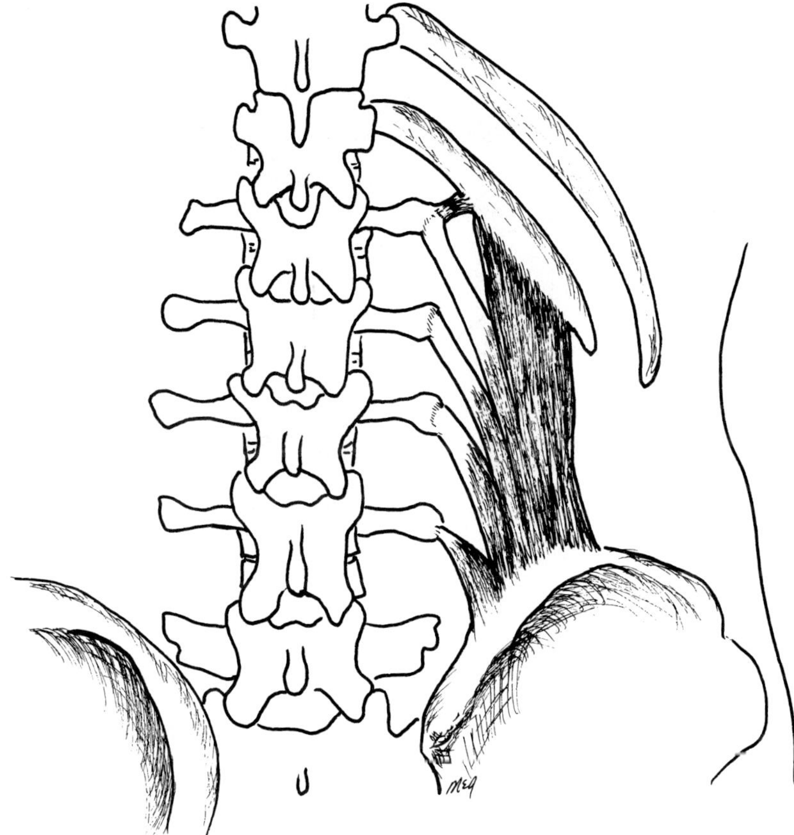

Figure 6.27. Quadratus lumborum, posterior view

*Innervation* Twelfth thoracic and first lumbar nerves.

*Action* Both sides: Stabilization of the lumbar spine. One side: Lateral flexion of the lumbar spine.

In addition to its importance as a stabilizer and lateral flexor, the quadratus lumborum is active in holding down the twelfth rib during periods of expiration.

**Trapezius** (trape'zius) **Part 1** All parts of the trapezius are discussed under the shoulder joint. Part 1 (fig. 6.28) is singled out for inclusion here because of its attachment to the cranium.

*Origin* Outer third of the clavicle.

*Insertion* Base of the skull.

*Innervation* Spinal assessory nerve.

*Action* Both sides: Extension and hyperextension of the atlantooccipital joint. One side: Rotation of the atlantoaxial joint to the opposite side.

Figure 6.28. Trapezius, posterior view

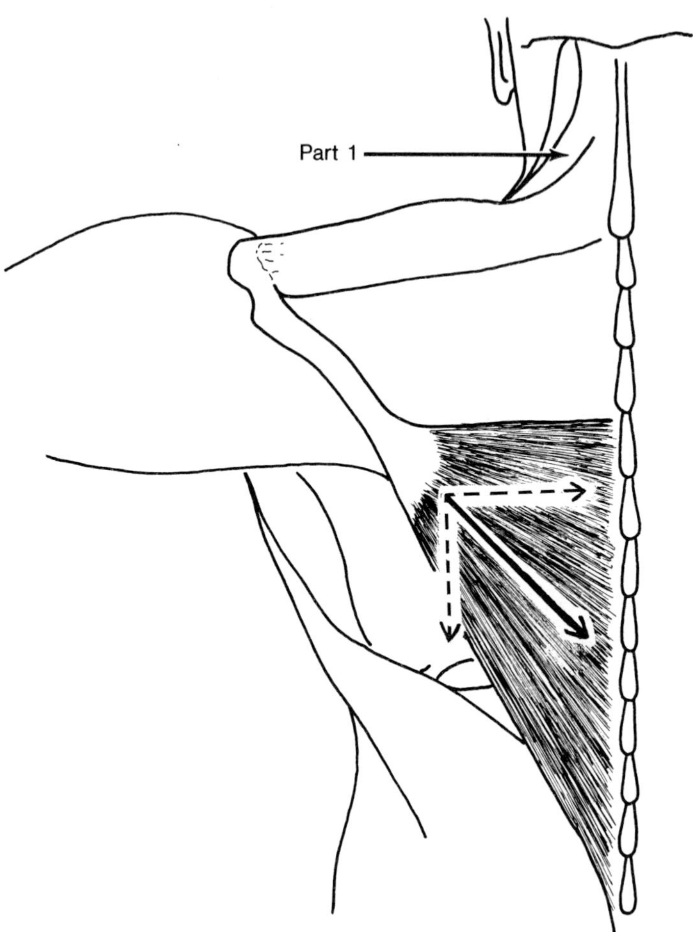


All parts of the trapezius are commonly known as scapula movers. When the scapula is stabilized, however, it forms an effective base from which part 1 of the trapezius can pull backwardly against the head.

### The Abdominals

The abdominal muscles are the rectus abdominis, external oblique, internal oblique, and transversalis abdominis. Because of their importance to the study of kinesiology, they will be considered separately, with the exception of the transversalis which is a respiratory muscle (see "Muscles of Respiration," chap. 10).

**Rectus Abdominis** (rec'tus abdom'inus) The rectus abdominis (fig. 6.29) is the most superficial of the abdominal muscles. It can be palpated between the sternum and the pubis.

*Origin* Crest of the pubis.

*Insertion* Cartilages of the fifth, sixth, and seventh ribs.

*Innervation* Seventh to twelfth intercostal nerves.

*Action* Both sides: Flexion of the spine. One side: Lateral flexion of the spine.

The two sides of the rectus abdominis are separated by a broad tendinous band called the *linea alba.* This band, together with the horizontal tendinous inscriptions of the muscle, give the rectus a rippled appearance which is clearly visible in lean persons.

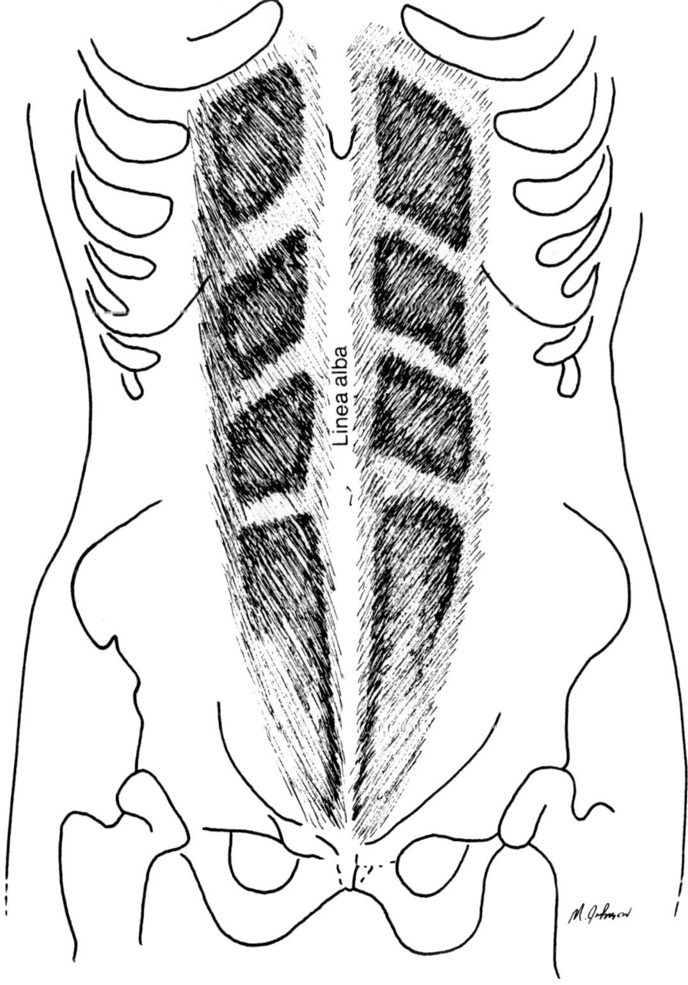


**Figure 6.29. Rectus abdominis, anterior view**

The primary action of the rectus abdominis is spinal flexion; it can contribute to lateral flexion but only in an assistive fashion because it is so near the sagittal axis. The muscle runs parallel to the vertical axis, and therefore cannot contribute to rotation.

**External Oblique** (exter'nal obli'que) The external oblique (fig. 6.30) is located on the front and side of the abdomen and is superficial in the area lateral to the rectus abdominis. It can be palpated by the finger tips when the hands are placed on the hips.

Figure 6.30. External oblique, lateral view

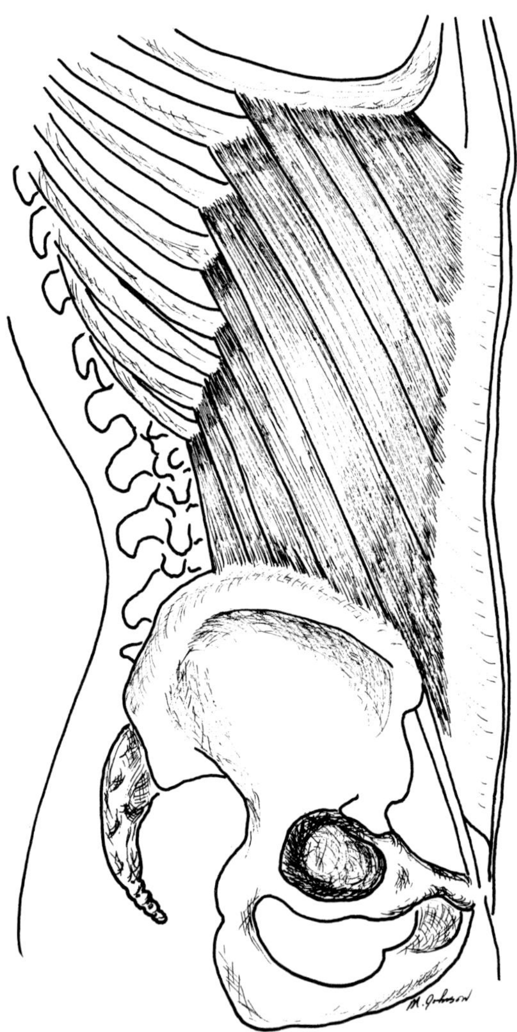

*Origin* Lower eight ribs by slips which interweave with those of the serratus anterior.

*Insertion* Anterior portion of iliac crest; crest of pubis via the linea alba.

*Innervation* Iliohypogastric, ilioinguinal and eighth to twelfth intercostal nerves.

*Action* Both sides: Flexion of the spine. One side: Lateral flexion of the spine and rotation to the opposite side.

The fibers of the external oblique are anterior and lateral to the frontal and sagittal axes respectively, and course diagonally downward toward the linea alba to form a *V*. When both sides are contracted together, tendencies to laterally flex and rotate are neutralized and the resultant action is that of spinal flexion. Contracting alone, each side of the muscle will laterally flex because of its relationship to the sagittal axis and/or will rotate the spine because of its diagonal line of pull. The action of rotation will be to the opposite side because the muscle's contraction will draw the ribs of the contracting side closer to the midline of the body.

**Internal Oblique** (inter'nal obli'que) The internal oblique (fig. 6.31) is located beneath the external oblique, and must be palpated through that muscle. The external oblique should first be relaxed on one side by rotating the spine to that side. The internal oblique can then be felt contracting beneath the relaxed external muscle.

*Origin* Lateral half of inguinal ligament; crest of the ilium; thoracolumbar fascia.

*Insertion* Linea alba; cartilages of lower four ribs.

*Innervation* Eighth to twelfth intercostal nerves; iliohypogastric and ilioinguinal nerves.

*Action* Both sides: Flexion of the spine. One side: Lateral flexion of the spine and rotation to the same side.

The actions of the internal oblique are accomplished in much the same manner as the external oblique. The direction of the fibers of the internal is opposite that of the external oblique, however, and as both sides of the muscle approach the linea alba, an inverted V is formed. In rotation, the ribs are pulled toward the iliac crest on that side, and the trunk is turned to that side. In flexion and lateral flexion, then, the two obliques are agonists; in the action of rotation, they are antagonists.

Figure 6.31. Internal oblique, lateral view

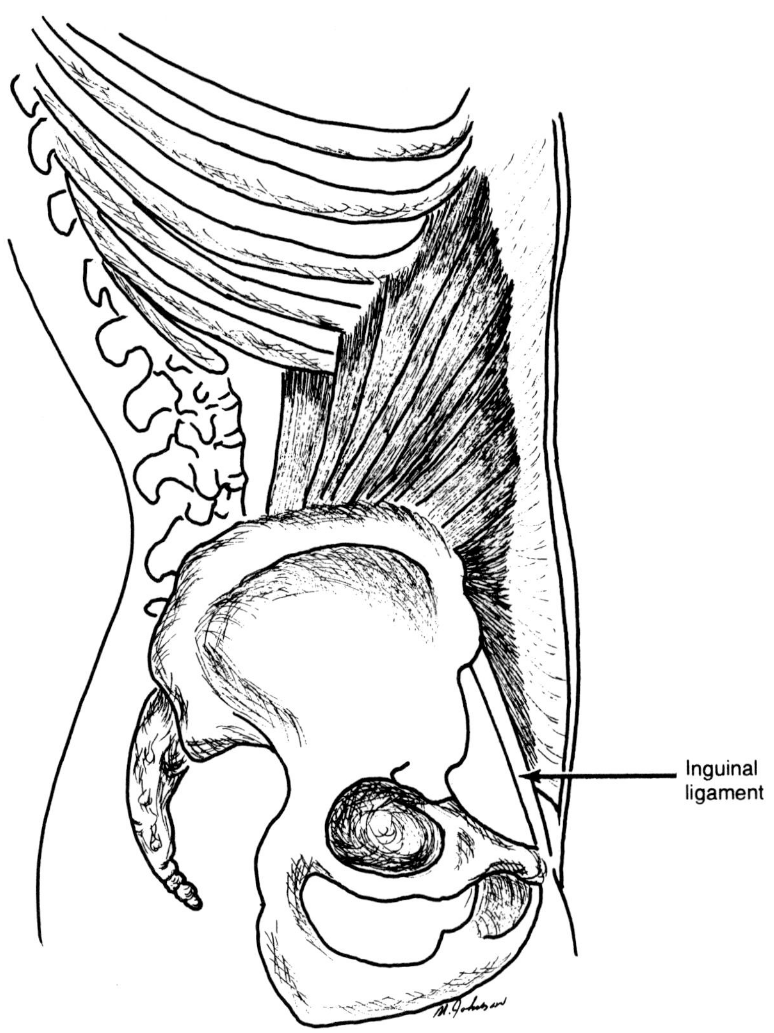


**Psoas Minor** (pso'as mi'nor, "p" is silent) The psoas minor (fig. 6.32) lies deep in the abdominal cavity. It cannot be palpated.

*Origin* Bodies of the last thoracic and first lumbar vertebrae.

*Insertion* Pectineal line of the pubis.

*Innervation* First lumbar nerve.

*Action* Both sides: Stabilization of the lumbar spine. One side: Lateral flexion of the lumbar spine.

The psoas minor is frequently missing on one or both sides, but when present it is capable of contracting to such a degree that it can cause lumbar scoliosis. The muscle is usually more prone to contracture in the female because of her wide pelvis.

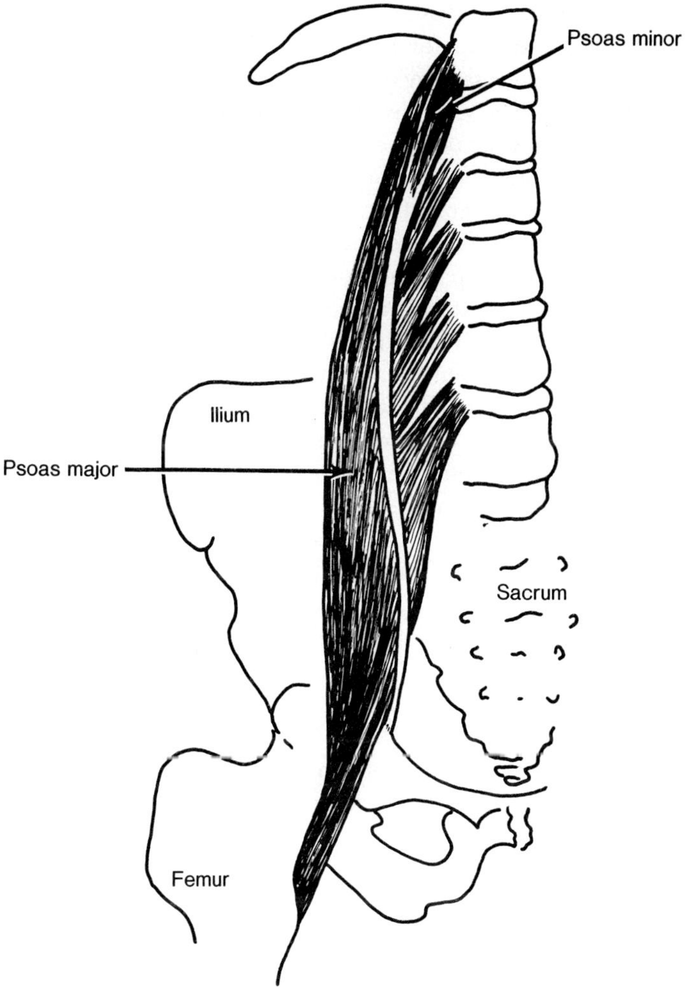

Figure 6.32. Psoas minor, anterior view

## Comments

The muscles of the spine and pelvic girdle are constantly at the mercy of the demands of upright posture. Poor body alignment, ill-conceived exercises, improper mechanics of lifting, pushing, and pulling can all contribute, to some degree, to their dysfunction. It would appear that every athlete should maintain constant watch over these muscles, for nothing is more debilitating to a sport or dance performance than acute back pain.

It is, perhaps, the athletes who incorporate extreme ranges of spinal movement in their respective movement repertoires who are most susceptible to muscular discomfort. Dancers and gymnasts are certainly included, and for both, the ability to hyperextend the spine is requisite to success. Since the spine is structured to allow for hyperextension, it may well be questioned that hyperextensive movements can cause such havoc. The answer would appear to lie, for both athletes, in the fact that aesthetic demands occupy a position of priority over kinetic requirements. Consider the dancer in arabesque position. A pleasing line will be achieved if both the spine and hip are hyperextended. If the hip is incapable of such flexibility, the dancer compensates by overextending the lumbosacral joint. Pain in the lower back is inevitable. The gymnast is no less the victum of lumbrosacral strain when "backbends" are included in routines. Lack of hip flexibility will, again, localize the arch in the lower back.

Other athletes are not immune to problems of the back. Mild scoliosis is quite common among those involved in sport because of overdevelopment of muscles on the preferred side of the body. Under the right (or wrong!) circumstances, a jump, or quick change of direction can cause painful spasm in the already shortened muscles.

It would be remiss, at this point, not to remind the reader that improper mechanics of force application are responsible for a high percentage of back problems. A generalization can be stated that may alleviate the problem: if the head is kept erect while lifting, pushing, and pulling, the muscular involvement will be safely delegated elsewhere. The erect head position will tend to keep the hips low and force the larger and stronger muscles of the hip and knee to carry out the task.

## Laboratory Experiences*

1. Have a partner lie supine on a table with hands on shoulders and hips and knees extended. Palpate the small of the back to detect whether it is contacting the table or whether it is arched upwardly. Ask the partner to press the small of the back to the table and palpate the abdominals. Which muscles are acting as agonists and which as antagonists, as this is done? Assume your partner is unable to press the back to the table. Which muscles should be strengthened and which should be stretched?

*It is difficult to explore fully the involvement of the abdominals in sports and dance without including the powerful hip flexors known as the iliopsoas. It is suggested that the student gain familiarity with that muscle complex (see chap. 7) so that the Laboratory Experiences will be more meaningful.

2. Having completed Experience 1 above, have your partner bend the knees so the feet can be placed flat on the table. Palpate the small of the back and notice that it is easily touching the table. Which muscles have been slackened by placing the legs in this new position?
3. Finallv, following the two experiences above, ask your partnear to straighten the legs and raise them briefly a few inches off the table. What happens to the small of the back? Why?
4. Place electrodes on the rectus abdominis of a partner and monitor the action potentials while such exercises as the cat back (on hands and knees while alternately hyperextending and flexing the spine), bent-knee sit up, head-raising while supine lying, and the basket-hang (bring knees to chin while hanging from a horizontal bar). Rank the exercises so they present a logical progression for the development of strength in the rectus abdominis.
5. Place electrodes on the superficial portion of the erector spinae of a partner. Have the partner begin in anatomical position and, slowly, touch the toes, return to the reference position, hyperextend the spine, and return to the reference position. When is the erector spinae active during these movements? What muscles, ligaments, and so on, are active when the erector spinae is silent?

# 7

# The Hip Joint

## Structure and Movements of the Hip Joint

As was noted in chapter 2, the hip joint represents the most striking example of the ball and socket point in the body (fig. 7.1). The globe-shaped head of the femur fits deeply into the acetabulum and is grasped tightly in place by a ring of fibrocartilage, the labrum, situated along the rim of the socket. The acetabulum is formed by the fusion of the pubis, the ischium, and the ilium.

Cartilaginous tissue completely covers the head of the femur except for a small interruption at the top of the head called the fovea. A large horseshoe-shaped portion of the acetabulum is also covered with cartilage, and is broadest along its upper part where it receives the greatest pressure from the femur during upright posture. These

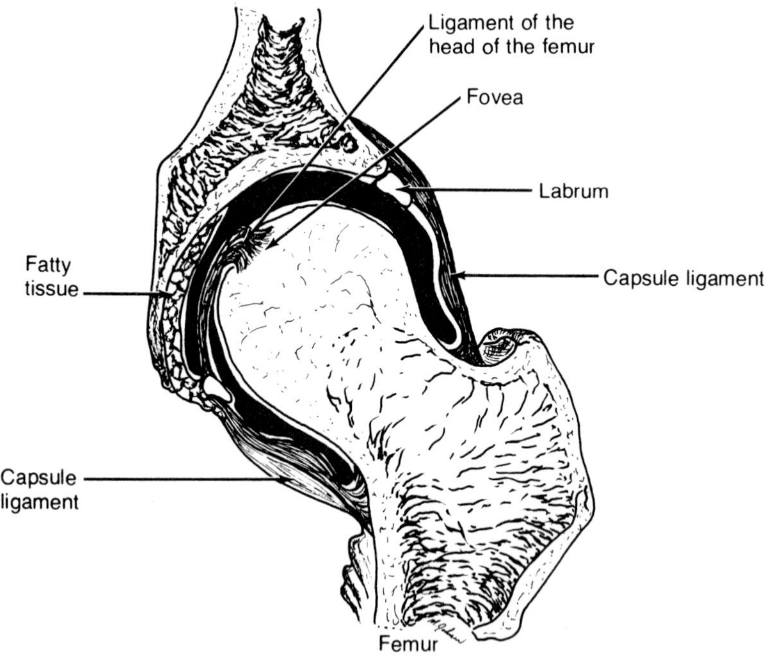


**Figure 7.1. The hip joint, cross section**

two sets of cartilage are intended to provide smooth articulating surfaces which can withstand wear and also provide some shock absorption.

The synovial capsule encloses the entire joint and is formed of a heavy fibrous material which is thickened in some of its portions to form ligamentous bands (figs. 7.2, 7.3). These bands, although seldom discernible from the rest of the capsule, are identified kinesiologically as ligaments and are named according to the bone from which they originate—the pubo-femoral, ischio-femoral, and ilio-femoral *(Y)* ligaments. All of the ligaments become taut when the hip is hyperextended; the pubo-femoral aids, additionally, in checking extreme abduction.

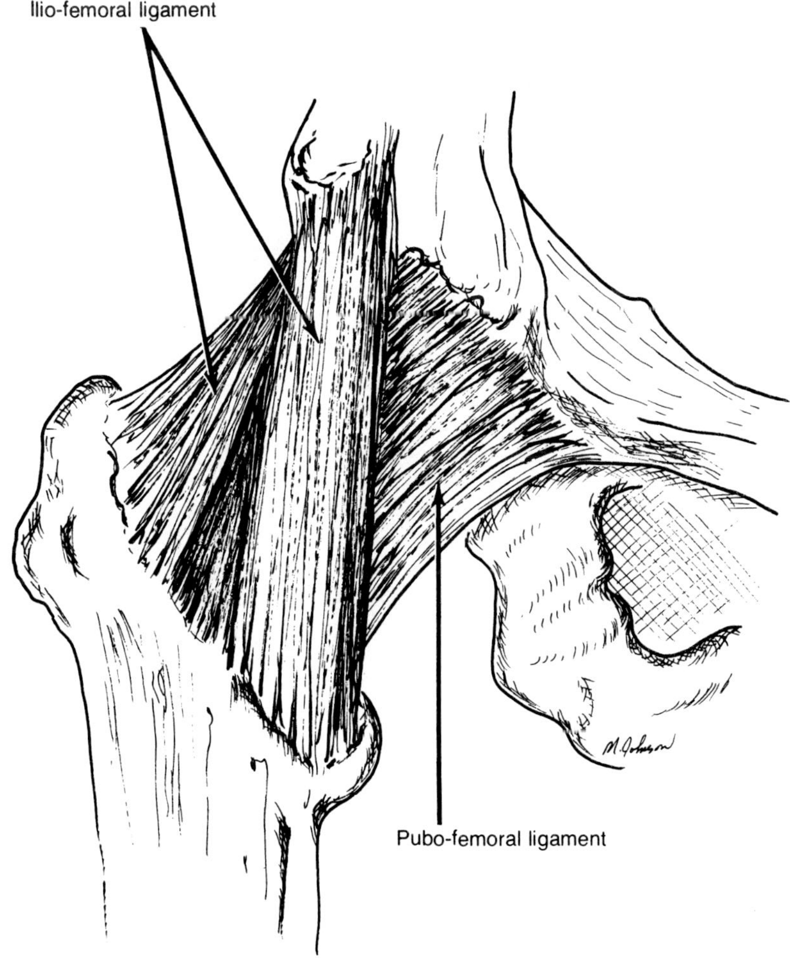


**Figure 7.2. Ligaments of the hip joint, anterior view**

Figure 7.3. Ligaments of the hip joint, posterior view

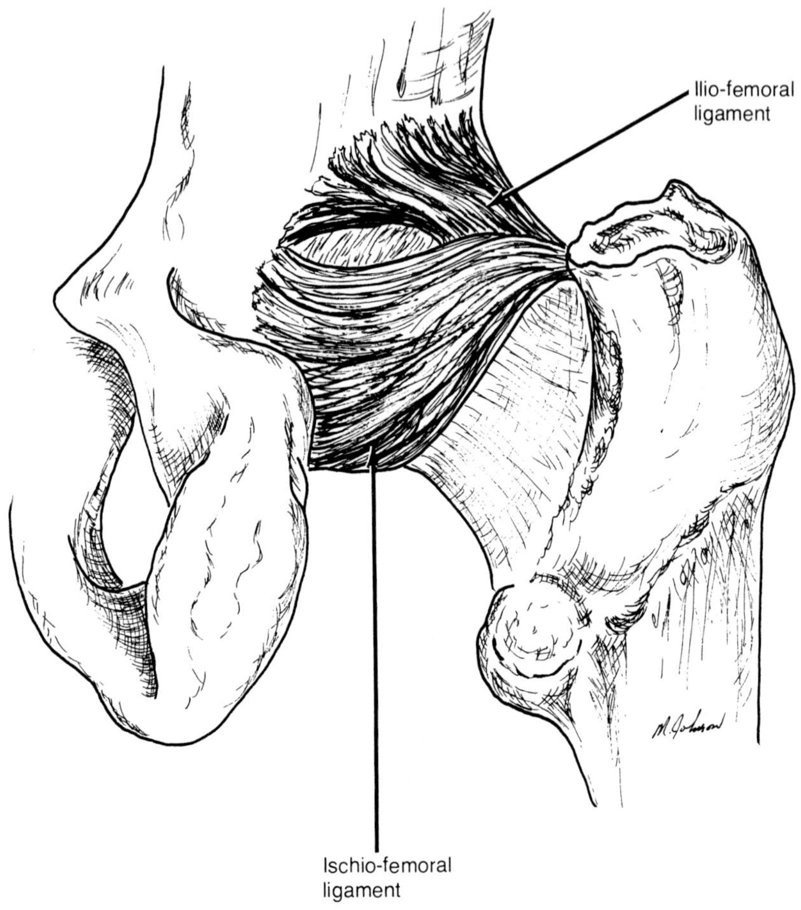


It has been mentioned that the fovea, a small portion of the head of the femur, is not covered with cartilage; rather, the fovea is the point of insertion of the ligament of the head of the femur. Its origin is along the floor of the acetabulum, and as it courses around the head of the femur, it carries blood supply to the area of the fovea. The tissues of this so-called ligament are too weak to provide the usual ligamentous function of joint stabilization, and therefore its true function in joint stabilization is uncertain.

The actions of the hip joint are those expected of a triaxial joint, and are shown in figure 7.4. A forward swinging of the femur around the frontal axis is known as flexion; backward swinging to the reference position is extension; and continued backward swing is hyperextension. Sideward movements of the femur around the sagittal axis are referred to as abduction if they are away from the body and adduction if they are toward the body. Twisting movements around the vertical axis are called inward and outward rotation.

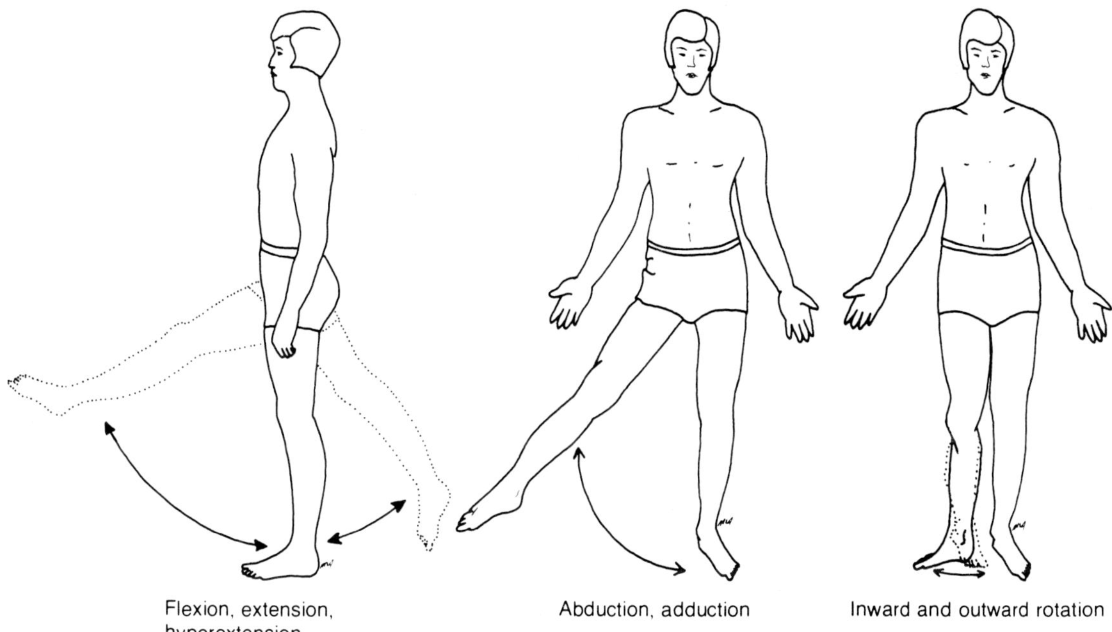


Figure 7.4. Movements of the hip joint

The hip joint is capable of performing an action in which the femur is placed in the horizontal plane and moved around the vertical axis (fig. 7.5). These movements are called horizontal abduction and horizontal adduction, and, as was the case with the shoulder joint, are not pure movements since they cannot be performed from the reference position without some preliminary movement such as flexion or abduction.

## Bone Markings

Anatomical landmarks pertinent to discussion of muscles of the hip are presented in figure 7.6. The student is urged to use them in conjunction with a skeleton.

## Musculature

The twenty-two muscles acting on the hip joint derive their various actions from their positions relative to the three axes of the joint. Muscles which pass anterior or posterior to the frontal axis will flex or extend (or hyperextend) the joint, whereas those which pass lateral

Figure 7.5. Horizontal abduction and horizontal adduction of the hip joint

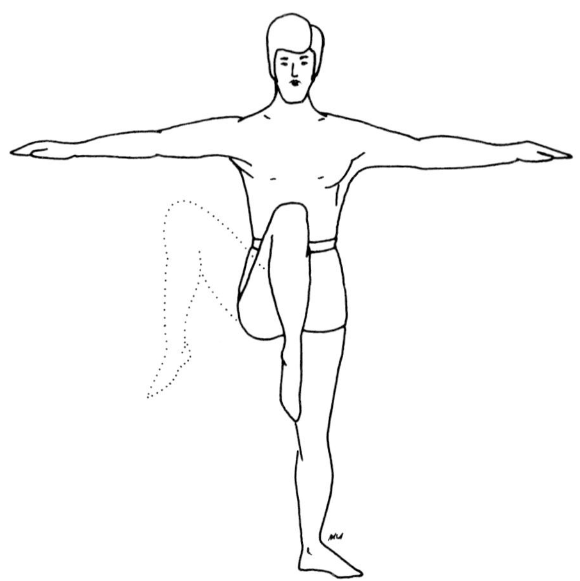

Figure 7.6. Bones of the pelvis and upper leg

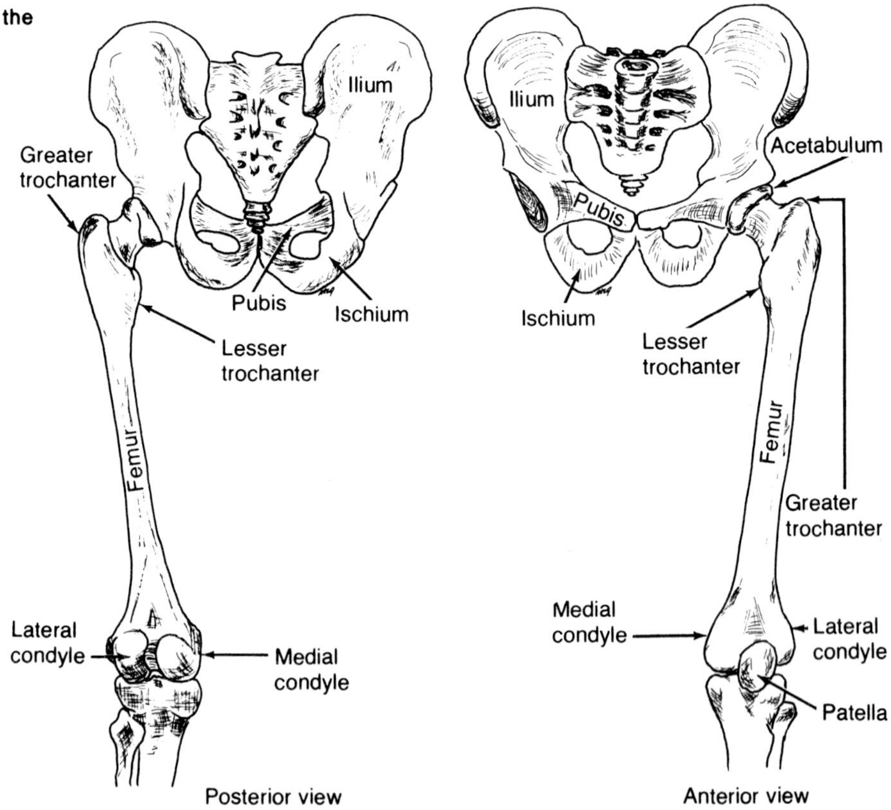

Ilium
Greater trochanter
Pubis
Ischium
Lesser trochanter
Femur
Lateral condyle
Medial condyle
Posterior view

Ilium
Acetabulum
Pubis
Ischium
Lesser trochanter
Femur
Greater trochanter
Medial condyle
Lateral condyle
Patella
Anterior view

or medial to the sagittal axis will abduct or adduct. Inward and outward rotation will be accomplished by muscles which originate on the pelvis and, as they course to their insertions on the femur, pass across the vertical axis. Muscles which contract to cause horizontal abduction and horizontal adduction will be those which cause abduction and adduction, since those are the muscles that will pass across the vertical axis when the femur is in the horizontal plane. Because all abductors are also horizontal abductors, and all adductors are also horizontal adductors, it has become practice to omit reference to horizontal abduction/adduction as a specific action and rather to infer it from stated abduction/adduction functions.

**Psoas** (pso'as)    The psoas (fig. 7.7), often described as two portions called the psoas major and psoas minor, lies deep in the abdominal cavity and cannot be palpated.

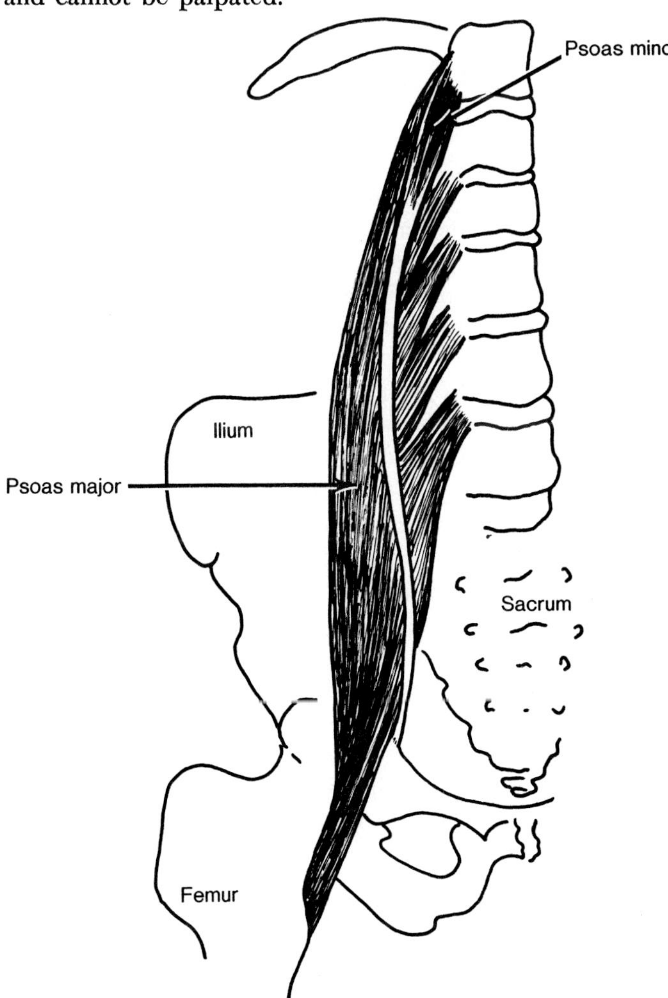


**Figure 7.7. The psoas, anterior view**

*Origin* Sides of the twelfth thoracic and all lumbar vertebrae and their intervertebral cartilages.

*Insertion* Lesser trochanter of the femur.

*Innervation* Femoral nerve.

*Action* Flexion of the hip.

The psoas is particularly effective during the initial part of hip flexion since the muscle is then long. As hip flexion progresses through the full range, the psoas becomes increasingly shorter and less effective. This is the basis for the reasoning which led to the bent-knee situp. Bending the knees while lying supine must be accompanied by hip flexion and thus the psoas, in shortened state, is made to be ineffective. The situp must now be performed by the abdominals as they flex the spine.

**Iliacus** (ili'acus) The iliacus (fig. 7.8) lies along the anterior surface of the ilium, the bone for which it is named. It canot be palpated.

*Origin* Anterior surface of the ilium and adjacent border of sacrum.

*Insertion* The tendon of the psoas superior to its attachment on the lesser trochanter.

*Innervation* Femoral nerve.

*Action* Hip flexion.

The iliacus and psoas major are frequently regarded by kinesiologists as a single muscle, the iliopsoas. Together, the two muscles are capable of exerting great strentgh to flex the hip, and are of considerable importance in athletic activities such as kicking and long jumping, during which the hip must be forcefully and quickly flexed.

**Rectus Femoris** (rec'tus fem'oris) The rectus femoris (fig. 7.9) lies on the anterior aspect of the thigh. It is a penniform muscle and is palpable midway between the hip and knee joints.

*Origin* By two heads, from the anterior inferior iliac spine, and the groove above the rim of the acetabulum.

*Insertion* Base of the patella.

*Innervation* Femoral nerve.

*Action* Flexion of the hip.

The rectus femoris, like the iliopsoas, crosses the hip joint anterior to the frontal axis of that joint to be a prime hip flexor. Its line of pull is very nearly parallel to the femur and does not provide for a long moment arm. Its contraction is, therefore, complementary to the power of the iliopsoas.

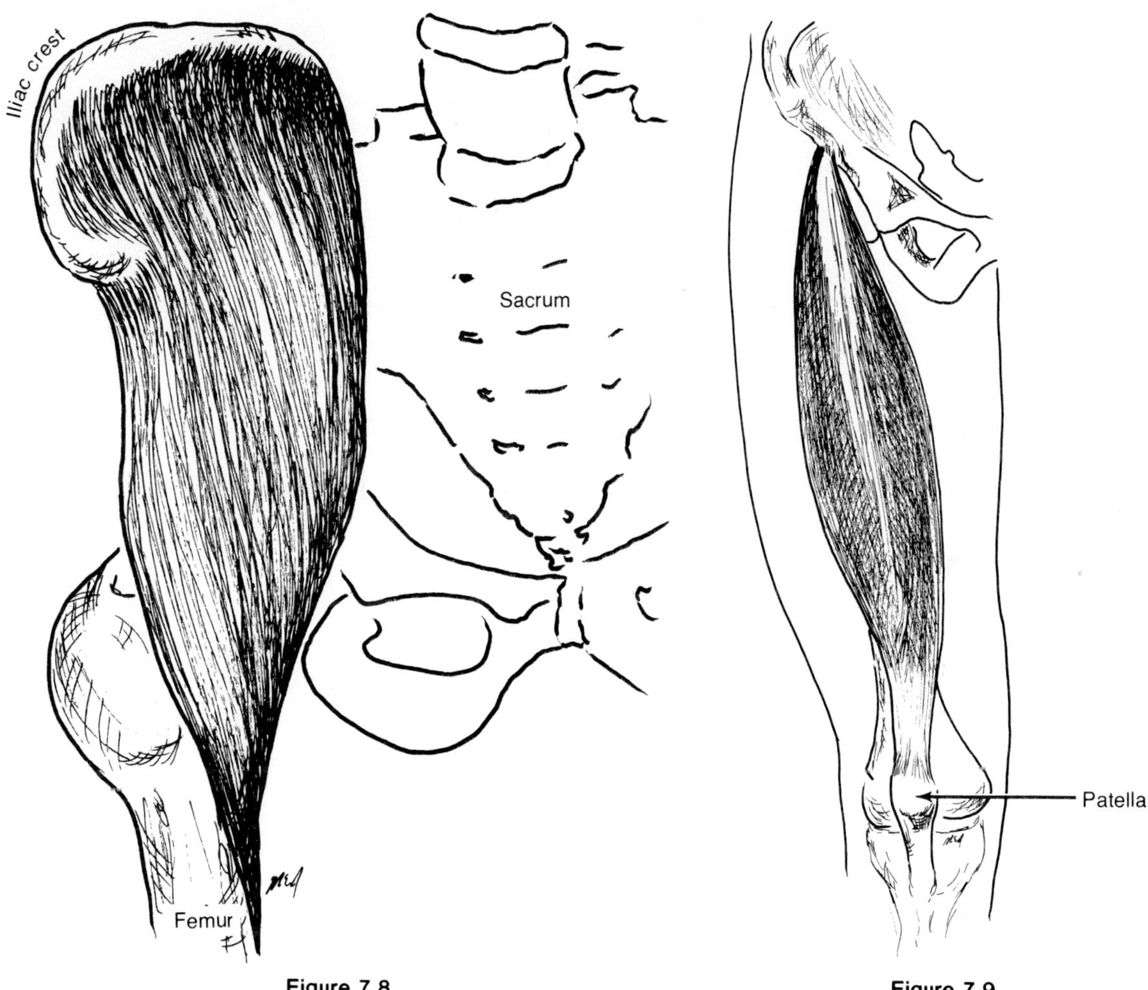


Figure 7.8

Figure 7.9

Figure 7.8. Iliacus, anterior view

Figure 7.9. Rectus femoris, anterior view

**Pectineus** (pectin'eus) The pectineus (fig. 7.10) is located just below the groin and is almost completely covered by the rectus femoris and sartorius. Palpation is difficult if not impossible because the muscle is easily confused with those muscles which cover or surround it.

*Origin* On the pubis between the iliopectineal eminence and the pubic tubercle.

*Insertion* On the medial aspect of the femur between the lesser trochanter and the linea aspera.

*Innervation* Femoral nerve.

*Action* Flexion and adduction of the hip joint.

Figure 7.10. Pectineus, anterior view

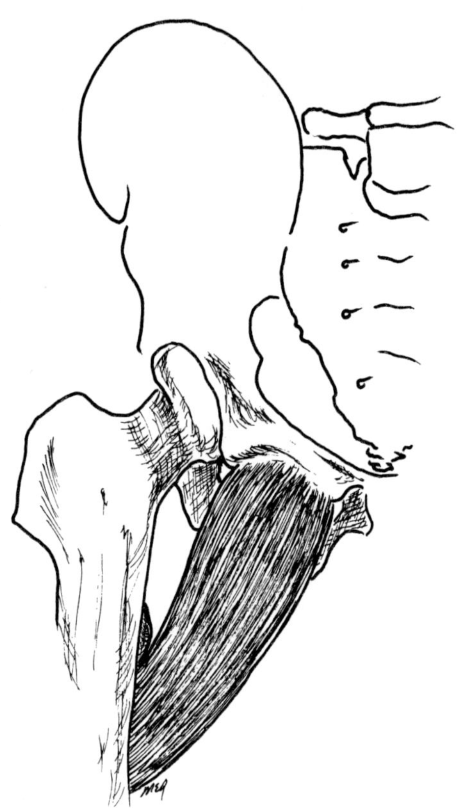

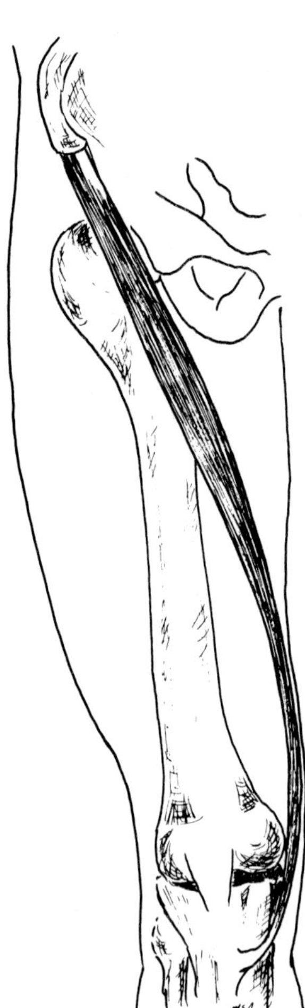

Figure 7.11. Sartorius, anterior view

The pectineus crosses the hip joint anterior to the frontal axis and inferior to the sagittal axis. It enjoys a relatively long moment arm to both axes as well as an advantageous angle of insertion. The muscle is, therefore, quite powerful in both flexion and adduction.

**Sartorius** (sarto'rius) The sartorius (fig. 7.11) is the longest muscle in the body. It is superficial as it courses diagonally medialward across the front of the thigh, but is difficult to palpate except in the area of its tendon of origin. Palpation can be accomplished during resisted flexion of the hip when the femur has been placed in a position of outward rotation. The superior portion of the muscle can be felt and observed just below the superior iliac spine. A dimple-like depression will be noted just lateral to the sartorius which separates it from the tensor fasciae latae.

*Origin* Anterior superior iliac spine and the adjacent portion of the notch distal to the spine.

*Insertion* Upper and medial aspect of the tibia.

*Innervation* Femoral nerve.

*Action* Flexion, abduction, and outward rotation of the hip joint.

The sartorius is a narrow band of muscle capable of great ability to shorten. It is more effective as a hip flexor than an abductor or outward rotator because its force arm is longest to the frontal axis. Its moment arm is quite short to the sagittal axis rendering it a weak abductor at best. The outward rotation function is similarly limited, and cannot be performed unless the knee is held in full extension, for otherwise the contraction of the muscle would be spent in moving the tibia.

**Tensor Fasciae Latae** (ten'sor fas'ciae la'tae) The tensor fasciae latae (fig. 7.12) is a small muscle located superficially on the anterior and lateral aspect of the upper thigh. It can be palpated lateral to the

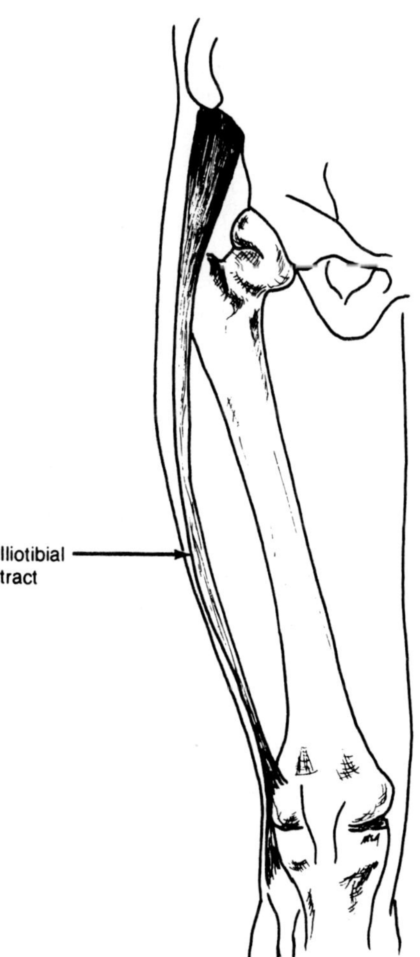


**Figure 7.12. Tensor fasciae latae, anterior view**

sartorius when the hip joint is flexed and outwardly rotated (see sartorius).

*Origin* The crest of the ilium near the anterior superior iliac spine.

*Insertion* The iliotibial tract of the fascia lata.

*Innervation* Superior gluteal nerve.

*Action* Tenses the fascia lata; through the fascia lata, the muscle flexes, abducts, and inwardly rotates the hip joint.

The tensor fasciae latae does not have a bony insertion; however, since the fascia lata extends down the lateral aspect of the thigh to attach to the tibia, the muscle is able to extend its action from tightening the fascia to moving the hip joint. The tensor passes to the anterior side of the frontal axis and to the lateral side of the sagittal axis, to become a flexor and abductor respectively. Its inward rotation function is weak and even debatable, since it and the fascia are nearly parallel to the femur as they course between the ilium and tibia. The muscle's ability to rotate inwardly would therefore be enhanced if the femur were already in a position of outward rotation.

**Gluteus Maximus** (glu'teus max'imus) The gluteus maximus (fig. 7.13) is a large buttocks muscle on the posterior aspect of the hip. It is easily observed and palpated.

*Origin* Posterior gluteal line of the ilium and the adjacent portion of the iliac crest; posterior and inferior surface of the sacrum; and the side of the coccyx.

*Insertion* Posterior aspect of femur below the greater trochanter; iliotibial tract of the fascia lata.

*Innervation* Inferior gluteal nerve.

*Action* Extension, hyperextension, and outward rotation of the hip joint.

The gluteus maximus is notoriously lazy during activities associated with daily living. It is perhaps for this reason that the muscle so easily loses its firmness and attracts fat deposits. The only prevention for such conditions appears to be through planned exercises which incorporate hyperextension and/or outward rotation of the hip. It should be noted however, that excessive contraction of the maximus may lead to unwanted bulk. *Turn-out,* the dancers' term for outward rotation, has been named as the cause of such hypertrophy of the maximus that range of motion can become restricted. In addition to turn-out, however, the musle "set" of the gluteus practiced by the dancer is probably equally responsible for the hypertrophy.

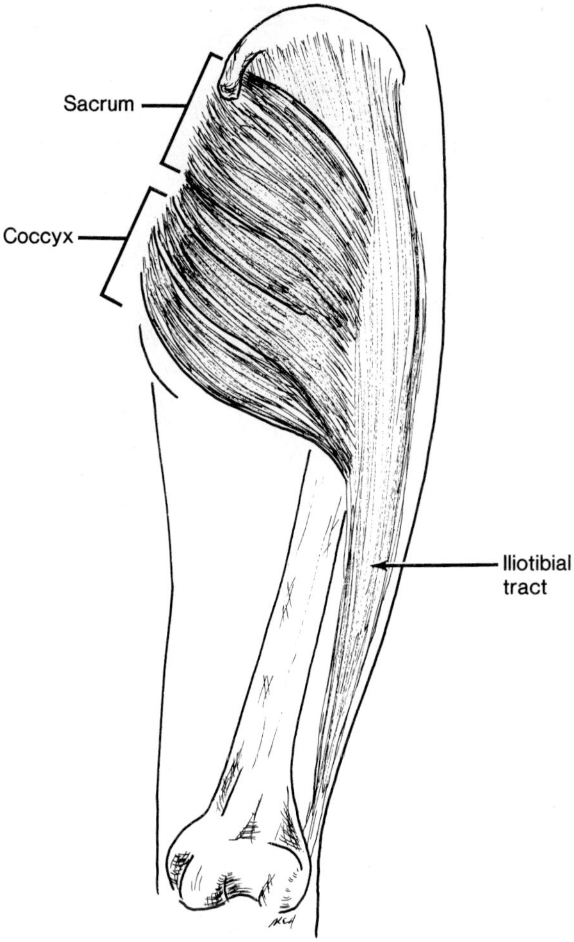

Figure 7.13. Gluteus maximus, posterior view

**Gluteus Medius** (glu'teus me'dius) The gluteus medius (fig. 7.14) is partially covered by the gluteus maximus and the tensor fasciae latae; it is superficial, just inferior to the iliac crest, and may be palpated there as the hip joint is abducted to raise the foot from the floor.

*Origin* Posterior surface of the ilium in the region bounded by the iliac crest, and the posterior and anterior gluteal lines.

*Insertion* Oblique ridge on the lateral aspect of the greater trochanter.

*Innervation* Superior gluteal nerve.

*Action* Abduction of the hip joint; anterior fibers flex and inwardly rotate; posterior fibers extend and outwardly rotate.

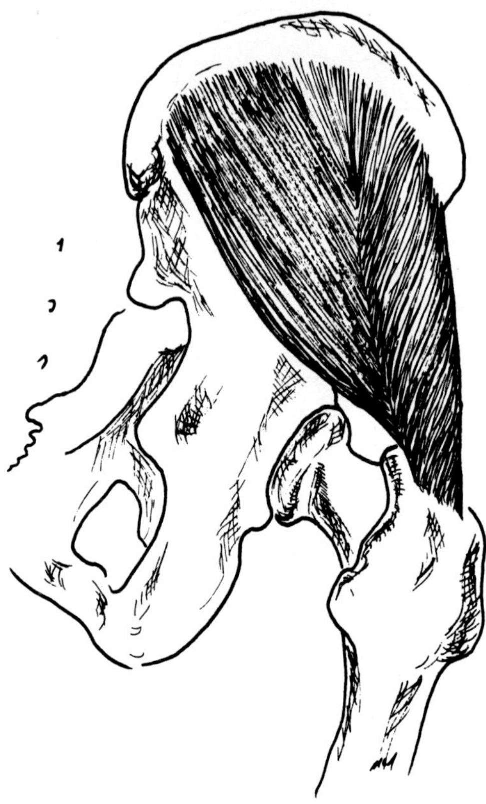

Figure 7.14. Gluteus medius, posterior view

Since all of the fibers of the gluteus medius pass the sagittal axis of the hip joint to the lateral side, the muscle is an excellent abductor. In addition, the angle of attachment of the medius on the greater trochanter approximates 90 degrees, affording superior mechanical advantage.

When the medius is viewed with respect to the frontal and vertical axes, it is seen that the middle portion of the muscle passes directly over these axes and is, therefore, nonfunctional in either frontal or horizontal plane movements of the femur. The anterior and posterior portions are, however, able to contribute to flexion/extension and inward/outward rotation since, by virtue of the size of the muscle, they are removed from the frontal and vertical axes. The gluteus medius and the deltoid are similar in their placement around the three axes of their respective ball-and-socket joints.

**Gluteus Minimus** (glu'teus min'imus) The gluteus minimus (fig. 7.15) is the smallest of the gluteal group and is covered by the gluteus medius. It cannot be palpated.

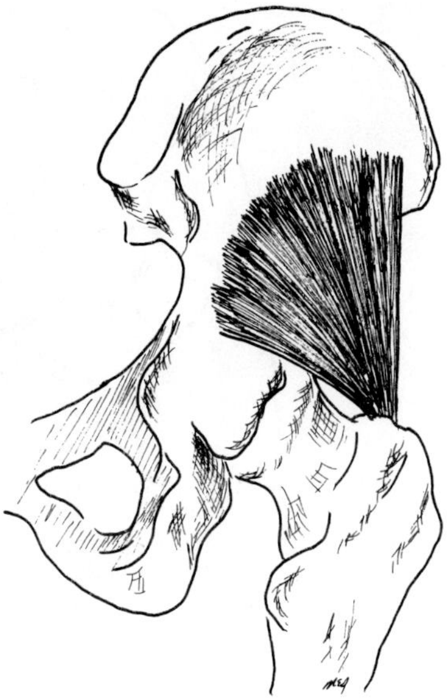

Figure 7.15. Gluteus minimus, posterior view

*Origin* Posterior surface of ilium between the anterior and inferior gluteal line, and from the edge of the greater sciatic notch.

*Insertion* Anterior border of the greater trochanter.

*Innervation* Superior gluteal nerve.

*Action* Abduction of the hip joint; anterior fibers inwardly rotate and aid in flexion; posterior fibers aid in outward rotation and extension.

The gluteus minimus and medius have similar relationships to the three axes of the hip joint and have, therefore, equivalent actions. The minimus, being smaller, is less powerful.

**Adductor Magnus** (adduc'tor mag'nus) The adductor magnus (fig. 7.16) is the largest of the adductor muscles and is located on the medial aspect of the thigh. It is difficult to palpate because of surrounding musculature; however, it may be isolated just medial to the gracilis at mid-thigh.

*Origin* Inferior ramus of the pubis and ischium, and inferior part of the ischial tuberosity.

*Insertion* Entire length of linea aspera, and supracondylar ridge, and adductor tubercle of the femur.

*Innervation* Obturator and sciatic nerves.

*Action* Adduction of the hip joint; upper portion aids in inward rotation and flexion; lower portion aids in outward rotation and extension.

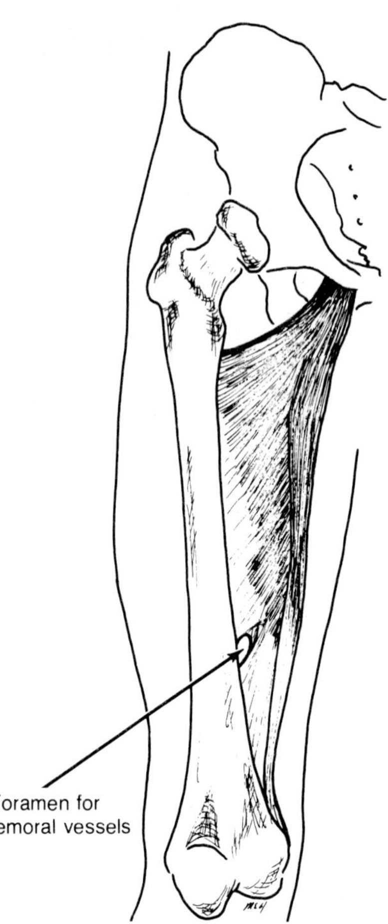


Figure 7.16. Adductor magnus, anterior view

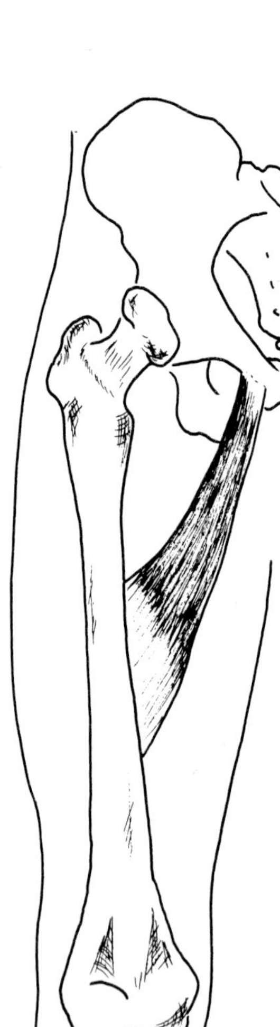

Figure 7.17. Adductor longus, anterior view

The adductor magnus, like the other adductors, fluctuates in its action on the femur according to postural states. For example, the magnus is active during inward rotation from a position of outward rotation. The muscle has little if any ability to inwardly rotate from the anatomical or fundamental reference position. Similarly, the ability of the upper magnus to flex the hip joint is enhanced if the femur is in positions of hyperextension or extension; and ability of the lower portion to extend is best when the hip joint has already been flexed. Regardless of posture, however, the magnus is well-placed to adduct, but tends to contribute to this action only when resistance is met.

**Adductor Longus** (adduc'tor lon'gus) The adductor longus (fig. 7.17) lies just medial to the pectineus and can be palpated at the medial aspect of the groin.

*Origin* Anterior surface of the pubis just below the crest.

*Insertion* Middle one-half of the linea aspera.

*Innervation* Anterior obturator nerve.

*Action* Adduction of the hip joint; aids in flexion and inward rotation.

The adductor longus is active in all stages of adduction regardless of whether the leg is resisted or unresisted. The ability of the muscle to flex or inwardly rotate is increased if the hip joint has previously been extended (or hyperextended) or outwardly rotated, respectively.

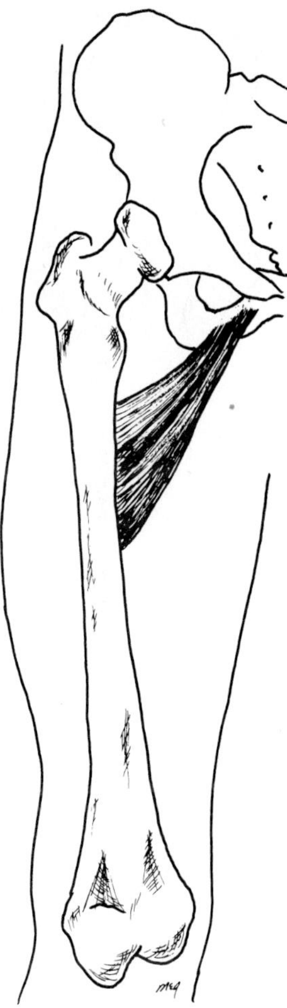

Figure 7.18. Adductor brevis, anterior view

**Adductor Brevis** (adduc'tor bre'vis) The adductor brevis (fig. 7.18) is the smallest of the adductors. It lies beneath the adductor magnus and adductor longus and cannot be palpated.

*Origin* Outer surface of pubis, on the inferior ramus.

*Insertion* Line from the lesser trochanter to the linea aspera including the upper portion of the linea aspera.

*Innervation* Anterior obturator nerve.

*Action* Adduction of the hip joint; aids in flexion and inward rotation.

The adductor brevis has a line of pull which is similar to that of the adductor longus and, therefore, responds in like fashion to movement of the femur.

**Gracilis** (gra'cilis) The gracilis (fig. 7.19) is a long and slender muscle located superficially along the inner thigh. It is difficult to palpate because it is easily confused with surrounding muscles; however, its tendon of insertion can usually be felt clearly. Begin the palpation in the middle of the posterior aspect of the knee, then move the fingers medially until the large tendon of the semitendinosus is encountered. If the fingers are moved slightly medially, the smaller tendon of the semimembranosus will be felt. The tendon of the gracilis lies just medial to the semimembranosus. Palpation may be facilitated by inwardly rotating the tibia against resistance.

*Origin* Inferior half of the symphysis and the superior half of the arch of the pubis.

*Insertion* Medial aspect of the tibia just below the condyle.

*Innervation* Anterior division of the obturator nerve.

*Action* Adduction of the hip joint; aids in flexion and inward rotation.

The gracilis is well located to be an adductor since it crosses the hip joint to the medial side of the sagittal axis. The muscle can be a weak flexor of the hip joint also, but only through the part of the flexion range in which the muscle courses anterior to the frontal axis.

Study of a skeleton will indicate that when the femur reaches a point at which it is approximately perpendicular to the trunk, the gracilis is no longer anterior to the axis but rather in line with it. If the femur is raised even higher, the gracilis will course posterior to the axis and will become an extensor.

That the gracilis will be an inward rotator is questionable since the two attachments of the muscle are aligned in parallel fashion with the femur regardless of the position of the thigh. If the gracilis does make a contribution to inward rotation, it would be under conditions of an outwardly rotated hip joint and an extended knee.

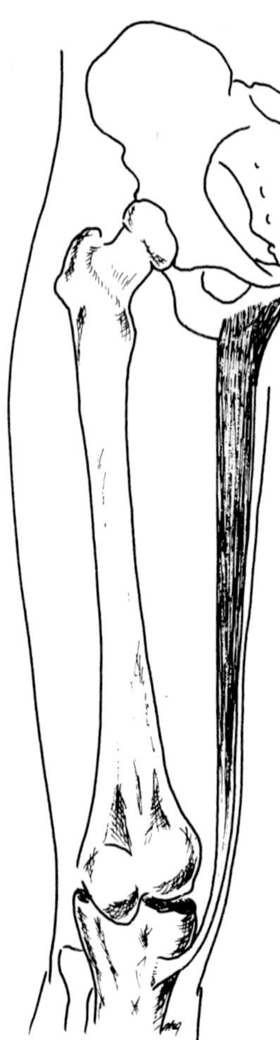

Figure 7.19. Gracilis, anterior view

**Semitendinosus** (semitendino'sus) The semitendinosus (fig. 7.20) is one of the hamstring muscles and is located superficially along the medial and posterior aspect of the thigh. It is most easily palpated in the area of its tendon of insertion as described under the gracilis.

*Origin* Medial facet of the ischial tuberosity by a common tendon with the long head of the biceps femoris.

*Insertion* Medial-anterior surface of the tibia just distal to the insertion of the gracilis.

*Innervation* Tibial portion of sciatic nerve.

*Action* Extension and hyperextension of the hip joint; aids in inward rotation and adduction.

The semitendinosus crosses the hip joint posterior to the frontal axis and, because of the tuberosity of the ischium, attaches at angles which afford it good mechanical advantage, especially through the range of extension.

The inward rotation function of the muscle follows from the fact that it wraps partially around the tibia as it inserts. If the knee is held extended, contraction of the muscle will assist the entire leg to rotate inwardly.

Comparison of the location of the semitendinosus with that of the sagittal axis of the hip joint will indicate that the muscle is an adductor. Its contribution is only assistive because of its short moment arm to the sagittal axis.

**Semimembranosus** (semimembrano'sus) The semimembranosus (fig. 7.21), a hamstring muscle, lies on the posterior aspect of the thigh. It is best palpated along its tendon of insertion as described under the gracilis.

*Origin* Lateral facet of the ischial tuberosity.

*Insertion* The medial and posterior aspect of the medial condyle of the tibia.

*Innervation* Tibial portion of the sciatic nerve.

*Action* Extension and hyperextension of the hip joint; aids in inward rotation and adduction.

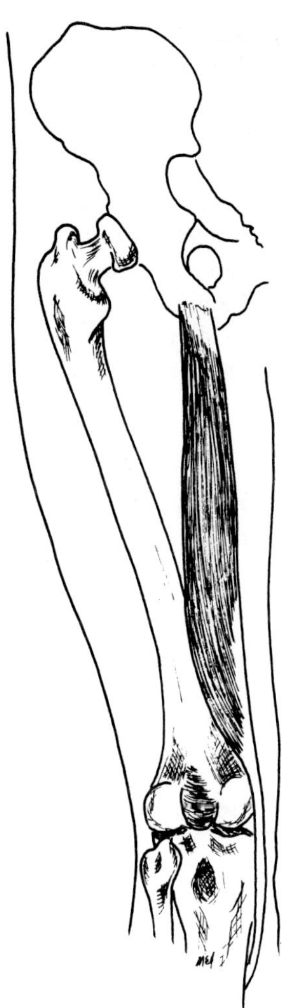

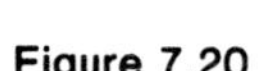

Figure 7.20

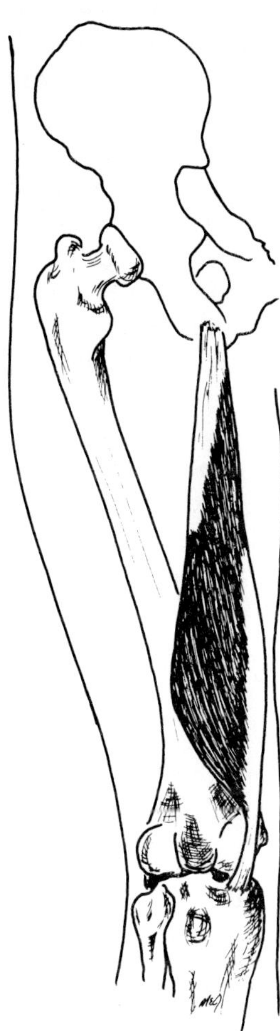

Figure 7.21

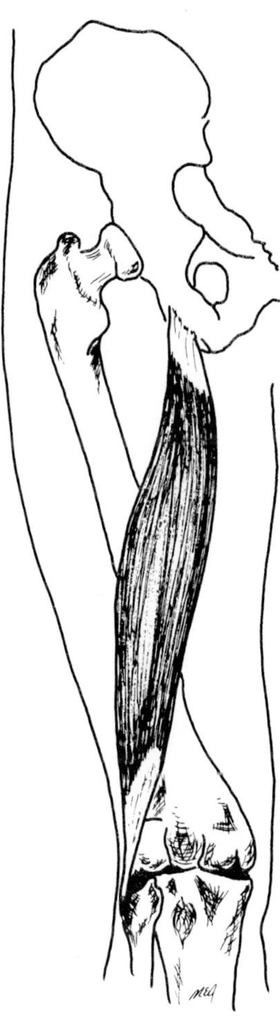

Figure 7.22

Figure 7.20. Semitendinosus, posterior view

Figure 7.21. Semimembranosus, posterior view

Figure 7.22. Biceps femoris, posterior view

The line of pull of the semimembranosus is very similar to that of the semitendinosus, with one exception—the origin of the membranosus is somewhat more lateral than that of the tendinosus. The membranosus is thus placed diagonally with respect to the vertical axis to aid in inward rotation.

**Biceps Femoris (long head)** (bi'ceps fem'oris) The long head of the biceps femoris (fig. 7.22) is located superficially on the lateral and posterior aspect of the thigh. It is best palpated in the region of its tendon of insertion as it crosses behind the knee on the lateral side. The biceps femoris is one of the three hamstring muscles.

*Origin* Medial facet of the ischial tuberosity.

*Insertion* Lateral condyle of the tibia and head of the fibula.

*Innervation* Tibial portion of sciatic nerve.

*Action* Extension and hyperextension of the hip joint; aids in outward rotation.

All of the hamstrings—the semitendinosus, semimembranosus, and biceps femoris—have essentially the same mechanical advantage in moving the femur through the range of extension and hyperextension. The biceps differs from the other hamstrings in its ability to rotate the hip joint because it crosses the vertical axis from inside to out, or from medial to lateral, and is therefore an outward rotator rather than an inward rotator.

**The Outward Rotators** Six muscles (fig. 7.23) lying deep in the pelvis have, as their primary action, the ability to rotate the hip joint outwardly. Although each is a specific muscle, it has become practice, in the study of kinesiology, to group them.

Figure 7.23. The outward rotators, posterior view

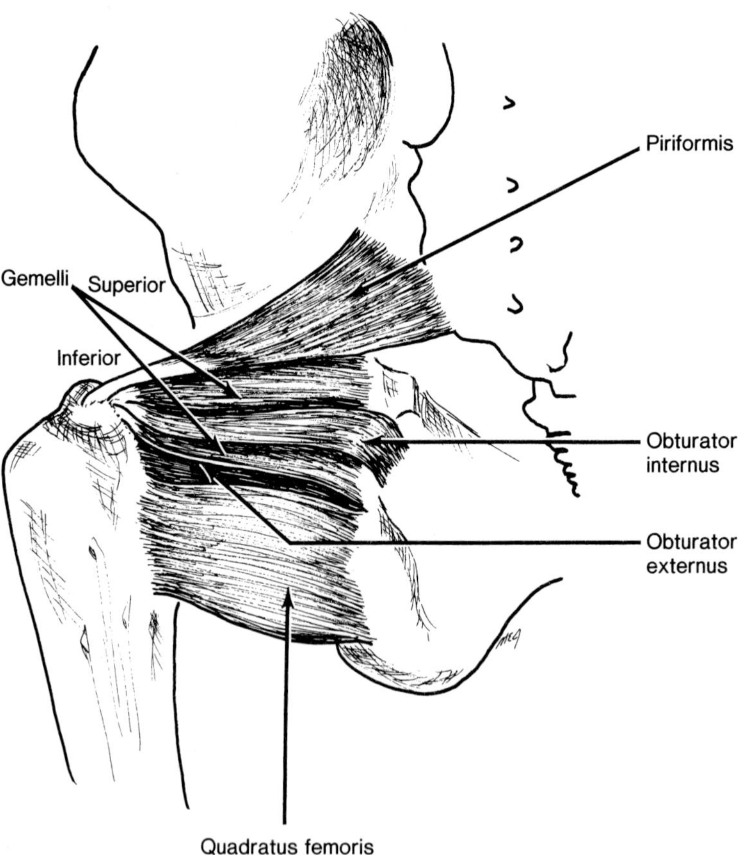

*Origin* Anterior and posterior surfaces of sacrum, and of the pelvis around the obturator foramen.

*Insertion* Greater trochanter of the femur.

*Innervation* Piriformis: First and second sacral nerves. Obturator internus: First and second sacral and fifth lumbar nerves. Obturator externus: Obturator nerve. Quadratus femoris: First sacral, and fourth and fifth lumbar nerves. Gamellus superior: A branch of the nerve to the obturator internus. Gamellus inferior: A branch of the nerve to the quadratus femoris.

*Action* Outward rotation of the hip joint; if the hip joint has been flexed, they act to horizontally abduct the joint.

## Comments

The twenty-two muscles of the hip comprise the largest muscle mass of the body. Their strength is required not only because of their function in weight-bearing but also because they must move the long, heavy third class lever represented by the lower leg. Most of the muscles are of the spurt type; those that cross the knee joint are shunt muscles and provide valuable stabilizing force at the hip joint. By this arrangement, they can, in addition, contribute to movement at two joints rather than one.

The two-joint function of the rectus femoris and hamstrings is an interesting one to consider. When the hip is flexed, the rectus is an agonist and the hamstrings are antagonists. During hip extension, the muscles reverse roles; the hamstrings become the agonists and the rectus functions as an antagonist. Flexion and extension of the knee involves like responsibilities of these muscles; for example, during knee flexion, the hamstrings are agonists and the rectus is an antagonist, and during extension, their muscle roles reverse. If both hip and knee movement are performed simultaneously, however, muscular responsibilities are more complicated. A place kick in soccer involves hip flexion and knee extension. The rectus must contract to flex the hip as well as extend the knee, and the hamstrings must relax to allow the leg to move as required. If the hamstrings lack the needed extensibility, they will limit the range of the leg, and their tension will be transferred to their origin, the ischial tuberosity. In response, the pelvic girdle will be pulled into backward tilt which will result in a hyperextension of the pelvis on the femur of the supporting leg. The iliofemoral or *Y* ligament checks this movement sharply and forcefully, and, in some instances, will actually pull the supporting leg off the ground.

Simultaneous execution of hip and knee flexion or hip and knee extension requires that both the hamstrings and rectus femoris be agonists at one joint and antagonists at the other. This would appear to be a contradictory situation since it is known that muscles, when they contract, tend to act as agonists at all joints they cross. The expected result is that the contracting rectus and hamstrings will neutralize each other at both joints and no motion will occur. Yet, that the muscles are apparently able to function cooperatively is demonstrated commonly in the execution of the vertical jump. Both muscle components contract sharply to project the body from the floor. The resulting actions of simultaneous hip and knee extension indicate that the hamstrings can exert more force than the rectus at the hip, but that the rectus is the more forceful of the two muscles at the knee. Study of the moment arms of the muscles at the two joints will confirm the conclusion; the moment arm of the hamstrings is longer at the hip than that of the rectus, whereas the moment arm of the rectus is the longer of the two at the knee.

## Laboratory Experiences

1. Stand with the feet spread side-to-side at approximately shoulder width. Shift the bulk of the weight to the left foot and, while holding this position, note the range of movement of the hips during their rotation to the left. Stand with the bulk of the weight on the right foot and, again, note the range of left rotation of the hips. You should find that the range is greater when the weight is on the right foot. Apply what you have found to the coaching of a batter in softball or baseball; to a golfer; to a softball pitcher; to a shot putter. In all of these sports, the hips represent the initial link in the movement chain. The degree to which they can be rotated is highly related to success in imparting force to the respective sports objects. Can you make a generalization regarding the timing of weight shift and the rotation of the hips?
2. Place electrodes on the gluteus maximus of a partner. Have your partner lie across a table while keeping the feet on the floor. Monitor the activity of the gluteus maximus as the leg is raised, with extended knee, to horizontal and then into hyperextension of the hip joint. During which portion of the movement is the gluteus maximus most active?
3. Have your partner place the foot back on the floor (see Experience #2) and apply resistance to the back of the ankle as the leg is raised. How does the activity of gluteus maximus compare with that found during the movement performed in Experience #2?

4. Monitor the electrical activity of the gluteus maximus as your partner pedals a bicycle which has touring handle bars, and one which has dropped handle bars. Do you note any difference in the two electromyograms?
5. Perform the palpations described in this chapter. After each, indicate an exercise or movement which will 1) strengthen the muscle involved, and 2) stretch that muscle.

# 8 The Knee Joint

## Structure and Movements of the Joint

The knee is the largest joint in the body and is actually comprised of three subjoints: two biaxial condyloid joints between the femur and tibia, and the nonaxial joint between the patella and the femur.

The two condyloid joints articulate the medial and lateral condyles of the femur with the medial and lateral condyles of the tibia (fig. 8.1). The menisci, crescent shaped discs of fibrocartilage, serve to deepen the tibial articulation with the condyles of the femur.

The synovial capsule of the knee is a strong and extensive membrane strengthened throughout by bands of tendons which cross the knee and by the fascia lata. The capsule is lined with a synovial membrane which begins at the proximal edge of the patella and extends distally to beneath the patellar ligament and the infrapatellar fat pad, then projects into the interior of the joint both superior and inferior to the menisci, and finally courses posteriorly to a position beneath the tendon of the popliteus. The cruciate ligaments are not included within the capsule.

Numerus bursae surround the knee joint. Some communicate with the joint capsule while others do not. Each bursa is located between tissues which would otherwise wear from friction.

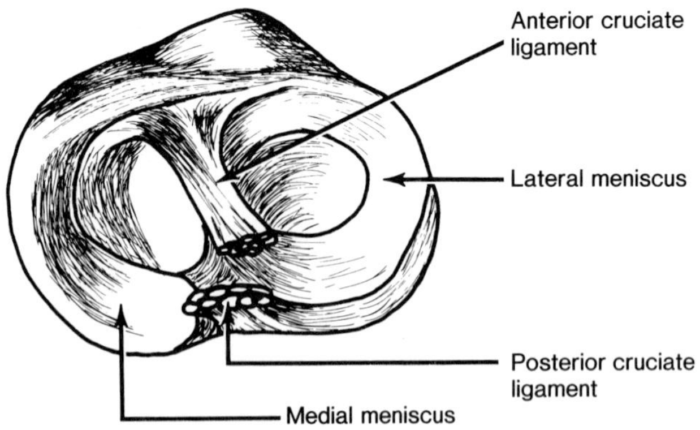


**Figure 8.1. Articulating surface of head of right tibia.**

The ligaments of the knee are the popliteals, collaterals, cruciates, coronary, transverse, and patellar (fig. 8.2). The popliteal ligaments, called the *oblique popliteal* and the *arcuate popliteal ligaments,* course between the posterior aspects of the femur and tibia, and between the lateral condyle of the femur and the articular capsule. The collateral ligaments, called the *medial* and *lateral collaterals* (or the *tibial and fibular collaterals*) join the medial condyles of tibia and femur, and lateral condyle of the femur with the head of the fibula, respectively. In the interior of the joint, the anterior and posterior cruciate ligaments divide the knee into right and left portions. The anterior cruciate joins the anterior intercondylar portion of the tibia with the posterior part of the intercondylar fossa of the femur, and the posterior cruciate runs between the posterior intercondylar region of the tibia with the anterior aspect of the intercondylar fossa of the femur.

The coronary ligaments connect the rims of the medial meniscus and lateral meniscus to the head of the tibia. The transverse ligament courses anteriorly between the two menisci, connecting their forward edges. It is sometimes absent. The patellar ligament is the mid-portion of the quadriceps femoris tendon which is extended from the patella to the tibial tuberosity.

Movements of the tibia around the femur are biaxial. Flexion and extension occur around the frontal axis and are caused by muscles which cross the joint posterior or anterior to that axis. Inward and outward rotation occur around the vertical axis and will be performed by muscles which insert on the medial or lateral aspect of the knee.

The joint between the patella and the femur is essentially of the gliding type, although the articulating surfaces of the joint do not match exactly. The articulation is further complicated by the presence of seven facets on the inner surface of the patella which are brought into contact with the femur as the knee joint is moved through its range of flexion/extension and inward/outward rotation.

## Bone Markings

The bone markings pertinent to the origins of the muscles of the knee joint have been presented in the preceeding chapter. Figure 8.3 displays only those markings concerned with the insertions of the several muscles.

Figure 8.2. Superficial tissues of right knee (a and b), deep tissues of right knee (c and d)

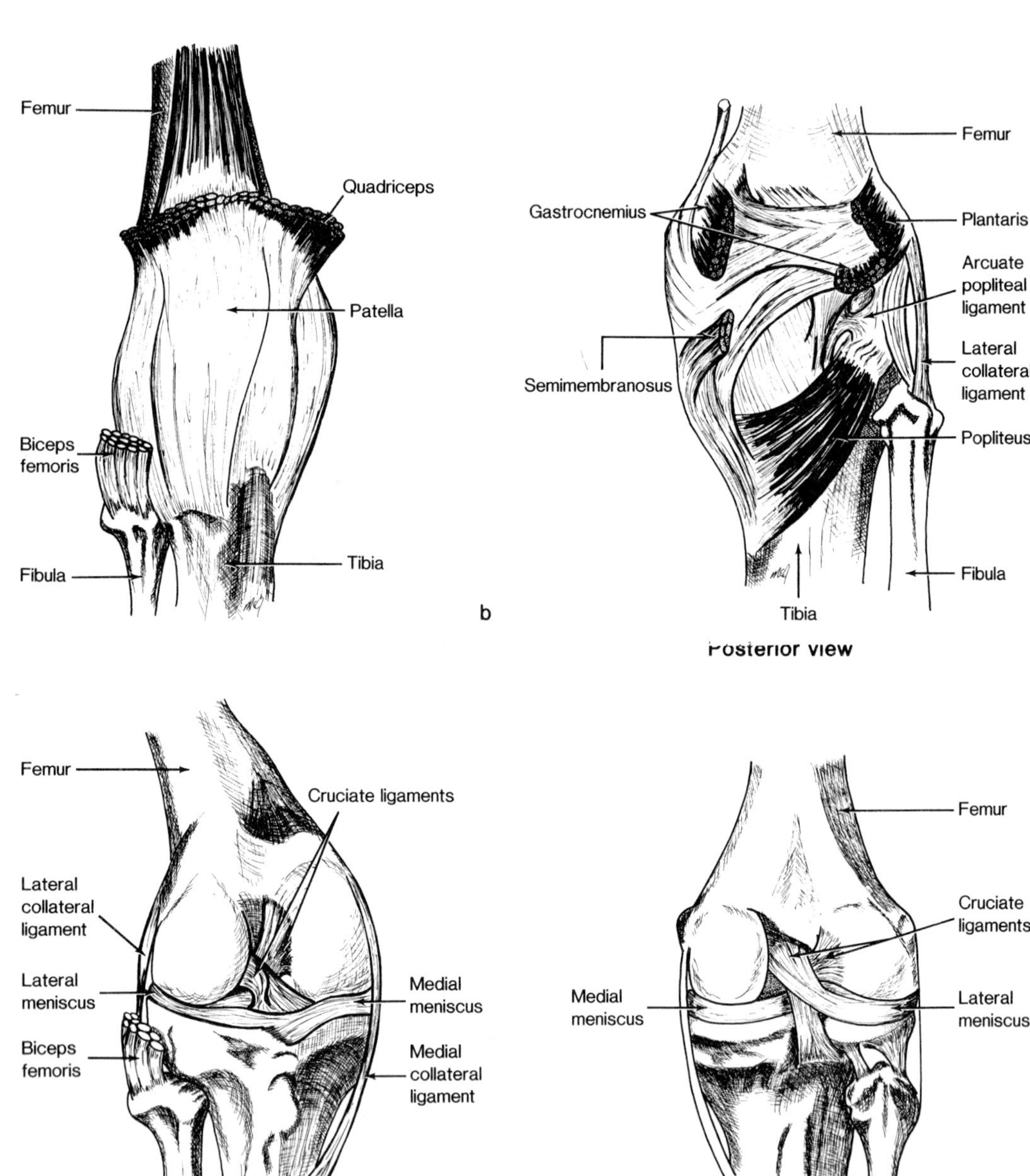

Lateral condyle

Intercondyloid eminence

Styloid process

Medial condyle

Tuberosity

Fibula

Tibia

Anterior view

**Figure 8.3. Proximal portion of the tibia and fibula**

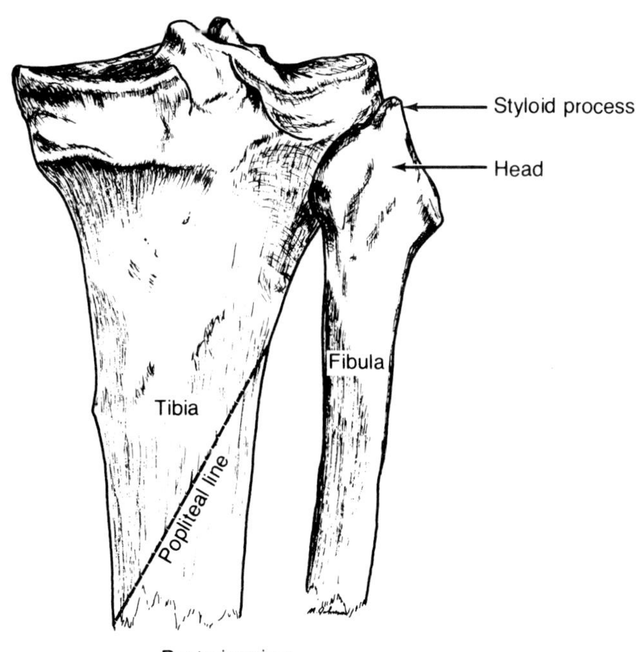


Posterior view

## Musculature

**Rectus Femoris** (rec'tus fem'oris)  The rectus femoris (fig. 8.4) lies on the anterior aspect of the thigh. It is a penniform muscle and is palpable midway between the hip and knee joints.

*Origin*  By two heads, from the anterior inferior iliac spine, and the groove above the rim of the acetabulum.

*Insertion*  Base of the patella.

*Innervation*  Femoral nerve.

*Action*  Extension of the knee joint.

Whereas the rectus femoris is a forceful mover of the hip joint, it is also an effective knee extensor. When both hip flexion and knee extension comprise an activity—as is the case with kicking—the muscle

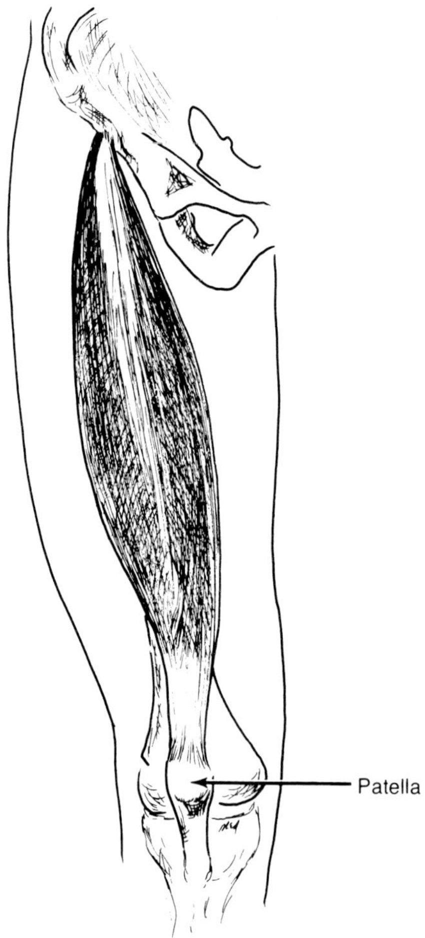


Figure 8.4. Rectus femoris, anterior view

contribution is second to none. When its power as a hip flexor is coupled with its force as a knee extensor, it is capable of generating great momentum in the foot.

**The Vasti** The vasti (fig. 8.5) are three muscles located on the front and sides of the thigh. They are the vastus lateralis, vastus medialis, and vastus intermedius (vas'tus latera'lis, vas'tus media'lis, and vas'tus interme'dius) which, together with the rectus femoris, form the muscle group known as the quadriceps femoris. The lateralis may be palpated at mid-thigh to the lateral side of the rectus femoris. The medialis is best palpated proximal and medial to the patella when the

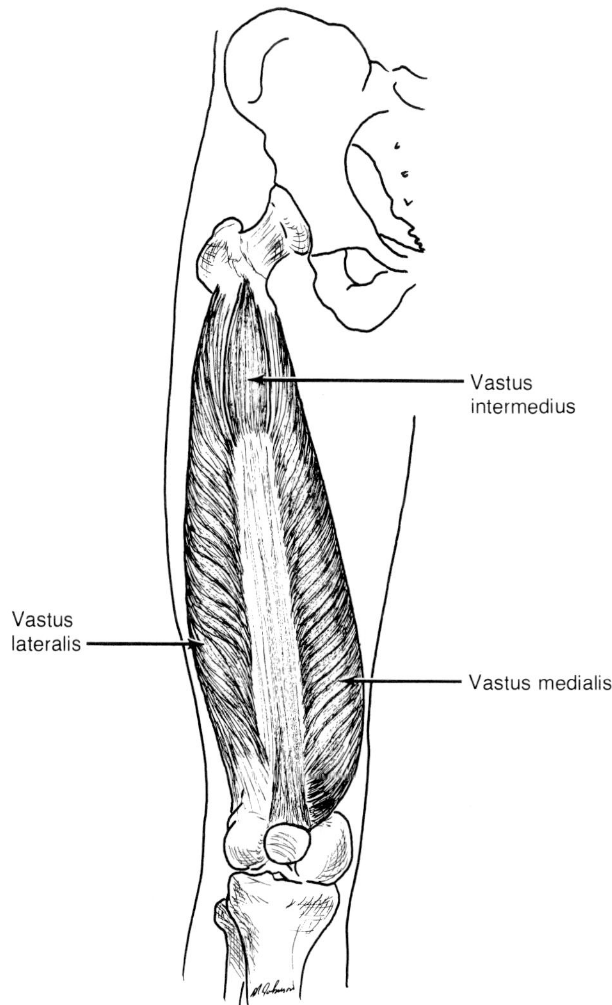


**Figure 8.5. The vasti muscles, anterior view**

knee is held in extension. The intermedius lies beneath the rectus femoris and cannot be palpated.

*Origin* Vastus lateralis: Lateral aspect of the femur extending from just below the greater tuberosity to and including the upper half of the linea aspera of the femur. Vastus medialis: Entire length of the linea aspera and supracondylar line of the femur. Vastus intermedius: Proximal two-thirds of the femur from its anterior and lateral surfaces.

*Insertion* All three vasti muscles insert on the patella through the tendon of the quadriceps femoris.

*Innervation* Femoral nerve.

*Action* All of the vasti extend the knee joint.

The lateralis and medius approach the patella and the tendon of the quadriceps femoris diagonally. Each requires the balancing pull of the other if a straight line of pull against the patella is to result. Since the intermedius is centered along the front of the thigh, it requires no neutralization. Its entire line of pull is directed optimally for knee extension.

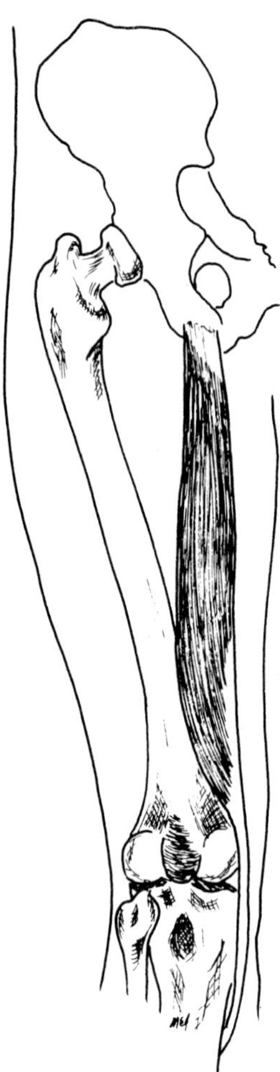

Figure 8.6. Semitendinosus, posterior view

**Semitendinosus** (semitendino'sus) The semitendinosus (fig. 8.6) is one of the hamstring muscles and is located superficially along the medial and posterior aspect of the thigh. It is most easily palpated in the area of its tendon of insertion as described under the gracilis (chap. 7).

*Origin* Medial facet of the ischial tuberosity by a common tendon with the long head of the biceps femoris.

*Insertion* Medial-anterior surface of the tibia just distal to the insertion of the gracilis.

*Innervation* Tibial portion of sciatic nerve.

*Action* Flexion and inward rotation of the knee.

The semitendinosus is not only posterior to the frontal axis as it crosses the knee joint but is also medial to the vertical axis. It is, therefore, a dual action muscle at the knee, performing both flexion and inward rotation. Its tendon of insertion with those of the sartorius and gracilis forms part of a broad tendinous structure called the pes anserinus.

**Semimembranosus** (semimembrano'sus) The semimembranosus (fig. 8.7), a hamstring muscle, lies on the posterior aspect of the thigh. It is best palpated along its tendon of insertion as described under the gracilis (chap. 7).

*Origin* Lateral facet of the ischial tuberosity.

*Insertion* The medial and posterior aspect of the medial condyle of the tibia.

*Innervation* Tibial portion of the sciatic nerve.

*Action* Flexion and inward rotation of the knee joint.

As one of the medial hamstring muscles, the semimembranosus crosses the knee joint posterior to the frontal axis and medial to the vertical axis. The resulting actions of the muscle are flexion and inward rotation, respectively.

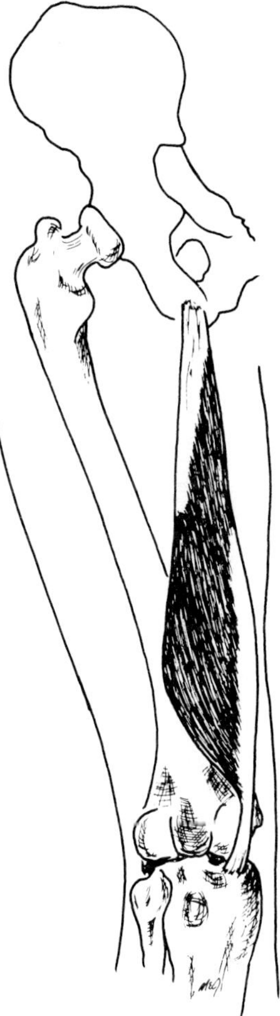

Figure 8.7. Semimembranosus, posterior view

**Biceps Femoris** (bi'ceps fem'oris) The biceps femoris (fig. 8.8) is comprised of a long head which crosses both the hip and the knee joints, and a short head which crosses the knee joint only. The muscle is the lateral hamstring and may be palpated on the posterior and lateral aspect of the thigh.

*Origin* Long head: Posterior aspect of ischial tuberosity. Short head: Lateral ridge of the linea aspera.

*Insertion* Both heads: Head of fibula and lateral condyle of tibia.

*Innervation* Long head: Tibial portion of sciatic nerve. Short head: Peroneal portion of sciatic nerve.

*Action* Flexion and outward rotation of knee joint.

The biceps femoris is the lateral hamstring and crosses the knee joint posterior to the frontal axis and lateral to the vertical axis. It joins the other hamstrings in knee flexion, but is one of the few muscles responsible for outward rotation of the tibia. In this latter action, the biceps femoris is extremely important to the integrity of the knee joint since it is the major muscle which will neutralize the inward rotation tendencies of the other knee flexors.

**Sartorius** (sarto'rius) The sartorius (fig. 8.9) is the longest muscle in the body. It is superficial as it courses diagonally medialward across the front of the thigh, but is difficult to palpate except in the area of its tendon origin. Palpation can be accomplished during resisted flexion of the hip when the femur has been placed in a position of outward rotation. The superior portion of the muscle can be felt and observed just below the superior iliac spine. A dimple-like depression will be noted just lateral to the sartorius which separates it from the tensor fasciae latae.

*Origin* Anterior superior iliac spine and the adjacent portion of the notch distal to the spine.

*Insertion* Upper and medial aspect of the tibia.

*Innervation* Femoral nerve.

*Action* Flexion and inward rotation of the knee joint.

The tendon of insertion of the sartorius wraps around the medial aspect of the upper tibia to attach nearly as far forward as the anterior crest. In addition to its ability to flex the knee, it is well-located to

Figure 8.8. Biceps femoris, posterior view

Figure 8.9. Sartorius, anterior view

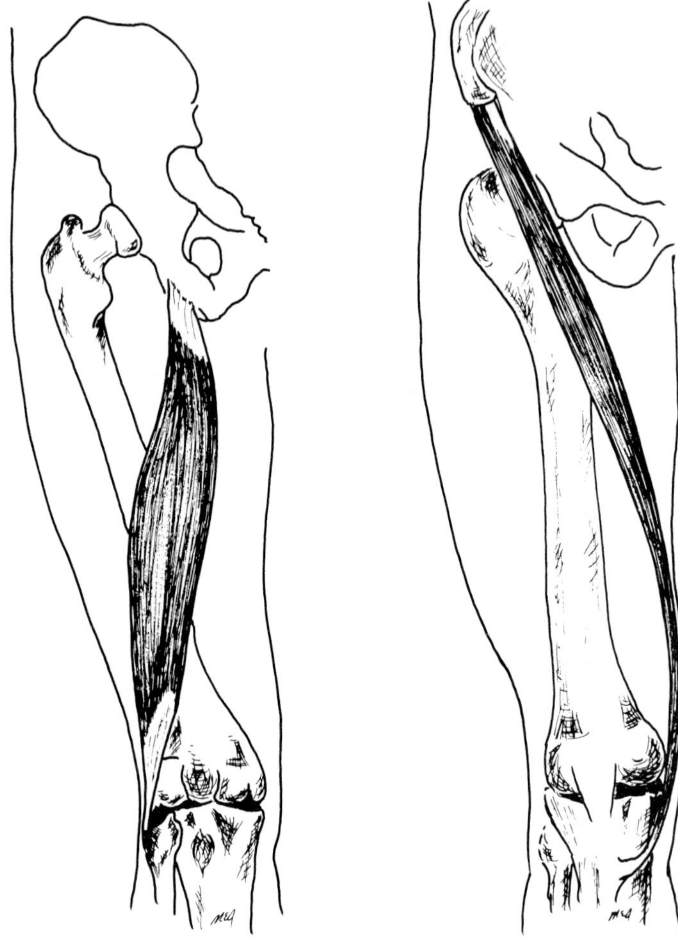

Figure 8.8

Figure 8.9

inwardly rotate by executing its unwrapping motion on the tibia. It should be noted that the muscle crosses anterior to the knee joint in a few individuals, and in such cases acts to extend the knee.

**Gracilis** (gra'cilis) The gracilis (fig. 8.10) is a long and slender muscle located superficially along the inner thigh. It is difficult to palpate because it is easily confused with surrounding muscles; however, its tendon of insertion can usually be felt clearly. Begin the palpation in the middle of the posterior aspect of the knee, then move the fingers medially until the large tendon of the semitendinosus is encountered.

If the fingers are moved slightly medially, the smaller tendon of the semimembranosus will be felt. The tendon of the gracilis lies just medial to the semimembranosus. Palpation may be facilitated by inwardly rotating the tibia against resistance.

*Origin* Inferior half of the symphysis and the superior half of the arch of the pubis.

*Insertion* Medial aspect of the tibia just below the condyle.

*Innervation* Anterior division of the obturator nerve.

*Action* Flexion and inward rotation of the knee joint.

The tendon of insertion of the gracilis passes posterior to the medial condyle of the femur, then curves around the medial condyle of the tibia to attach to the proximal tibia on its medial surface. At its insertion, it is above the tendon of the semitendinosus and below that of the sartorius; these three tendons of insertion form the structure known as the pes anserinus.

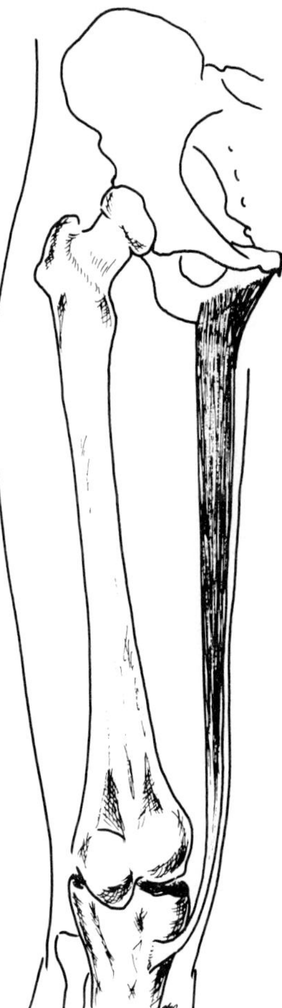

Figure 8.10. Gracilis, anterior view

**Popliteus** (poplite'us) The popliteus (fig. 8.11) is a small muscle located deep on the posterior surface of the knee. It cannot be palpated.

*Origin* Anterior and lateral portion of the lateral condyle of the femur; head of fibula; lateral meniscus; and oblique popliteal ligament.

*Insertion* Posterior surface of the tibia, proximal to the popliteal line.

*Innervation* Tibial nerve.

*Action* Flexion and inward rotation of tibia.

Resolution of the line of pull of the popliteus yields a vertical or flexion component, and a horizontal or rotational component. If the tibia is free to move, contraction of the popliteus will flex and inwardly rotate the knee joint by moving the tibia. If the tibia is held stationary, as it would be while standing, contraction of the muscle will pull against the femur and lateral meniscus to initiate the unlocking action of the knee which must occur at the beginning of flexion.

**Gastrocnemius** (gastrocne'mius) The gastrocnemius (fig. 8.12) is the large superficial muscle located on the posterior aspect of the lower leg. It may be palpated and observed easily as the ankle is moved through dorsi- and plantar flexion.

*Origin* By two heads, from the posterior surfaces of the two femoral condyles.

*Insertion* Posterior aspect of calcaneus through the Achilles tendon.

Figure 8.11. Popliteus, posterior view

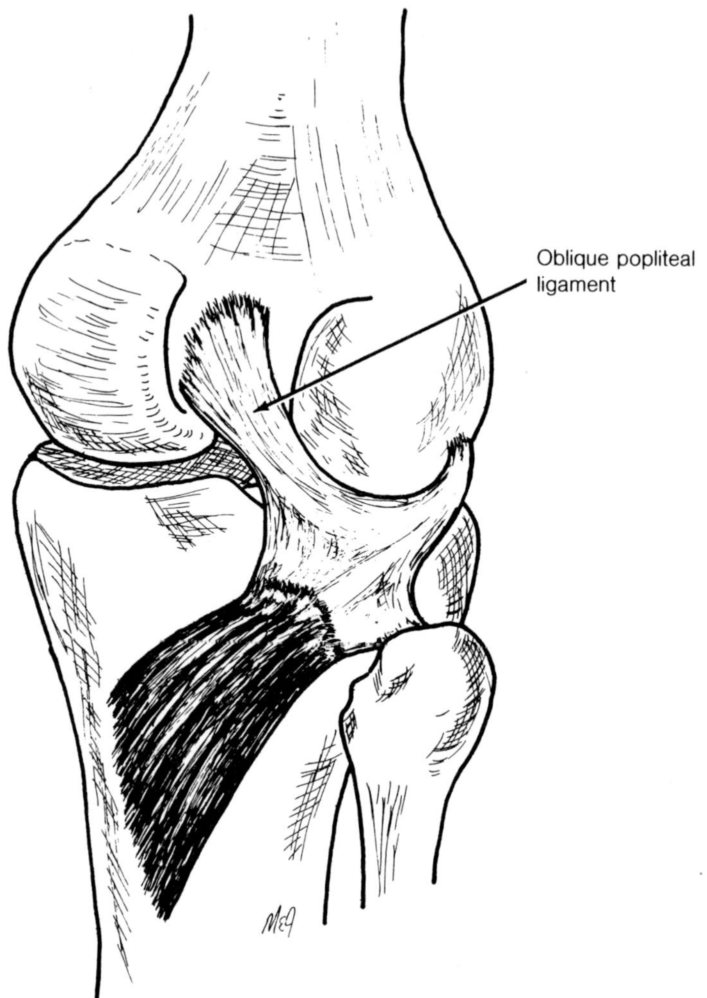


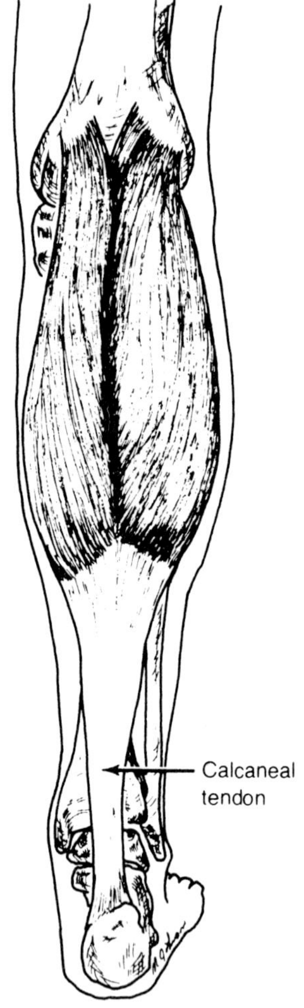


Figure 8.12. Gastrocnemius, posterior view

*Innervation* Tibial nerve.

*Action* Aids in flexion of the knee joint.

The contribution of the gastrocnemius to knee flexion is only assistive because, despite the fact that it does cross the knee posterior to the frontal axis, it is rather close to it and does not exhibit a long moment arm.

**Plantaris** (planta'ris) The plantaris (fig. 8.13) is poorly developed in man and is missing in some. The muscle lies between the gastrocnemius and the soleus. It cannot be palpated.

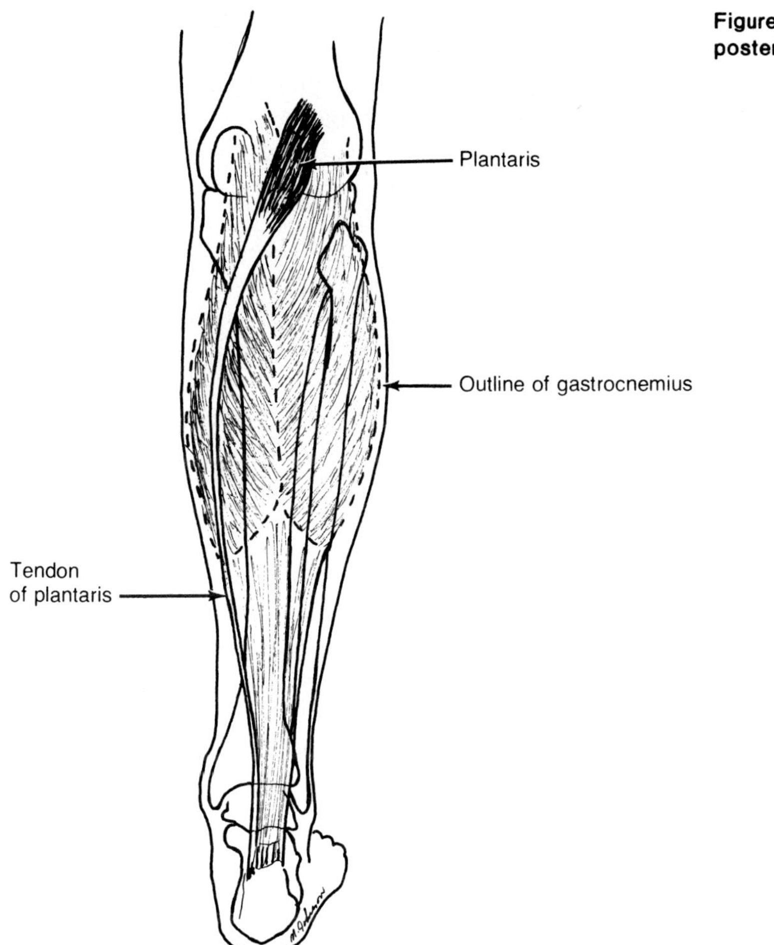


**Figure 8.13. Plantaris, posterior view**

*Origin* Distal portion of the linea aspera of the femur; oblique popliteal ligament of the knee joint.

*Insertion* Posterior surface of calcaneus.

*Innervation* Tibial nerve.

*Action* Weak assistant for knee flexion.

## Comments

The knee joint has become a major topic of conversation among those involved in athletics and dance. The high incidence of injury has focused attention of performers, trainers, coaches, and physicians alike on the joint and, as a result, innumerable conceptions—and misconceptions—have flourished and spread. Most of these have not been verified by research, so it becomes of extreme importance to learn the anatomical and mechanical aspects of the knee joint in order to form a sound and practical basis for prevention of injury.

Consideration of the composite actions of the joint should be the initial step. When the knee is flexed, the ligaments are lax, and the tibia is allowed to rotate around its long axis; when it is extended, the ligaments and the bony structure of the joint prohibit tibial rotation. Since, in the course of sport and dance performance, the knee is in the flexed position far more often than it is in extension, it follows that an effort should be made to ensure that the musculature of the knee, its last line of defense, be maintained at peak strength so that it can act to check excessive and injurious twisting of the tibia. The task of selecting appropriate exercises is a simple one; all of the muscles which cross the knee joint are either flexors or extensors; they may have added abilities to rotate the tibia, but all will be involved in moving the lower leg around the frontal axis. One needs only to ensure therefore, that strength-gaining exercises be performed during both flexion and extension. Care must be taken, however, not to overly strengthen either set of muscles. A ratio of four to three, or four to two, of extensor strength to flexor strength, is satisfactory. It is noted, additionally, that the musculature of the knee should be held in contraction if there is possibility of an impending blow to the knee. For example, football players must be taught to maintain tension in the thigh muscles after the tackle until they are sure that no late hits can occur.

Joint action between the patella and femur is also important to this discussion. The vastus medialis and lateralis exert opposite forces on the patella. If one muscle is stronger than the other, the patella will be pulled off-center when the quadriceps are contracted. Comparable strength in the two muscles can be achieved by exercising the knee joint through its full range of extension.

As a second step toward the prevention of injury, one must consider normal ranges of motion of the knee joint. The reader is urged to determine the maximum amount of flexion, extension, inward and outward rotation of which the joint is capable when it is unencumbered by the body weight. Use of these ranges as guidelines when body weight is superimposed will result in conservative but preventative allowances. For instance, when the knee is fully flexed by drawing the foot from the floor toward the buttocks, the angle between the upper and lower leg will be approximately 30 degrees. During full knee bends, however, the knee is forced, by the body weight, to flex to the point at which the femur and tibia are almost parallel: surely, the possibility of overstretching the ligaments is a real one. If the knee bends are performed only to the 30-degree point, however, possibility of causing trauma will be largely negated. Similarly, it can be established that the joint can hyperextend only minimally from muscular contraction alone. Assumption of positions of upright posture which require the knee to hyperextend farther than this point can carry the risk of injury.

## Comments on Two-Joint Muscles

There are several muscles of the human body that cross two or even more joints as they course between their origins and insertions. Many of these are found in the lower arm and leg and are discussed in those chapters. Such muscles are typically arranged in order to cause the same action at all the joints they cross. For example, the flexor digitorum profundus crosses four major joints, causing all of them to flex. The extensor digitorum longus crosses some five joints, causing extension of each. The basic mechanics of these muscles reside in their domino-like action of moving the most distal bony segment first followed, in turn, by the next-most distal segment, and so on. Because of the sameness of their actions at the joints they cross, they can easily be overstretched or overshortened and will, therefore, be compromised in attaining certain positions demanding strength.

The two-joint muscles of the upper leg deserve special attention in that they cause opposite movements of the joints they cross. The hamstrings (biceps femoris, semitendinosus, and semimembranosus) are active as hip extensors and knee flexors. The rectus femoris, antagonistic to the hamstrings, causes hip flexion and knee extension. The cooperation of these muscles must be quite precise during locomotor movements as well as during any movement that requires motion at the hip and/or the knee.

These muscles have been the focus of numerous kinesiological and biomechanical studies. Their cooperative activities during gait, running, squatting, and other such movements have been explored and, whereas each investigator has supplied us with more information than we had previously, we have been unable to unlock the secret of success.

Emerging from the research that has been done are some conclusions and postulations that are of interest to performers and coaches alike. The first regards the discomfort of contracting these muscles when they are at their shortest lengths. Knee extension accompanied by hip flexion places the rectus femoris at its shortest length. If the muscle is contracted strongly while the leg is in this position, a heavy, painful cramp will often occur. A rather common situation in which these conditions are found is on a so-called "quadriceps bench" on which a person sits and lifts weights with one or both legs. Overly heavy weights held at full extension of the knee can easily cause the onset of a cramp, especially if the trunk is inclined forward.

A similar condition can be seen in the hamstrings when the knee is flexed and the hip extended. One need only to stand on one foot and attempt to touch the buttocks with the opposite foot while pressing down against it with the hand. Verification will be both immediate and vivid.

Just as these muscles can be shortened by selective placements of the hip and knee joints, they can also be lengthened. The rectus femoris reaches its most extreme length during knee flexion with hip hyperextension—that position in which runners find themselves after "toe-off" of each stride. Running with maximum effort early in the season is accompanied all too frequently by tears of the rectus femoris. One should be cautious, also, about changing from smooth-soled shoes to cleated shoes. Cleated shoes provide for more ground friction; however, they also require more effort to remove them from the ground—an effort provided by the hamstrings. Increased contraction of the hamstrings after toe-off causes, in turn, increased knee flexion and hip hyperextension. Unless a gradual change to the new footwear is made, chances for a tear in the rectus femoris are very good indeed.

The hamstrings are placed at their greatest length when the knee is extended with the hip flexed. Such a position is reached during the "sit and reach" exercise—an exercise that is performed for the purpose of stretching the hamstrings. Although this extreme position is not reached during all of our sport and dance techniques, it is approximated by long jumpers, hurdlers, and runners, to name a few. Since hamstring tears occur so often during these activities, it would only seem logical to maintain these muscles at a length that will accommodate such stresses. Exercise programs do not appear to solve the total problem, however. Athletes and dancers alike can work diligently to achieve extreme flexibility of the hip joint only to be faced, at the wrong moment, with a devastating muscle tear. The answer to this worrisome problem is not yet known, but perhaps a postulation is in order. It has been noted by the author that hamstring tears tend to accompany a change in the position of the trunk of runners while they are in full stride. While trunk lean is associated with sprinting speed, it must be controlled or the athlete will fall. At periods of maximum velocity of running, no further acceleration is possible. Trunk lean must be lessened for control of the center of mass. If the lessening takes place quickly (rather than gradually), the rectus femoris is stretched equally as rapidly and, in its attempt to respond to the stretch, contracts to cause sudden knee extension—a condition that seems to be abhorent to the hamstrings. Result—a muscle tear. All of this is pure speculation. It is clear that more research must be done if we are to eliminate this insidious problem from the world of movement.

## Laboratory Experiences

1. Sit on a bench or table that is high enough to allow your feet to be off the floor and have a partner attach a 10-kilogram weight boot to your right foot. Gradually relax the muscles which cross the right knee as you palpate the space between the femur and tibia. You should notice a widening of the joint space and a feeling of tension in the collateral ligaments when the musculature has been completely relaxed. On the basis of what you have found, make a conclusion regarding the appropriate use of a weight boot in rehabilitation of the knee.
2. Sit in a chair which is low enough to allow you to flex the hip and knee joints to approximately 90 degrees when the foot is flat on the floor. Perform inward and outward rotation of the knee joint as you palpate each set of agonists. The palpations may be enhanced if a partner applies resistance at the ankle joint.
3. Place electrodes on the three superficial muscles comprising the quadriceps and monitor their electrical activity as the knee joint is moved, against resistance, from 90 degrees of flexion to full extension. During what portion of the movement is each muscle active?
4. While continuing to monitor the electrical activity of the quadriceps, perform a knee bend to the point at which the back of the thigh and the calf touch, then return to standing position. Now perform a knee bend to the full squat position and, while in that position, allow the quadriceps to relax. Return to standing position. From a comparison of the two sets of electromyograms, determine 1) whether one knee bend elicits more activity than the other; 2) why the full squat is potentially dangerous to the knee joint.
5. Use an isokinetic measuring device to determine the maximum strength of a partner's knee extensors and knee flexors. Calculate the ratio of flexors to extensors. Does this ratio hold true for other members of the class?
6. Stand with the spine extended and heels on the floor. Slowly flex the knee joint while being careful to perpendicularly align the hip joint with the foot. How much flexion of the knee joint is allowed by surrounding musculature? Which muscle is acting as the major limiting factor to increased flexion?

# 9 The Ankle and Foot

The ankle and foot have developed in man to provide for two functions—static weight-bearing and propulsive weight-bearing. More than thirty joints between and amoung the twenty-six bones of the foot attest to the intricacy of the foot structure.

The ankle joint, or talocrural joint (fig. 9.1), is formed through the articulation of the tibia and fibula with one of the tarsal bones, the

**Figure 9.1. Bones of the lower leg and foot**

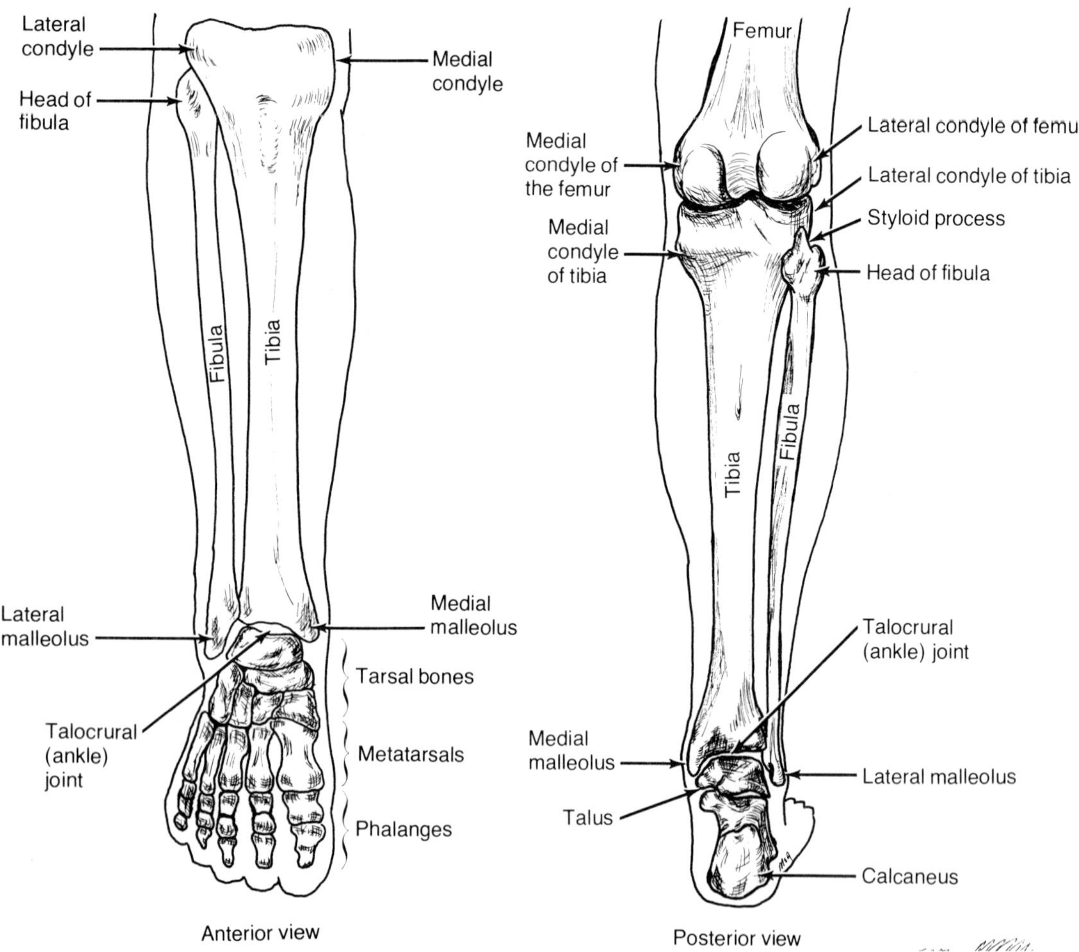

talus. The talus articulates with a second tarsal bone, the calcaneus, to form the subtalar joint and with a third tarsal bone, the navicular, to comprise the talocalcaneonavicular joint. Through the calcaneocuboid articulation, the calcaneus communicates with a fourth tarsal, the cuboid. This joint, together with that between the talus and navicular form an S shaped articulation called the *midtarsal joint.* The navicular articulates with the remaining tarsals, the three cuneiforms, through the cuneonavicular joint, as well as the cuboid by the cuboideonavicular joint. Between the cuneiforms are the intercuneiform joints; the third cuneiform communicates with the cuboid through the cuneocuboid joint. All of the joints between the tarsals are referred to collectively as the *intertarsal joints* (fig. 9.2).

The three cuneiforms and the cuboid articulate with the bases of the five metatarsals by the tarsometatarsal joints. The metatarsals articulate, in turn, with the phalanges by the metatarsophalangeal

**Figure 9.2. Bones of the foot**

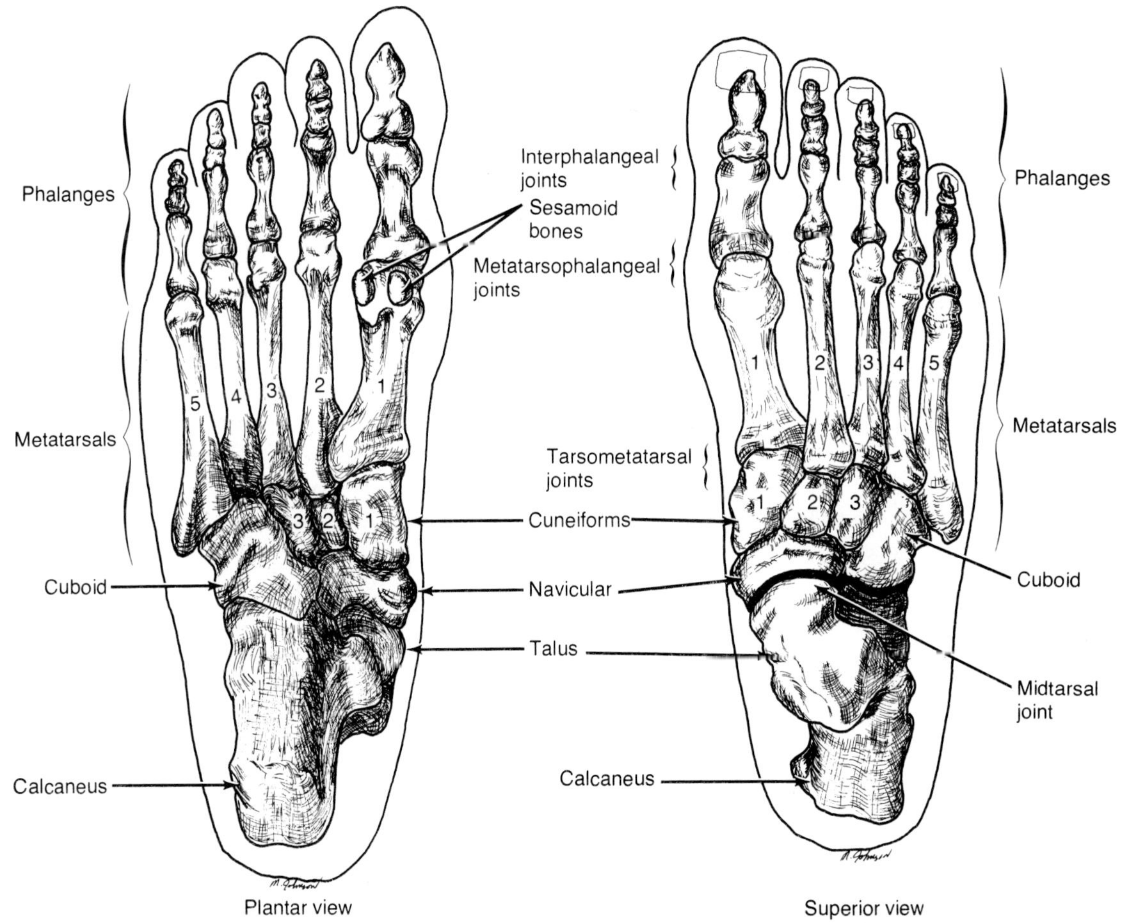

joints. Joints between the phalanges are referred to as the *interphalangeal joints* (fig. 9.2). The metatarsals also articulate between themselves, at their bases, through joints called *intermetatarsal joints.*

## Bone Markings

Figures 9.1 and 9.2 present the bone markings referred to in the discussion of origins and insertions of the muscles. The illustrations should be used in conjunction with a skeleton.

## Joints of the Ankle and Foot

### Talocrural Joint

The talocrural joint is formed by the tibia and its malleolus, the fibula and its malleolus, and the inferior transverse ligament, which together present a receptacle for the talus. Unlike their proximal joint, the tibia and fibula are bound tightly together, and having no synovial capsule, form a cartilaginous joint. The talocrural joint, itself, is a hinge joint and is surrounded by a joint capsule which is thin and membranous. As a hinge joint, there is a single axis of rotation passing (approximately) through the two malleoli (fig. 9.3). Movements of the joint are designated as *dorsiflexion* (raising the foot toward the anterior surface of the leg) and *plantar flexion* (lowering the foot as when "pointing the toes").

Four ligaments connect the bones of the joint (fig. 9.4). Three of these are located on the lateral aspect of the joint and are the anterior and posterior talofibular ligaments, and the calcaneofibular ligament. As their names imply, they course betwen the fibula and the talus, and fibula and calcaneous, respectively. The large, triangular deltoid ligament connects the tibial malleolus with the talus, calcaneous, and navicular bones.

### Intertarsal Joints

The subtalar joint is the aritculation between the talus, calcaneus, and navicular. It is synovial and nonaxial, and affords only gliding motion. Connecting the two bones are anterior, posterior, lateral, medial, and interosseus talocalcaneal ligaments, the dorsal talonavicular ligament, and the joint capsule.

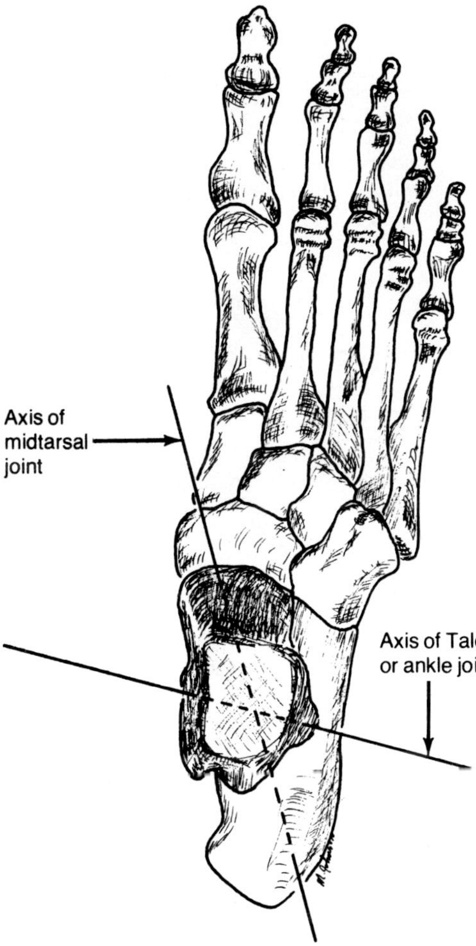

Figure 9.3. Axes of rotation of ankle and foot, superior view

The midtarsal joint, a double articulation including part of the subtalar joint, communicates the calcaneus with the cuboid, and the talus with the navicular. The joint permits a type of rotational movement by which the foot can be slightly dorsi- or plantar-flexed while simultaneously being inverted (sole being turned inwardly) or everted (sole being turned outwardly). It is interesting to note that neither inversion nor eversion can be performed without an accompanying amount of adduction or abduction of the foot around the heel. Because of this, some kinesiologists use the terms *supination* and *pronation* to describe the combination movements of adduction/inversion and abduction/eversion, respectively. Those terms will not be employed in this text, however, since they are so frequently construed to connote

**Figure 9.4. Ligaments of the ankle and foot**

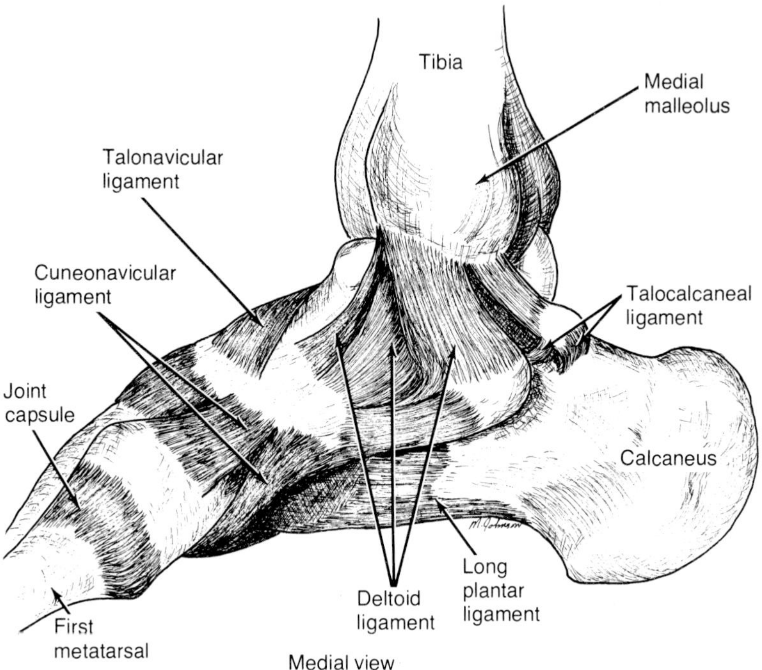


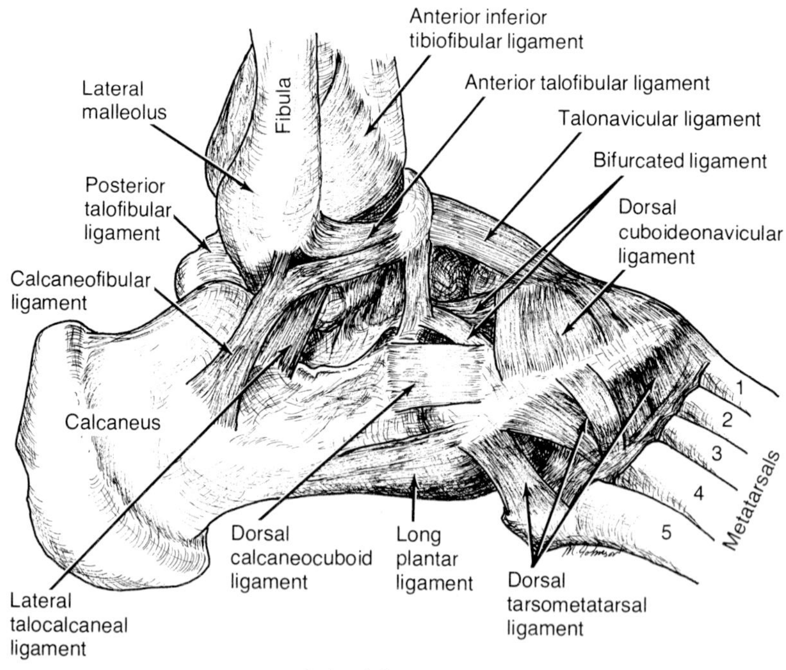

pathological conditions. Rather, inversion and eversion will be used with the understanding that adduction and abduction occur simultaneously. The axis of rotation (fig. 9.3) takes an approximate direction from a lateral-posterior point on the heel to the articulation between the navicular and first cuneiform. This junction may be located easily by palpating the end of the medial malleolus, then moving the fingers about four centimeters toward the toes until a groove is felt between the prominent navicular bone and the cuneiform.

The ligaments of the midtarsal joint (figs. 9.4, 9.5) are the dorsal talonavicular and calcaneocuboid ligaments, part of the bifurcated ligament, and the long and short plantar ligaments. In addition, the plantar calcaneonavicular ligament, also called the *spring ligament,* spans the joint to support the head of the talus. This ligament is broad,

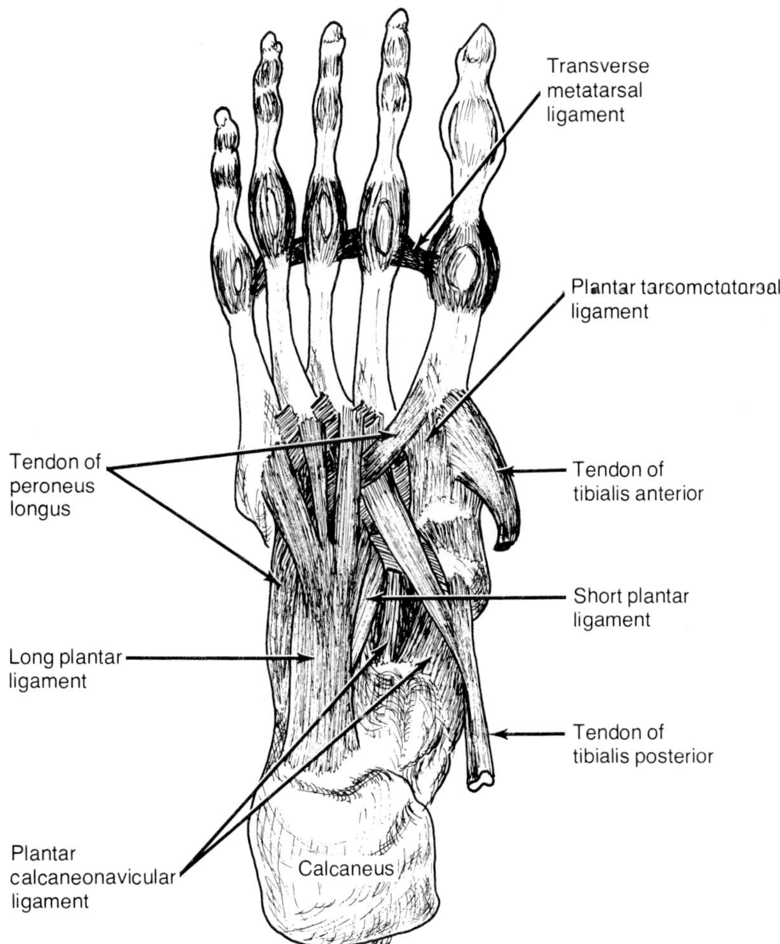


**Figure 9.5. Ligaments of the plantar aspect of the foot**

thick, and considerably elastic to provide for shock absorption. Improper foot mechanics can cause a permanent stretch in the ligament resulting in the lowered arch associated with flat feet.

The remaining intertarsal articulations are the cuneonavicular, cuboideonavicular, intercuneiform, and cuneocuboid joints. They are all synovial gliding joints, and are reinforced by dorsal and plantar ligaments, and in the case of the latter three joints, by interosseus ligaments.

### Tarsometatarsal and Intermetatarsal Joints

These are all nonaxial and synovial joints which permit only a slight gliding motion between the bones. Dorsal, plantar, and interosseus ligaments span the articulations.

The heads of the metatarsals are connected by the transverse metatarsal ligament. This ligament is a narrow band which holds the bones in some proximity when the foot bears weight.

### Interphalangeal Joints

The interphalangeal joints are synovial hinge joints which permit only flexion and extension. Plantar and collateral ligaments connect the bones. The great toe has a single interphalangeal joint; the four lesser toes have two such joints.

## Musculature

The muscles of the ankle and foot are divided into two groups, extrinsic and intrinsic. Extrinsic muscles originate in the lower leg or just above the knee and insert distal to the ankle. Intrinsic muscles originate and insert in the foot. In describing the actions of the muscles, the axis which passes through the two malleoli will be referred to as the *axis of the ankle;* the axis around which inversion and eversion are performed will be called the *midtarsal axis.*

### Extrinsic Muscles

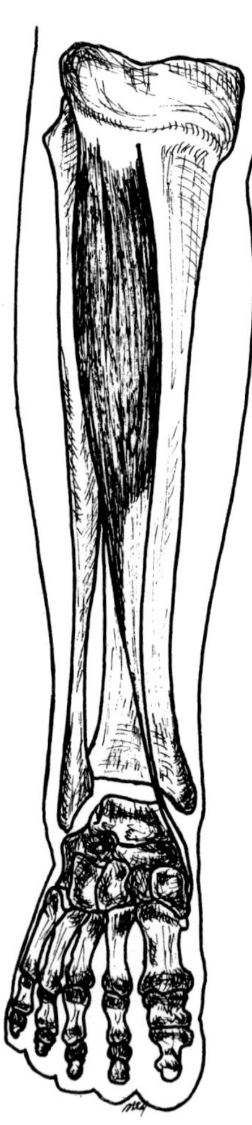

Figure 9.6. Tibialis anterior, anterior view

**Tibialis Anterior** (tibia'lis ante'rior) The tibialis anterior (fig. 9.6) is located on the anterior aspect of the lower leg. It can be palpated just lateral to the tibia and can be followed across the ankle almost to its insertion. Palpation is enhanced if the foot is dorsiflexed and inverted.

*Origin* Upper two-thirds of the lateral tibia and adjacent portion of the interosseus membrane which connects the tibia and fibula.

*Insertion* Medial and plantar surface of first cuneiform and base of first metatarsal.

*Innervation* Deep peroneal nerve.

*Action* Dorsiflexion of the ankle joint; inversion of the midtarsal joint.

The tendon of the tibialis anterior, which begins about two-thirds of the way down the leg, crosses the ankle joint anterior to the axis of the ankle and medial to the axis of the midtarsal joint. The muscle is, thus, an important one in both of its actions. The inversion action disappears, however, when the foot is held in plantar flexion. This is probably because forceful plantar flexion is accompanied by a certain amount of medial movement of the front of the foot—just enough to place the insertion of the muscle in line with the axis of the midtarsal joint. This medial movement is termed, by dancers, *sickling of the foot,* and is deplored as being unattractive and undisciplined. Dismay is loudly voiced when it is realized after viewing slow motion film of leaps and other body elevations from the floor, that sickling is an unavoidable part of vertical projection.

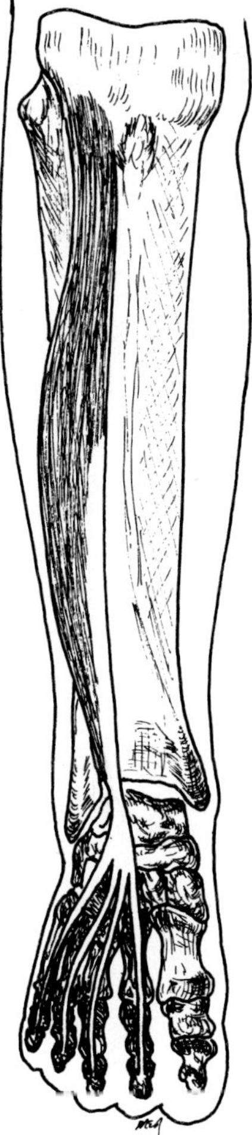

Figure 9.7. Extensor digitorum longus, anterior view

**Extensor Digitorum Longus** (exten'sor digito'rum lon'gus) The extensor digitorum longus (fig. 9.7) is located on the lateral and anterior aspect of the leg. It is best palpated where its tendon divides into four slips just distal to the ankle joint.

*Origin* Upper three-fourths of the anterior fibula; lateral condyle of the tibia; adjacent portions of the interosseus membrane between the tibia and fibula.

*Insertion* Second and third phalanges of the four lesser toes.

*Innervation* Deep peroneal nerve.

*Action* Extension of the interphalangeal and metatarsophalangeal joints of the four toes; dorsiflexion of the ankle; eversion of the midtarsal joint.

The primary function of the muscle is extension of the interphalangeal joints; however, the muscle does cross the ankle and midtarsal joints, and must be examined for its contribution to their movements. These can best be explained by noting that the muscle crosses the ankle anterior to the axis of that joint and lateral to the axis of the midtarsal joint. The moment arm is long to each axis indicating the importance of the muscle in both dorsiflexion and eversion.

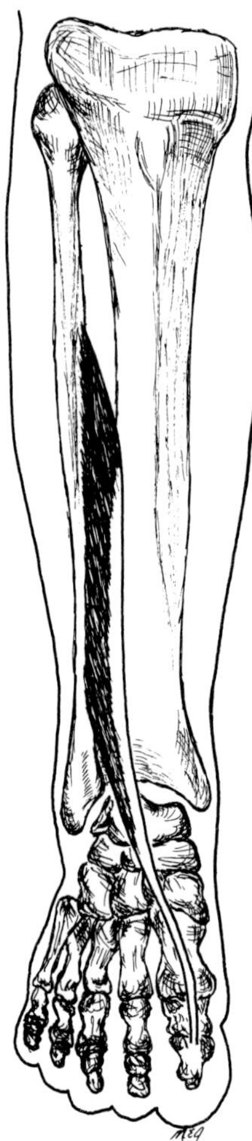

Figure 9.8. Extensor hallucis longus, anterior view

**Extensor Hallucis Longus** (exten'sor hal'lucis lon'gus) The extensor hallucis longus (fig. 9.8) is located between the extensor digitorum longus and the tibialis anterior in the lower part of the leg. Its tendon can be palpated on the dorsum of the ankle as the great toe is raised and lowered.

*Origin* Middle half of the anterior fibula and adjacent portions of the interosseus membrane between the tibia and fibula.

*Insertion* Base of the distal phalanx of the great toe.

*Innervation* Deep peroneal nerve.

*Action* Extends the interphalangeal and metatarsophalangeal joints of the great toe; dorsiflexion of the ankle joint.

Movement of the great toe is the primary function of the extensor hallucis longus; however, since it is anterior to the axis of the ankle, it also functions as a dorsiflexor. The muscle has been variously reported as both an everter and an inverter of the midtarsal joint. Examination of its location indicates that it lies on or very near the axis of the midtarsal joint and makes negligible conributions to either eversion or inversion.

**Peroneus Tertius** (perone'us ter'tius) The peroneus tertius (fig. 9.9) appears to be a part of the extensor digitorum longus and is often described as the fifth tendon of that muscle. It is difficult to distinguish from the extensor digitorum longus but may be palpated on the dorsum of the foot proximal to the prominent base of the fifth metatarsal.

*Origin* Distal third of the anterior fibula and adjacent portions of the interosseus membrane between the tibia and fibula.

*Insertion* Dorsal surface of the base of the fifth metatarsal.

*Innervation* Deep peroneal nerve.

*Action* Dorsiflexion of the ankle joint; eversion of the midtarsal joint.

The line of pull of the peroneus tertius is similar to that of the extensor digitorum longus as the latter muscle crosses the ankle and midtarsal joints. It can be credited therefore, with the same actions.

**Peroneus Longus** (perone'us lon'gus) The peroneus longus (fig. 9.10) is located on the lateral aspect of the lower leg. Its tendon is easily palpated above and slightly behind the lateral malleolus as the foot is held in eversion.

*Origin* Head and upper two-thirds of fibula; occasionally from the lateral condyle of the tibia.

*Insertion* Lateral surface of the first cuneiform and adjacent portion of the first metatarsal.

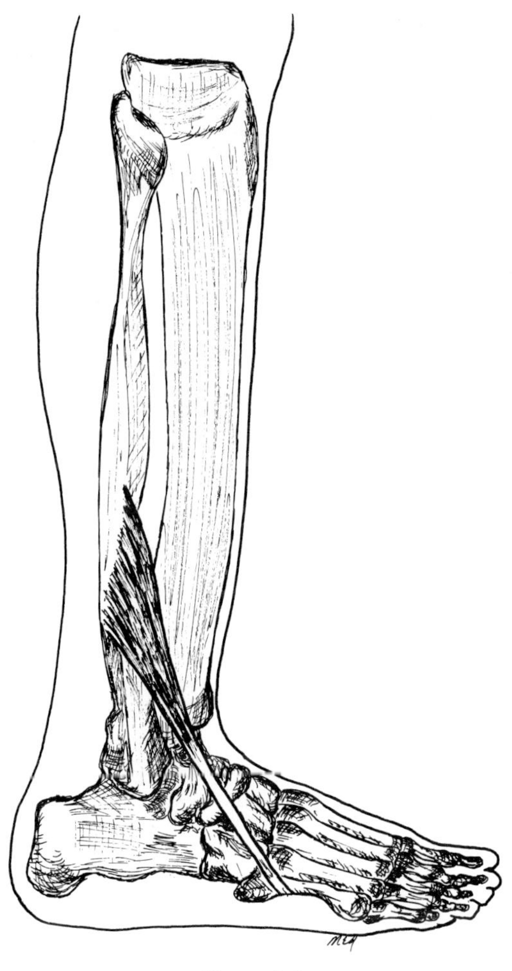

Figure 9.9

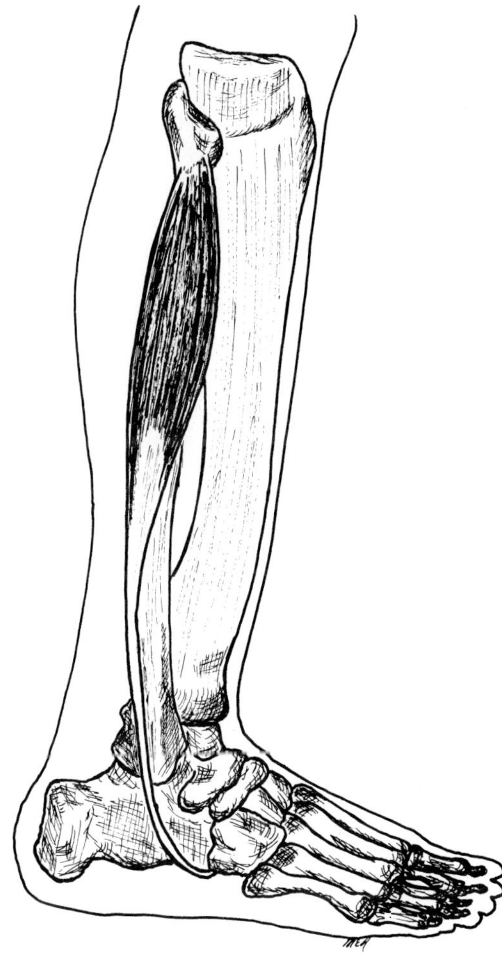

Figure 9.10

Figure 9.9. Peroneus tertius, lateral view

Figure 9.10. Peroneus longus, lateral view

*Innervation* Superficial peroneal nerve.

*Action* Eversion of the midtarsal joint; aids in plantar flexion of the ankle joint.

The tendon of the peroneus longus changes direction twice before its insertion. From its downward run on the outside of the leg, it passes behind the lateral malleolus, using that bony prominence as a pulley around which the tendon passes to direct itself toward the toes. It maintains this direction until it reaches the cuboid where it finds a groove that turns it at an approximate right angle to pass diagonally across the sole of the foot to attach near the tibialis anterior. Through its progress, the muscle passes the midtarsal joint lateral to the axis with a long moment arm. It passes close but posterior to the axis of the ankle and hence can contribute only assistively to plantar flexion.

**Peroneus Brevis** (perone'us bre'vis) The peroneus brevis (fig. 9.11) is shorter and smaller than the peroneus longus. It lies beneath the latter muscle and cannot be palpated except where its tendon approaches the prominent base of the fifth metatarsal.

*Origin* Distal two-thirds of the fibula.

*Insertion* Lateral side of the base of the fifth metatarsal.

*Innervation* Superficial peroneal nerve.

*Action* Eversion of the midtarsal joint; aids in plantar flexion of the ankle joint.

The line of pull is similar to that of the peroneus longus, and the resulting actions are essentially the same as those of that muscle.

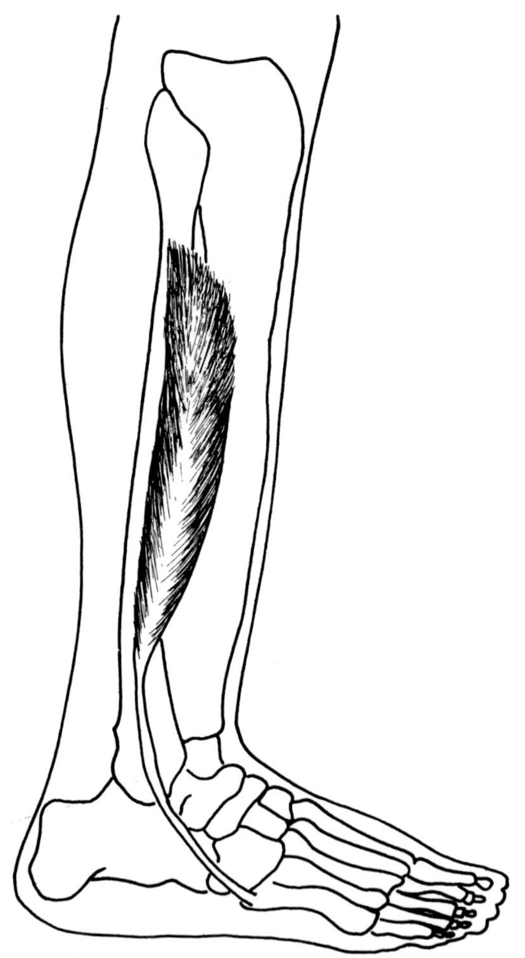

Figure 9.11. Peroneus brevis, lateral view

**Gastrocnemius** (gastrocne'mius) The gastrocnemius (fig. 9.12) is the large superficial muscle on the posterior portion of the lower leg. It is often referred to as the *calf muscle,* and is easily palpated between the knee and heel.

*Origin* By two heads, from the posterior surfaces of the condyles of the femur.

*Insertion* Posterior surface of the calcaneus by the calcaneal (Achilles) tendon.

*Innervation* Tibial nerve.

*Action* Plantar flexion of the ankle joint.

The calcaneus, by virtue of its posterior projection, offers optimum insertion for the gastrocnemius by way of the calcaneal tendon. The moment arm of this muscle is the longest it can be from the axis of the ankle and this, paired with the muscle's large size, allows for forceful plantar flexion. The gastrocnemius is not recruited, however, during standing at ease but only when ankle motion is required. The gastrocnemius may aid weakly in inversion of the midtarsal joint since the calcaneal tendon attaches to the calcaneus just medial to the axis of that joint. The moment arm is extremely short, however, and any contribution to inversion is so overshadowed by the ability of the gastrocnemius to plantar flex that it is considered negligible. Its action as an inverter can be seen well through slow-motion photography. Films exposed in a camera situated to record the front view of runners will show that the foot inverts immediately after it leaves the ground. The gastrocnemius accompanied by the soleus are the major muscles involved in providing thrust to the ground for each running step. Their attachment to the lateral side of the inversion axis is responsible for the brief pidgeon-toed look of the foot. This same phenomenon can be seen, also, during the vertical jump. The strong contraction of the gastrocnemius and soleus manifests itself first in forceful plantar flexion to elevate the body and then in inversion (or in the dancers' terminology, "sickling") when ground contact is lost.

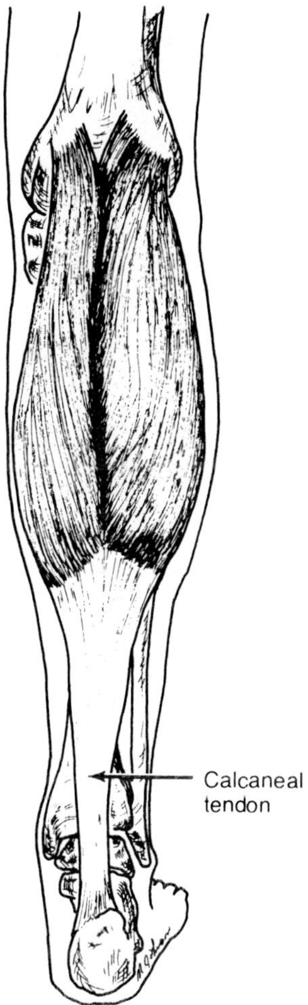


Figure 9.12. Gastrocnemius, posterior view

**Soleus** (so'leus) The soleus (fig. 9.13) is located beneath the gastrocnemius except along its lower and lateral aspect where a portion protrudes and may be palpated.

*Origin* Upper posterior surface of the fibula, tibia, and interosseus membrane.

*Insertion* Posterior surface of the calcaneus by means of the calcaneal (Achilles) tendon.

Figure 9.13. Soleus, posterior view

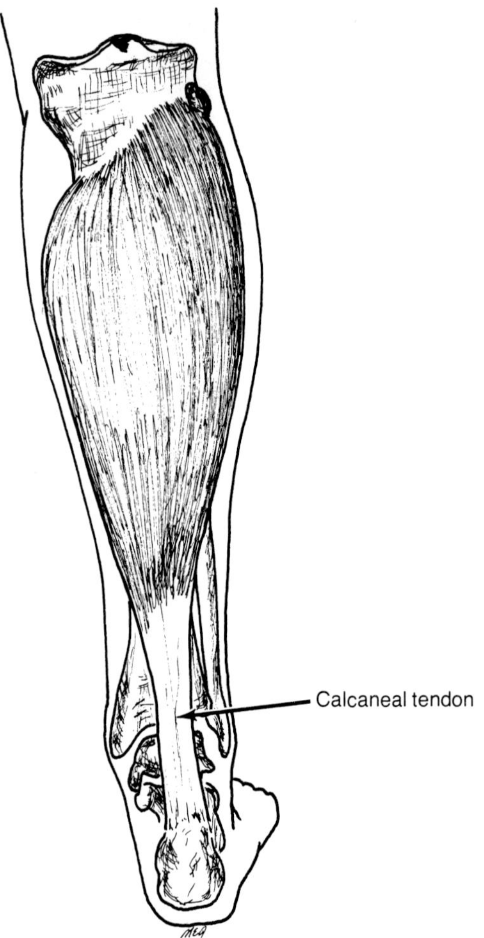


*Innervation* Tibial nerve.

*Action* Plantar flexion of the ankle joint.

The soleus is an associate of the gastrocnemius and with that muscle forms the muscular unit called the triceps surae. The muscular activity of the soleus differs from the gastrocnemius only in that the soleus is involved more constantly in static standing.

**Plantaris** (planta'ris) The plantaris (fig. 9.14) is a small muscle located deep in the back of the knee. Its tendon runs between the gastrocnemius and soleus; it cannot be palpated.

*Origin* Distal portion of the linea aspera and oblique popliteal ligament.

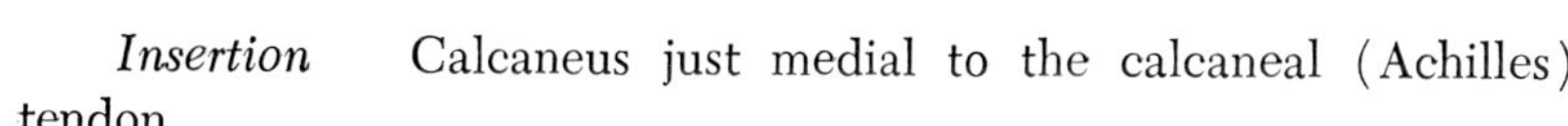


Figure 9.14. Plantaris, posterior view

*Insertion* Calcaneus just medial to the calcaneal (Achilles) tendon.

*Innervation* Tibial nerve.

*Action* Aids in plantar flexion of the ankle joint.

The plantaris has the same moment arm to the axis of the ankle that the soleus and gastrocnemius do, since their tendons insert side by side; however, the small size of the plantaris enables it to contribute only weak assistance to plantar flexion.

**Flexor Digitorum Longus** (flex'or digito'rum lon'gus) The flexor digitorum longus (fig. 9.15) is located deep on the back of the lower leg. It cannot be palpated.

*Origin* Posterior surface of the tibia from just below the popliteal line.

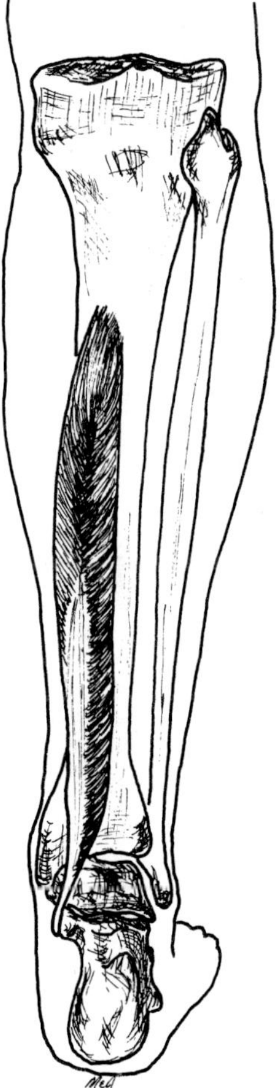

Figure 9.15. Flexor digitorum longus, posterior view

*Insertion* Base of distal phalanges of four lesser toes.

*Innervation* Tibial nerve.

*Action* Flexion of the interphalangeal and metatarsophalangeal joint of the four lesser toes; plantar flexion of the ankle joint; inversion of the midtarsal joint.

The responsibility of the flexor digitorum longus is primarily that of moving the toes; however, it contributes also to the movement of the other joints it crosses. The muscle runs posterior to the axis of the ankle and medial to the midtarsal axis to be a plantar flexor and inverter, respectively.

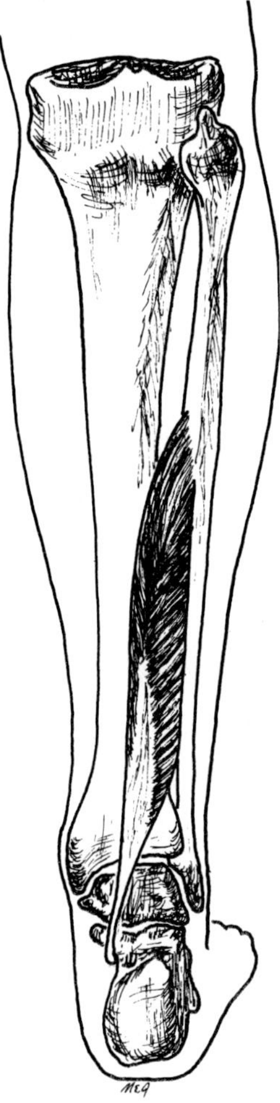

Figure 9.16. Flexor hallucis longus, posterior view

**Flexor Hallucis Longus** (flex'or hal'lucis lon'gus) The flexor hallucis longus (fig. 9.16) is located to the lateral side of the flexor digitorum longus deep in the back of the leg. It cannot be palpated.

*Origin* Lower two-thirds of the posterior surface of the fibula and the distal portion of the interosseus membrane between the tibia and fibula.

*Insertion* Base of the distal phalanx of the great toe.

*Innervation* Tibial nerve.

*Action* Flexion of the interphalangeal and metatarsophalangeal joints of the great toe; plantar flexion of the ankle joint; inversion of the midtarsal joint.

The tendon of the flexor hallucis longus crosses the axis of the ankle and midtarsal joints just to the posterior side of the tendon of the flexor digitorum longus; hence, the two muscles function similarly on those joints. The major responsibility of the muscle is, however, movement of the great toe.

**Tibialis Posterior** (tibia'lis poste'rior) The tibialis posterior (fig. 9.17) lies beneath the triceps surae on the back of the lower leg. It cannot be palpated.

*Origin* Posterior surface of upper two-thirds of the tibia, medial surface of upper two-thirds of the fibula, and adjacent portion of interosseus membrane between the tibia and fibula.

*Insertion* Tuberosity of the navicular with fibrous slips to the calcaneus, cuboid, the three cuneiforms, and the bases of the second through fourth metatarsals.

*Innervation* Tibial nerve.

*Action* Plantar flexion of the ankle joint; inversion of the midtarsal joint.

The tendon of the tibialis posterior crosses the ankle and midtarsal joints, with the tendons of the flexor digitorum longus and the flexor hallucis longus, and functions with them at these joints. These three muscles are often referred to as the *Tom, Dick and Harry* muscles: *Tom* for tibialis posterior, *Dick* for flexor digitorum longus, and *Harry* for flexor hallucis longus.

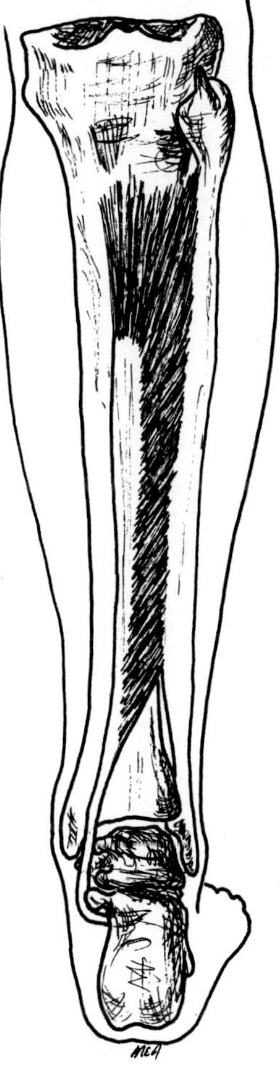
Figure 9.17. Tibialis posterior, posterior view

## Intrinsic Muscles

The intrinsics of the foot lie in one dorsal layer and four plantar layers. The muscles of the plantar aspect are covered by a strong layer of fibrous tissue called the plantar fascia or plantar aponeurosis. It attaches to the medial tubercle of the calcaneus and spreads toward the heads of the metatarsals where is divides into five slips and attaches to the skin and the tendons of the flexor muscles. It supports the foot during all forms of weight-bearing and, with the ligaments of the foot, is a primary contributor to its arched contour.

### *The First Plantar Layer*

**Flexor Digitorum Brevis** (flex'or digito'rum bre'vis) The flexor digitorum brevis (fig. 9.18) lies immediately beneath the central portion of the plantar aponeurosis. It cannot be palpated.

*Origin* Tuberosity of the calcaneus and the central part of the plantar aponeurosis.

*Insertion* By four tendons which divide distally to insert on the sides of the middle phalanges of the four lesser toes.

*Innervation* Medial plantar nerve.

*Action* Flexion of the proximal interphalangeal joints and metatarsophalangeal joints of four lesser toes.

**Abductor Hallucis** (abduc'tor hal'lucis) The muscle is located to the medial side of the flexor digitorum brevis (fig. 9.19). It cannot be palpated.

*Origin* Tuberosity of the calcaneus, the flexor retinaculum, and the plantar aponeurosis.

*Insertion* Tibial side of the base of the proximal phalanx of the great toe.

*Innervation* Medial plantar nerve.

*Action* Abduction of the metatarsophalangeal joint of the great toe.

Figure 9.18. Flexor digitorum brevis, plantar view

Figure 9.19. Abductor hallucis, plantar view

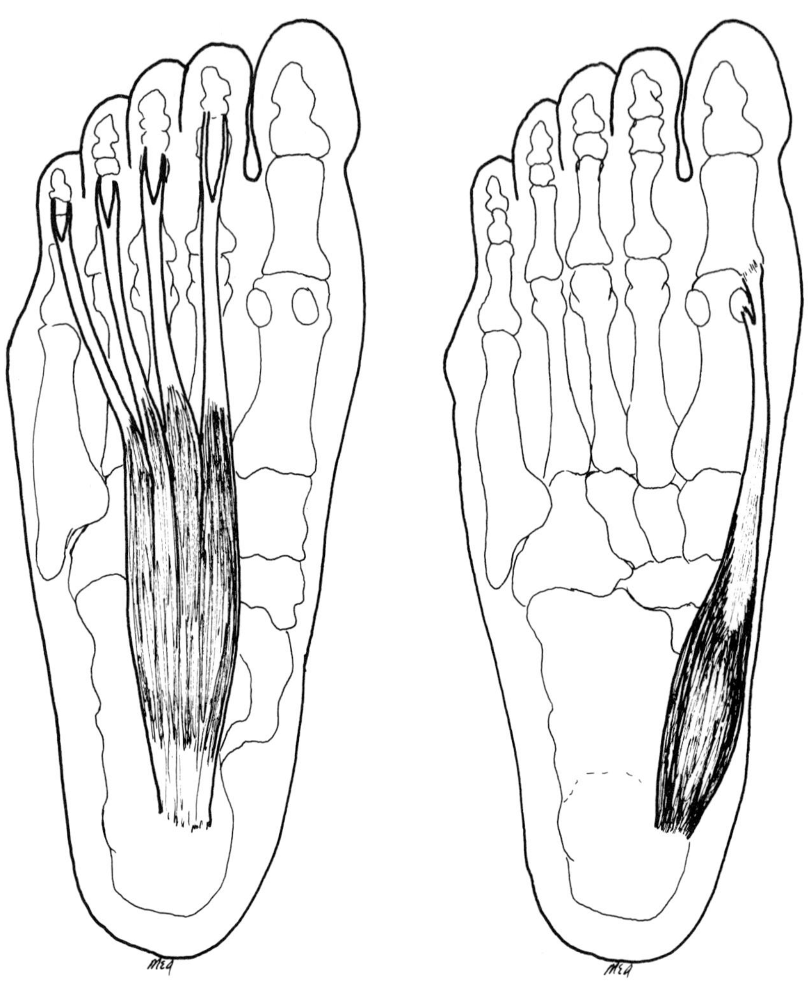

**Abductor Digiti Minimi** (abduc'tor dig'iti min'imi) The abductor digiti minimi (fig. 9.20) is located along the lateral side of the foot beneath the plantar aponeurosis. It cannot be palpated.

*Origin* Tuberosity and plantar surface of the calcaneus and plantar aponeurosis.

*Insertion* Fibular side of the base of the first phalanx of the little toe.

*Innervation* Lateral plantar nerve.

*Action* Abduction of the metatarsophalangeal joint of the little toe.

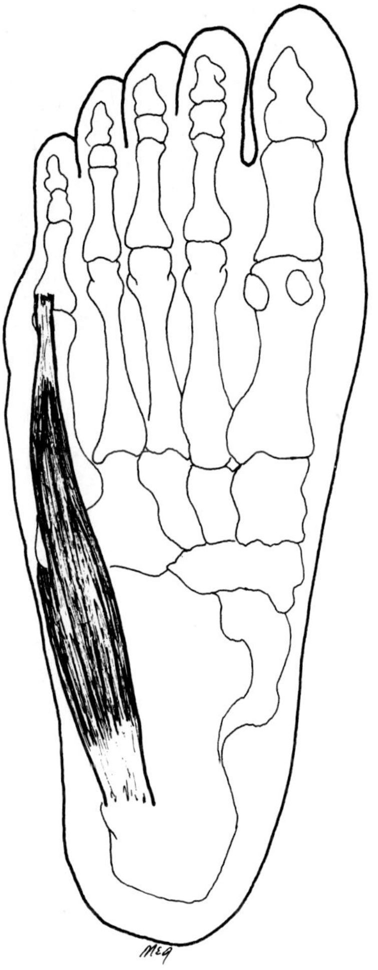

Figure 9.20. Abductor digiti minimi, plantar view

## *The Second Plantar Layer*

**Quadratus Plantae** (quadra'tus plan'tae) The quadratus plantae (fig. 9.21) is beneath the muscles of the first layer but is separated from them by a plantar nerve and blood vessels.

*Origin* By two heads, from the tibial and fibular surfaces of the calcaneus.

*Insertion* Tendon of the flexor digitorum longus just before it divides.

*Innervation* Lateral plantar nerve.

*Action* Through the tendon of the flexor digitorum longus, flexion of the distal interphalangeal joints of the four lesser toes.

Figure 9.21. Quadratus plantae and lumbricales, plantar view

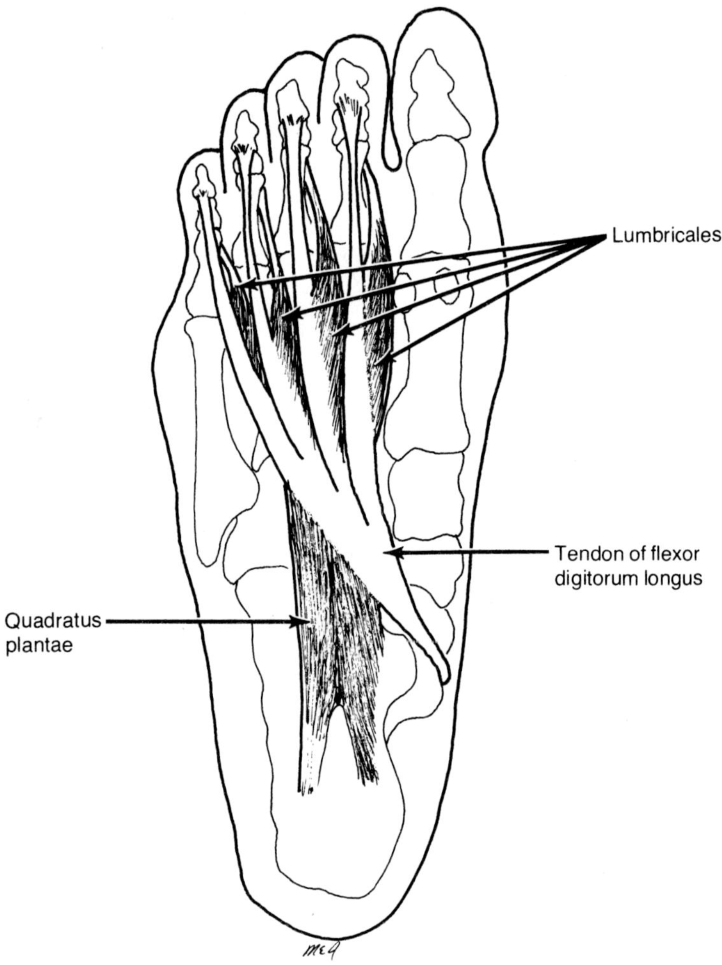


**Lumbricales** (lumbrica'les) The lumbricales (fig. 9.21) are four small muscles located in conjunction with the tendons of the flexor digitorum longus. They are numbered from the tibial side of the foot.

*Origin* Tendons of the flexor digitorum longus.

*Insertion* After passing to the tibial side of the four lesser toes, the muscles insert on the tendons of the extensor digitorum longus.

*Innervation* Medial and lateral plantar nerves.

*Action* Through the tendons on which the muscles originate and insert, they flex the metatarsophalangeal joints of the four lesser toes and extend the interphalangeal joints of these toes.

### *The Third Plantar Layer*

**Flexor Hallucis Brevis** (flex'or hal'lucis bre'vis) The flexor hallucis brevis (fig. 9.22) is sometimes described as the first plantar interosseus. It is analogous to the flexor pollicis brevis in that respect.

*Origin* Cuboid and third cuneiform bones.

*Insertion* By two heads, to the sides of the base of the proximal phalanx of the great toe.

*Innervation* Medial plantar nerve.

*Action* Flexion of the metatarsophalangeal joint of the great toe.

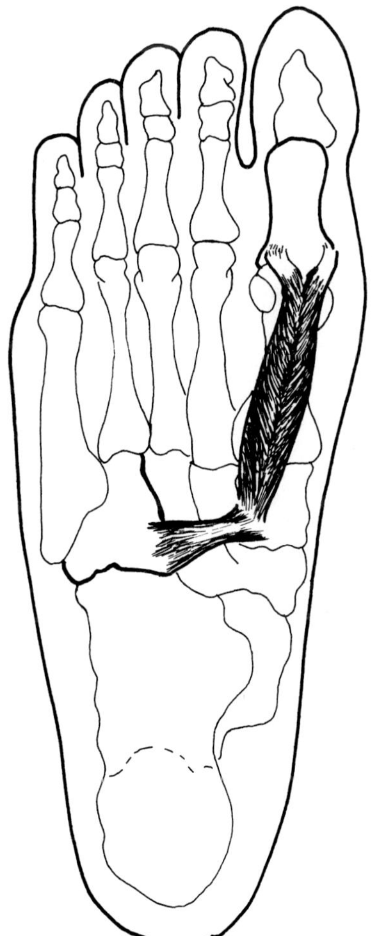

Figure 9.22. Flexor hallucis brevis, plantar view

**Adductor Hallucis** (adduc'tor hal'lucis) The adductor hallucis (fig. 9.23) is characterized by two widely separated heads. Except for its common tendon of attachment, it would appear to be two muscles.

*Origin* Oblique head: Base of second through fourth metatarsals. Transverse head: Metatarsophalangeal ligaments of the third through fifth toes.

*Insertion* Fibular side of the base of the proximal phalanx of the great toe.

*Innervation* Lateral plantar nerve.

*Action* Adduction of the metatarsophalangeal joint of the great toe.

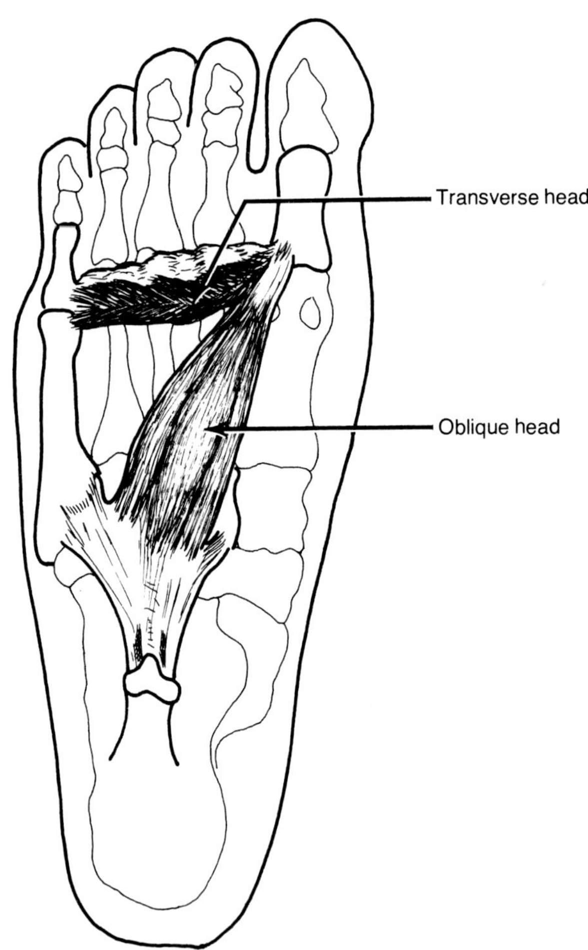


Figure 9.23. Adductor hallucis, plantar view

**Flexor Digiti Minimi Brevis** (flex'or dig'iti min'imi bre'vis) The flexor digiti minimi brevis (fig. 9.24) lies along the metatarsal of the little toe. It resembles an interosseus muscle.

*Origin* Base of the fifth metatarsal.

*Insertion* Lateral side of the base of the first phalanx of the little toe.

*Innervation* Lateral plantar nerve.

*Action* Flexion of the metatarsophalangeal joint of the little toe.

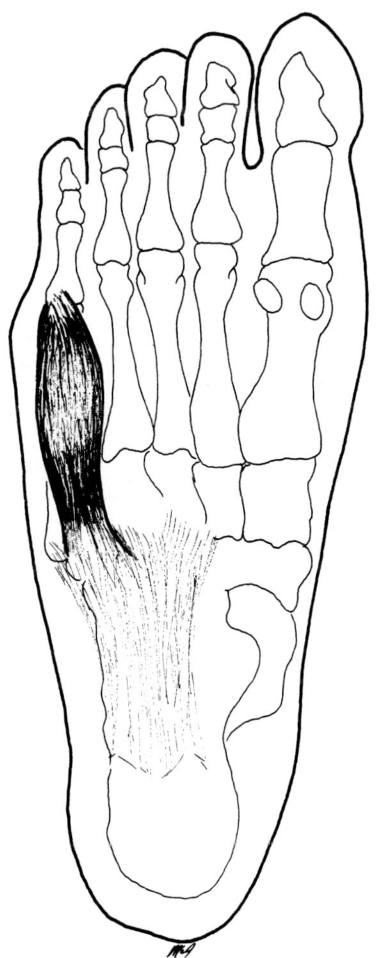

Figure 9.24. Flexor digiti minimi brevis, plantar view

## *The Fourth Plantar Layer*

**The Dorsal Interossei** (dor'sal interos'sei) The dorsal interossei (fig. 9.25) are four small muscles occupying the spaces between the metatarsals. They are numbered from the tibial side of the foot.

*Origin* Each muscle originates by two heads from the sides of adjacent metatarsals.

*Insertion* Bases of proximal phalanges of the four lesser toes, and the tendons of the extensor digitorum longus as shown in figure 9.25.

*Innervation* Lateral plantar nerve.

*Action* Abduction of third and fourth metatarsophalangeal joints, and tibial and fibular deviation of that joint of the second toe; flexion of the metatarsophalangeal joints and extension of the interphalangeal joints of the second, third, and fourth toes.

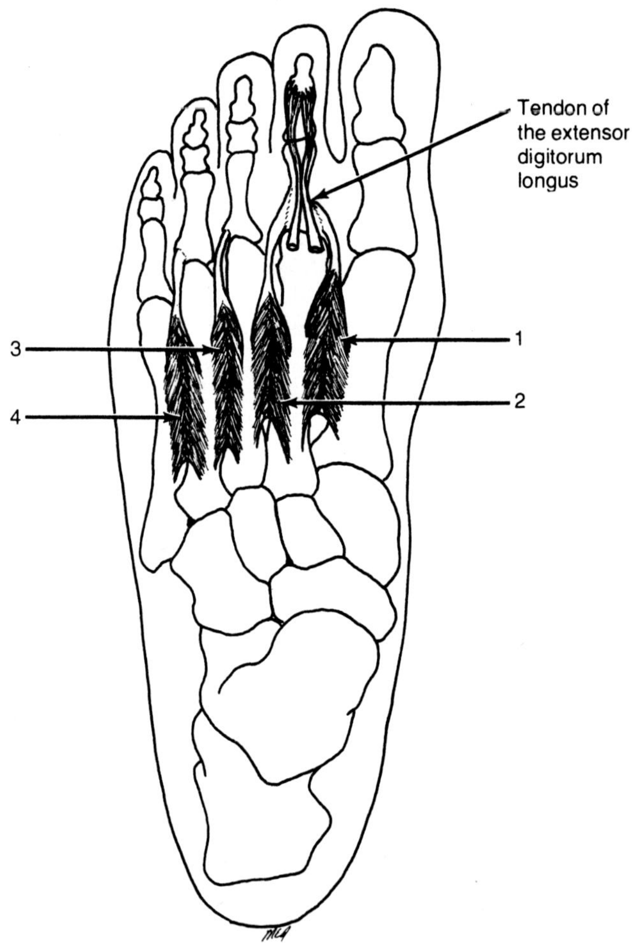


Figure 9.25. Dorsal interossei, dorsal view

**Plantar Interossei** (plan'tar interos'sei) The plantar interossei (fig. 9.26) are three small muscles which lie beneath the third, fourth, and fifth metatarsals. They are numbered from the tibial side of the foot.

*Origin* Tibial side of the third through fifth metatarsals.

*Insertion* Tibial sides of the bases of the first phalanges of the third through fifth toes.

*Innervation* Lateral plantar nerve.

*Action* Adduction of the metatarsophalangeal joints of the third, fourth, and fifth toes; flexion of the metatarsophalangeal joints and extension of the interphalangeal joints of those toes.

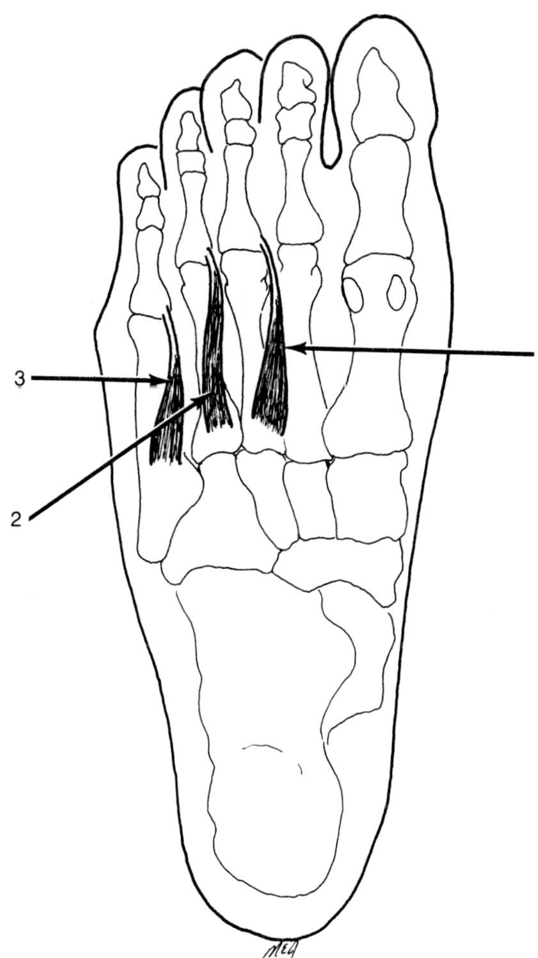


Figure 9.26. Plantar interossei, plantar view

## The Dorsal Layer

**Extensor Digitorum Brevis** (exten'sor digito'rum bre'vis) The extensor digitorum brevis (fig. 9.27) is the only intrinsic muscle on the dorsum of the foot. It is superficial in some of its parts but is difficult to palpate because it is easily confused with the long extensor.

*Origin* Lateral surface of the distal portion of the calcaneus.

*Insertion* By four tendons, to the base of the proximal phalanx of the great toe, and the tendons of the extensor digitorum longus of the second, third, and fourth toes.

*Innervation* Deep peroneal nerve.

*Action* Extension of the metatarsophalangeal joints of the first through the fourth toes.

**Figure 9.27. Extensor digitorum brevis, dorsal view**

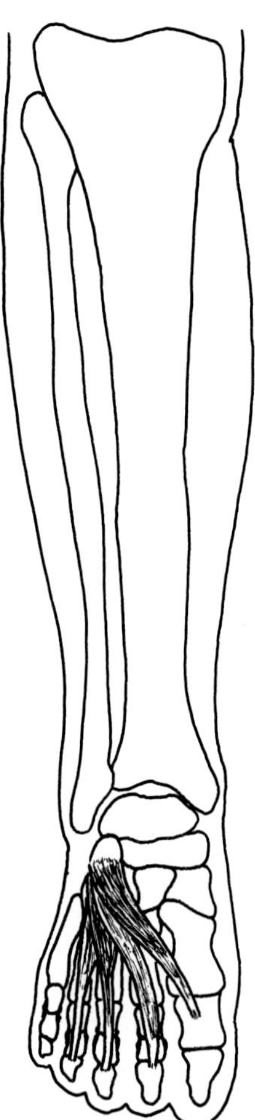

## Comments

It is surprising that the ankle and foot have not received more attention from the worlds of sport and dance. Dance is, perhaps, more to be complimented than sport, for it has voiced concern for the young dancer who is put on pointe before proper calcification of the foot has occurred, and for dancers who must perform, barefooted, on floors sealed with varnish and other such "nonslip" surfaces. Nevertheless, discussion relating to an anatomy of this portion of the body has largely been neglected—a curious omission since the preponderance of our activities are initiated by the foot on its supporting surface.

So little research has been completed which relates to the ankle and foot that it is difficult, or impossible, to state any generalizations; however, a few isolated examples may suffice as "takeoff" points on which relevant movement concepts can be built. One such example concerns the frequent alternation between footwear with low heels (or no footwear at all) and footwear comprising the popular two- or three-inch heel. While wearing the low-heel shoes, or with no shoes, the foot enjoys maximum contact with the floor, and the weight of the body is spread over its total surface. Shoes with higher heels cause the body weight to be localized over the metatarsophalangeal joints, and especially over the second of these joints since the second metatarsal is the longest of the five. There is frequent soreness in the ball of the foot below the head of that metatarsal because of underlying bruised tissue. This problem may be encountered, also, by those dancers who, after several months of inactivity, attempt to regain peak ability in a day or two. Since so many of the activities in dance are performed on half-pointe, the effect on the foot is the same as that from wearing high-heeled shoes.

A difficulty of the same origin often befalls those individuals who habitually wear shoes with high heels, and suddenly note, with alarm, that they cannot place their heels on the floor. The triceps surae and other plantar flexors have shortened in response to the carriage demanded by the shoes.

Sprains of the ankle joint are quite common among performers in sports and dance, and most of these occur from forceful inversions of the ankle. Study of the ligamentous structure will indicate, however, that the ankle is better protected from this type of sprain than from eversion sprains, because there are more lateral than medial ligaments. It must follow that the foot is more prone to accidental inversion than eversion—a conclusion that will be verified when the weight-bearing surface of the foot is examined. Since the weight of the body is spread along the lateral margin of the foot, only a slight miscue in stepping can result in weight placement to the outside of the foot—the inversion sprain. A gross misplacement is required, however, for the weight line to exceed the foot's medial margin and cause an eversion sprain. Unfortunately, the added ligamentous protection against inversion sprains can be somewhat obscured by inappropriate choice of sports shoes. A generalization is offered—if one can look down upon the top of the shoe while the foot is bearing weight, he should be able to see the sole projecting along the entire circumference of the forepart of the shoe. Otherwise, the foot can too easily roll laterally over the sole and sprain may result.

## Laboratory Experiences

1. Examine the ankle mechanism on a human skeleton and note that one of the malleoli is longer than the other. Keeping this in mind, visualize the ankle joint in an inversion sprain and in an eversion sprain. In which of the two sprains will the tarsal bones of the foot be made to contact a malleolus? Which of the two sprains is seen more commonly? Do you agree that most inversion accidents result in sprains while most eversion accidents result in fractures to the fibula?
2. Draw an outline of your foot on a piece of paper. Make a mark on the outline directly below each malleolus, and below the joint space between the navicular and first cuneiform bones. Finally, make a mark slightly lateral to the line of insertion of the gastrocnemius. Join the two malleoli marks with a straight line, and then join the remaining two marks with a straight line. The result should be a large *X* on the diagram which represents the two axes of the ankle joint. Label each quadrant-like area according to the movement of the ankle which will occur if a muscle in that quadrant contracts. For example, the medial-anterior quadrant should be labeled dorisflexion and inversion.
3. Palpate the tendons of the extrinsic muscles of the foot as they cross the ankle joint and locate them as precisely as possible on the diagram completed in Experience #2. Does your drawing show agreement with the actions stated in this chapter for the muscles concerned? Can you determine, from your drawing, whether the muscles will be relatively weak or strong movers according to their relationships to the two axes?
4. Examine the metatarsals of a human skeleton. Which metatarsal is longest? Now, rise on your toes (half-pointe) and note that the area of the ball of the foot which supports the greatest weight is under

the first and second metatarsals. Further examination of the skeleton will indicate that the first metatarsal is considerably larger than the second; the force of the body weight transmitted through the first metatarsal is thus spread over a larger area than is the case with the second metatarsal. Can you now determine why the ball of the foot under the second metatarsal often becomes sore and tender after wearing shoes with elevated heels? or after running or dancing with bare feet?

# 10 Muscles of Respiration

The thorax, as a unit, comprises the sternum, the costal cartilages, the ribs, and the thoracic vertebrae (fig. 10.1). The sternum consists of three portions—manubrium, body, and xiphoid process—which are joined by fibrocartilage and fibrous tissue. The manubrium supports the two clavicles through synovial joints of a modified ball-and-socket nature (see chap. 2) and articulates with the first rib by means of an immovable cartilaginous joint. The body of the sternum articulates with the costal cartilages of the second through the seventh ribs; these joints are synovial and nonaxial. The xiphoid process is the smallest of the three portions and is a thin, long cartilage which gradually ossifies with age.

The ribs are pliable bony arches which form the major part of the thorax. The first seven are designated *true ribs* because they articulate, through their costal cartilages, with the sternum. The lower five ribs are called *false ribs* and of these, the last two, being free at their anterior ends, are termed the *floating ribs*. The ribs have in common the characteristics of vertebral and sternal extremities, and a body. The vertebral extremity presents a tubercle which articulates with the transverse process of its thoracic vertebra, a head which articulates with the bodies of two adjacent vertebrae, and a flattened portion lateral to the head called *the neck*. Both articulations of the vertebral extremity are synovial and of the gliding type. The sternal extremity presents a shallow concavity into which the costal cartilage is inserted. The body of the rib is the bony expanse between the two extremities and is characterized by the internal and external surfaces, superior and inferior borders, and a point of sharpest curvature called the angle.

Movements of the thorax are mainly those of the ribs and are described as *elevation* and *depression*. These movements occur in conjunction with the breathing movements of inspiration and expiration. During inspiration, the ribs are elevated to enlarge the size of the thorax. During expiration, if breathing is at resting levels, the muscles relax and gravity depresses the ribs. No muscular contraction is required unless the expiration is forced. In this event, activity of the abdominals and rib depressors is required.

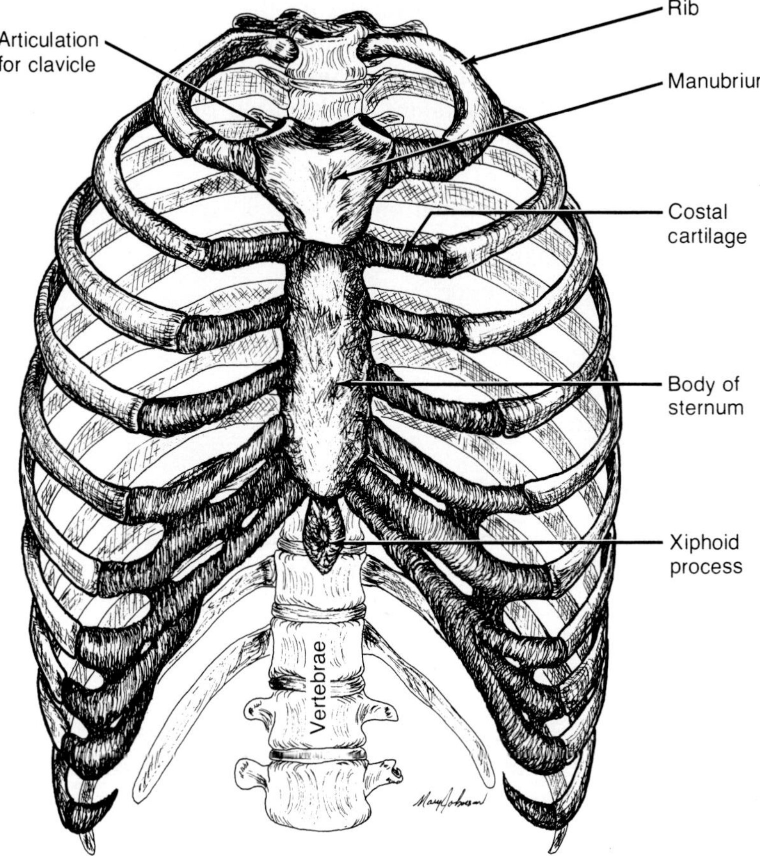


**Figure 10.1. The thorax, anterior view**

## Muscles of the Thorax

The muscles acting on the thorax during resting respiration are:

Diaphragm
External Intercostals
Internal Intercostals

Additional recruitment of the following muscles is necessary during forced inspiration:

Sternocleidomastoid
Levators costarum
Scaleni
Serratus posterior superior
Pectoralis minor
Trapezius Part 1
Levator scapulae
Rhomboids

These muscles combine actions to elevate the clavicle, scapula, and ribs in order to further increase the size of the thorax beyond that required by resting respiration. All of these muscles, with the exception of the serratus posterior superior, are discussed fully in chapters devoted to the shoulder joint or the spine and will not be duplicated in this chapter.

Muscles recruited to action during forced expiration are:

Internal intercostals
Serratus posterior inferior
Transversus abdominis
Transversus thoracis
Rectus abdominis
External oblique
Internal oblique
Quadratus lumborum

These muscles join in depressing the rib cage beyond that which is possible because of the passive depression accomplished by gravity, and the elasticity of the relaxed muscles of inspiration. Only the first four muscles listed above will be discussed in this section since the others have been covered fully under muscles of the spine.

**The Diaphragm** (di'aphragm) The diaphragm (fig. 10.2) is the dividing muscle between the thoracic and abdominal cavities. It is tendinous along its dome and muscular along its sides. It cannot be palpated.

*Origin* Like a circular rim, from the upper two lumbar vertebrae, the lumbar fascia, the inner portions of the last six ribs around to the inner surface of the xiphoid process of the sternum.

*Insertion* The central tendon which forms the dome of the muscle.

*Innervation* Phrenic nerve.

*Action* Depression of the central tendon which in turn increases the diameter of the thorax.

**External Intercostals** (exter'nal intercos'tals) The external intercostals are eleven thin sheets of fibers located between the ribs (fig. 10.3). They can be palpated on lean individuals anterior to the serratus anterior.

*Origin* Inferior border of the ribs.

*Insertion* Superior border of the rib below that of the rib of origin.

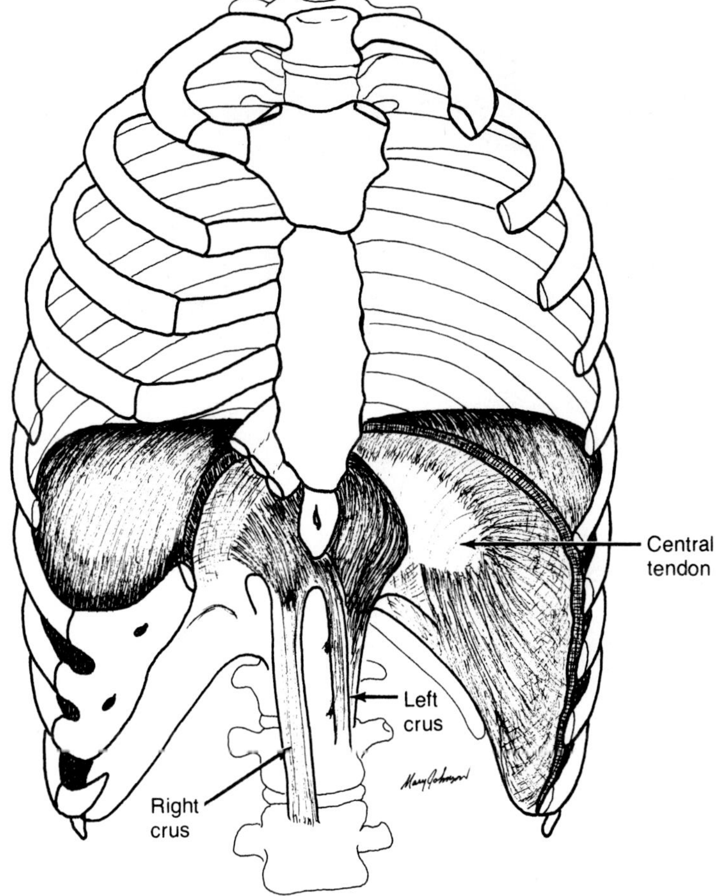


**Figure 10.2. Diaphragm, anterior view**

*Innervation* Intercostal nerves.

*Action* Elevation of the ribs thereby increasing the size of the thorax.

**Internal Intercostals** (inter'nal intercos'tals) The internal intercostals (fig. 10.3) are eleven sheets of muscular fibers located just beneath the external intercostals. The direction of their fibers is at right angles to that of their external counterparts. They cannot be palpated.

*Origin* Inner surface of a rib or its costal cartilage.

*Insertion* Superior surface of the rib below that of the origin.

*Innervation* Intercostal nerve.

*Action* Slight contraction during resting respiration; depression of the ribs during forced expiration in order to decrease the size of the thorax.

Figure 10.3. Intercostals, anterior view

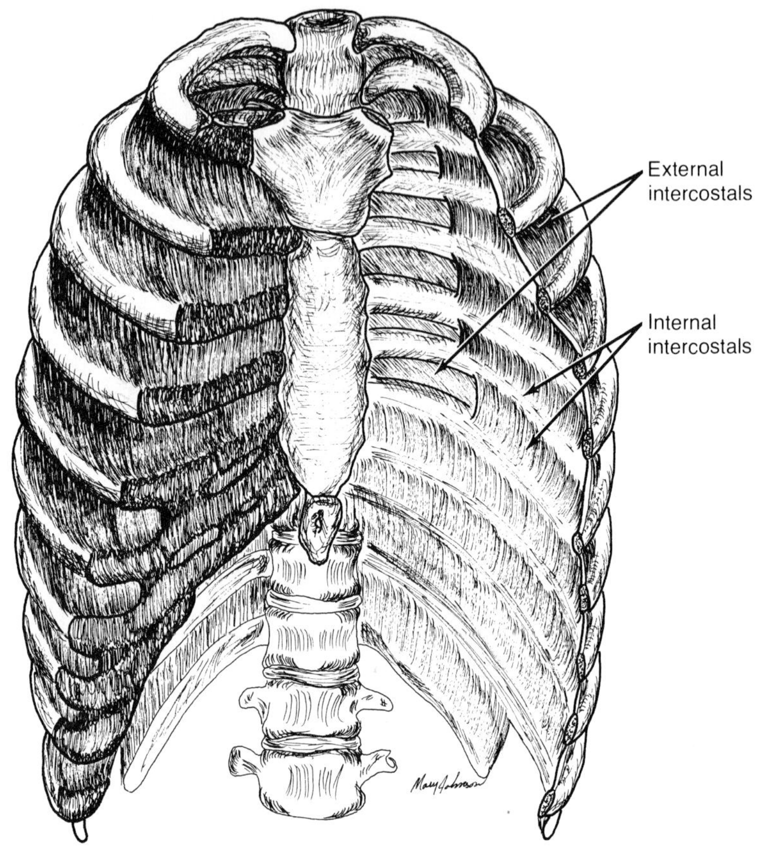


**Serratus Posterior Superior** (serra'tus poste'rior supe'rior) This muscle is comprised of a flat sheet of muscle fiber located beneath the scapula (fig. 10.4). It cannot be palpated.

*Origin* Posterior portion of the ligamentum nuchae; spinous processes of the last cervical and first two or three thoracic vertebrae.

*Insertion* Superior borders of the second through the fifth ribs in the vicinity of their angles.

*Innervation* First four thoracic nerves.

*Action* Elevation of the ribs on which the muscle is inserted, increasing the size of the thorax.

**Serratus Posterior Inferior** (serra'tus poste'rior infe'rior) The serratus posterior inferior (fig. 10.4) is located in the middle of the back. It is a second-layer muscle, lying beneath the trapezius and latissimus dorsi, and cannot be palpated.

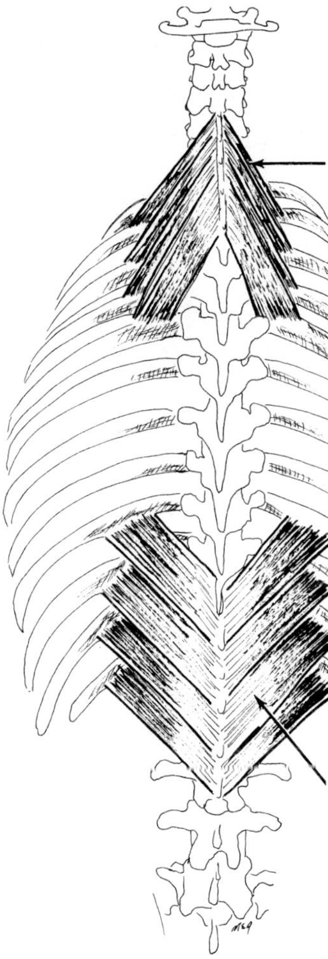

Figure 10.4. The serratus posterior muscles, posterior view



*Origin* Spinous processes of last two thoracic and first two or three lumbar vertebrae.

*Insertion* Inferior borders of lower four ribs in the vicinity of their angles.

*Innervation* Ninth to twelfth thoracic nerves.

*Action* Depression of the ribs on which the muscle inserts, acting mainly to neutralize the inward pull of the diaphragm.

**Transversus Abdominis** (transver'sus abdom'inis) The transversus abdominis (fig. 10.5) is the deepest of the abdominal muscles. It cannot be palpated.

Figure 10.5. Transversus abdominis, lateral view

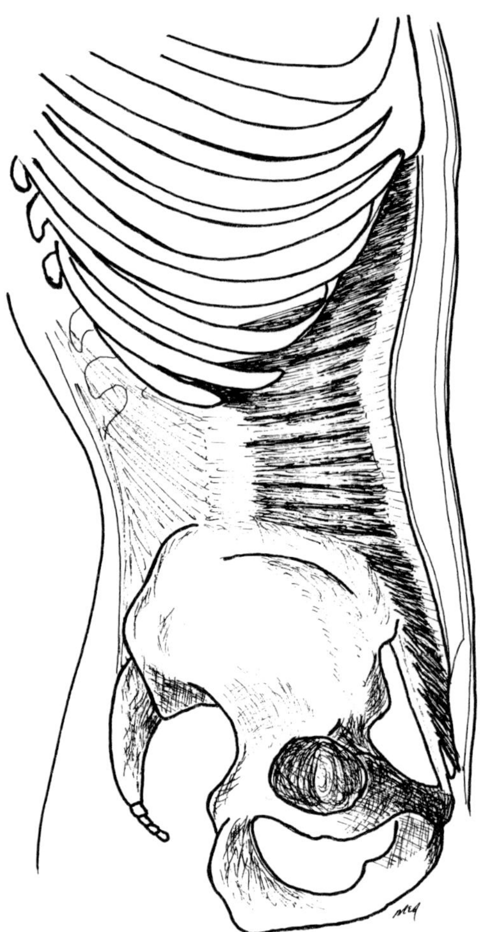

*Origin* Lateral portion of the inguinal ligament; inner portion of the iliac crest; thoracolumbar fascia; inner surfaces of last six ribs.

*Insertion* Linea alba.

*Innervation* Seventh to twelfth intercostal nerves; iliohypogastric and ilioinguinal nerves.

*Action* Compresses the abdomen during forced expiration.

**Transversus Thoracis** (transver'sus thora'cis) The transversus thoracis is a thin sheet of muscle and tendon located on the inner surface of the anterior wall of the thorax. It cannot be palpated.

*Origin* Posterior third of inner surface of the sternal body and xiphoid process; costal cartilages of last three or four true ribs.

*Insertion* Costal cartilages of second through sixth ribs.

*Innervation* Intercostal nerve.

*Action* Depresses the anterior portions of the ribs on which the muscle inserts, decreasing the size of the thorax.

## Comments

Respiration, when the body is at rest, involves low muscular activity. During exercise, however, the rib cage must be expanded to greater dimensions, and activity of the involved musculature increases surprisingly. The athlete, who, in the process of performing his sport, requires increased circumference of the thorax to accommodate his air-filled lungs, exhibits activitly in the muscles which are associated with forced inspiration. The expiration phase of thorax movement is, largely, a passive one, therefore the muscles of forced expiration are not recruited. Any muscle which is continuously active tends to hypertrophy. So it is with the muscles of inspiration, and since these muscles are located primarily in the region of the neck, they give rise to the thickness so frequently noted there.

## Laboratory Experiences

1. Palpate the sternocleidomastoid during forced inspiration. What degree of involvement in respiration do they have?
2. Determine, through palpation or electromyography the involvement of the superficial abdominal muscles during resting and forced expiration. What sports might entail the recruitment of the superficial abdominals to affect efficient respiration?

# Bibliography for Part 1


American Physical Therapy Association. "Focus on the lower back." *Physical Therapy* 59 (1979):965-1076.

Arnheim, D. D., and Schlaich, J. *Dance Injuries*. St. Louis: The C. V. Mosby Company, 1975.

Asmussen, E. "Movement of man and study of man in motion: A scanning review of the development of biomechanics." In *Biomechanics V-A,* ed. P. V. Komi. Baltimore: University Park Press, 1976.

Barham, N. J., and Wooten, E. P. *Structural Kinesiology*. New York: Macmillan Company, 1973.

Basmajian, J. V. *Muscles Alive*. 3rd ed., Baltimore: The Williams & Wilkins Company, 1974.

Brantigan, O. C. *Clinical Anatomy*. New York: McGraw-Hill Book Company, 1963.

Broer, M. R. *Efficiency of Human Movement*. 2d ed. Philadelphia: W. B. Saunders Company, 1966.

Brunnstrom, S. *Clinical Kinesiology*. 3d ed. Philadelphia: F. A. Davis Company, 1972.

Clayson, S. J.; Newman, I. M.; Debevec, D. F.; Anger, R. W.; Skowland, H. V.; and Kottke, F. J. "Evaluation of mobility of hip and lumbar vertebrae of normal young women." *Archives of Physical Medicine and Rehabilitation* 43 (1962):1-8.

Close, J. R. *Motor Function in the Lower Extremity*. Springfield, Ill.: Charles C Thomas Publisher, 1964.

Crowe, P.; O'Connell, A. L.; and Gardner, E. B. "An electromyographic study of the role of the abdominal muscles and certain hip flexors during sit-ups." Report presented at the National Convention of the American Association for Health, Physical Education, and Recreation, Minneapolis, Minn., 1963.

deVries, H. A. "Muscle tonus in postural muscles." *American Journal of Physical Medicine* 44(1965):275-91.

DeSousa, O. M.; DeMoraes, J. L.; and Vieria, F. L. deM. "Electromyographic study of the brachioradialis muscle." *Anatomical Record* 139 (1961):125-31.

Duvall, E. N. *Kinesiology: The Anatomy of Motion*. Englewood Cliffs, N.J.: Prentice-Hall, 1959.

Eaton, R. G. *Joint Injuries of the Hand*. Springfield, Ill.: Charles C Thomas Publisher, 1971.

Edington, D. W., and Edgerton, V. R. *The Biology of Physical Activity*. Boston: Houghton Mifflin Company, 1976.

Evans, F. G. *Biomechanical Studies of the Musculo-Skeletal System*. Springfield, Ill.: Charles C Thomas Publisher, 1961.

Featherstone, D. F. *Dancing Without Danger*. Cranbury, N.J.: A. S. Barnes & Company, 1970.

Fischer, F. J., and Houtz, S. J. "Evaluation of the function of the gluteus maximus muscle." *American Journal of Physical Medicine* 47:(1968): 182-91.

Flint, M. M. "An electromyographic comparison of the function of the iliacus and the rectus abdominis muscles." *Journal of American Physical Therapy Association* 45(1965):248-52.

Floyd, W. F., and Silver, P. H. S. "Electromyographic study of patterns of activity of the anterior abdominal wall muscles in man." *Journal of Anatomy* 84(1950):132-45.

Freedman, L., and Munro, R. R. "Abduction of the arm in the scapular plane; scapular and glenohumeral movements." *Journal of Bone and Joint Surgery* 48A(1966):1503-10.

Giannestras, N. J. *Foot Disorders Medical and Surgical Management.* 2d ed. Philadelphia: Lea & Febiger, 1973.

Goss, C. M. *Gray's Anatomy of the Human Body.* 29th ed. Philadelphia: Lea & Febiger, 1973.

Harris, M. L. "Flexibility," (Review of Literature). *Journal of American Physical Therapy Association* 49(1969):491-601.

Hlavac, H. F. *The Foot Book.* Mountain View, Calif.: World Publications, 1977.

Herman, R., and Bragin, S. J. "Function of the gastrocnemius and soleus muscles." *Journal of American Physical Therapy Association* 47(1967): 105-13.

Hopper, B. J. *The Mechanics of Human Movement.* New York: American Elsevier Publishing Company, 1973.

Holland, G. J. The physiology of flexibility; a review of the literature. In *Kinesiology Review.* Washington, D.C.: American Association of Health, Physical Education, and Recreation, 1968.

Hollinshead, W. H. "Anatomy of the spine." *Journal of Bone and Joint Surgery* 47A(1965):209-15.

———. *Functional Anatomy of the Limbs and Back.* 3d ed. Philadelphia: W. B. Saunders Company, 1969.

House, E. L., and Pansky, B. *A Functional Approach to Neuroanatomy,* 3rd ed. New York: McGraw-Hill Book Company, 1979.

Inman, V. T. "The shoulder as a functional unit." *Journal of Bone and Joint Surgery* 44A(1962):977-78.

Inman, V. T.; Saunders, J. B. deC. M.; and Abbott, L. C. "Observations on the function of the shoulder joint." *Journal of Bone and Joint Surgery* 26(1944):1-30.

Jensen, C. R., and Schultz, G. W. *Applied Kinesiology.* New York: McGraw-Hill Book Company, 1970.

Kendall, H. O.; Kendall, F. P.; and Wadsworth, G. E. *Muscles Testing and Function* 2d ed. Baltimore: The Williams & Wilkins Company, 1971.

Kent, B. "Functional anatomy of the shoulder complex." *Journal of American Physical Therapy Association* 51(1971):867-88.

Klein, K. K. "The knee and the ligaments." *Journal of Bone and Joint Surgery* 44A(1962):1191-92.

Klein, K. K., and Allman, F. L. *The Knee in Sports.* Austin, Tex.: Jenkins Publishing Company, 1969.

LaBan, M. M.; Raptou, A. D.; and Johnson, E. W. "Electromyographic study of function of iliopsoas muscle." *Archives of Physical Medicine and Rehabilitation* 46(1965):676-79.

Larson, R. F. "Forearm positioning on maximal elbow-flexor force." *Journal of American Physical Therapy Association* 49(1969):748-56.

Lewis, R. W. *The Joints of the Extremities.* Springfield, Ill.: Charles C Thomas Publisher, 1955.

Logan, G. A., and McKinney, W. C. *Kinesiology.* Dubuque, Iowa: Wm. C. Brown Company Publishers, 1970.

Lucas, G. L. *Examination of the Hand.* Springfield, Ill.: Charles C Thomas Publisher, 1972.

MacConail, M. A., and Basmajian, J. V. *Muscles and Movements: A Basis for Human Kinesiology.* Baltimore: The Williams & Wilkins Company, 1969.

McCraw, L. W. "Effects of variations of forearm position in elbow flexion." *Research Quarterly* 35(1964):504-10.

Merrifield, H. H. "An electromyographic study of the gluteus maximus, the vastus lateralis and the tensor fasciae latae." *Dissertation Abstracts* 21 (1961):1833.

Michele, A. A. *Iliopsoas Development of Anomalies in Man.* Springfield, Ill.: Charles C Thomas Publisher, 1962.

Morris, C. B. "The measurement of the strength of muscle relative to the cross section." *Research Quarterly* 19(1948):295-303.

Quiring, D. P., and Warfel, J. H. *The Head, Neck, and Trunk.* 2d ed. Philadelphia: Lea and Febiger, 1960.

-----. *The Extremities.* 2d ed. Philadelphia: Lea and Febiger, 1960.

Partridge, M. J., and Walters, C. E. "Participation of the abdominal muscles in various movements of the trunk in man." *Physical Therapy Review* 39(1959):791-800.

Pauly, J. E. "An electromyographic analysis of certain movements and exercises. I. Some deep muscles of the back." *Anatomical Record* 155 (1966):223-34.

Pauly, J. E.; Rushing, J. L.; and Scheving, L. E. "An electromyographic study of some muscles crossing the elbow joint." *Anatomical Record* 159(1967):47-53.

Perrott, J. W. *Structural and Functional Anatomy.* 3rd ed. Great Britain: Edward Arnold, Ltd., 1977.

Pocock, G. S. "Electromyographic study of the quadriceps during resistive exercise." *Journal of American Physical Therapy Association* 43(1963): 427-34.

Rasch, P. J., and Burke, R. K. *Kinesiology and Applied Anatomy.* 5th ed. Philadelphia: Lea and Febiger, 1974.

Root, M. L.; Orien, W. P.; and Weed, J. H. *Normal and Abnormal Function of the Foot,* vol. 2. Los Angeles: Clinical Biomechanics Corporation, 1977.

Root, M. L.; Orien, W. P.; Weed, J. H.; and Hughes, R. J. *Biomechanical Examination of the Foot,* vol. 1. Los Angeles: Clinical Biomechanics Corporation, 1971.

Shevlin, M. G.; Lehmann, J. F.; and Lucci, J. A. "Electromyographic study of the function of some muscles crossing the glenohumeral joint." *Archives of Physical Medicine and Rehabilitation* 50(1969):264-70.

Singleton, M. C. "Functional anatomy of the shoulder." *Journal of American Physical Therapy Association* 46(1966):1043-51.

Singleton, M. C., and LeVeau, B. F. "The hip joint: structure, stability, and stress." *Journal of American Physical Therapy Association* 55(1975): 957-73.

Steindler, A. *Kinesiology of the Human Body Under Normal and Pathological Conditions.* Springfield, Ill.: Charles C Thomas Publisher, 1955.

Subotnick, S. I. *Podiatric Sports Medicine.* Mount Kisco, N.Y.: Futura Publishing Company, Incorporated, 1975.

Subotnick, S. I. *The Running Foot Doctor*. Mountain View, Calif.: World Publications, 1977.

Sweigard, L. E. *Human Movement Potential: Its Ideokinetic Facilitation*. New York: Dodd, Mead & Company, 1974.

Walters, C. E., and Partridge, M. J. "Electromyographic study of the differential action of the abdominal muscles during exercise." *American Journal of Physical Medicine* 36(1957):259-68.

Wheatley, M. S., and Jahnke, W. D. "Electromyographic study of the superficial thigh and hip muscles in normal individuals." *Archives of Physical Therapy* 31(1951):508-22.

Williams, M., and Lissner, H. *Biomechanics of Human Motion*. Philadelphia: W. B. Saunders Company, 1962.

**PART 2**

# Mechanical Aspects of Human Motion

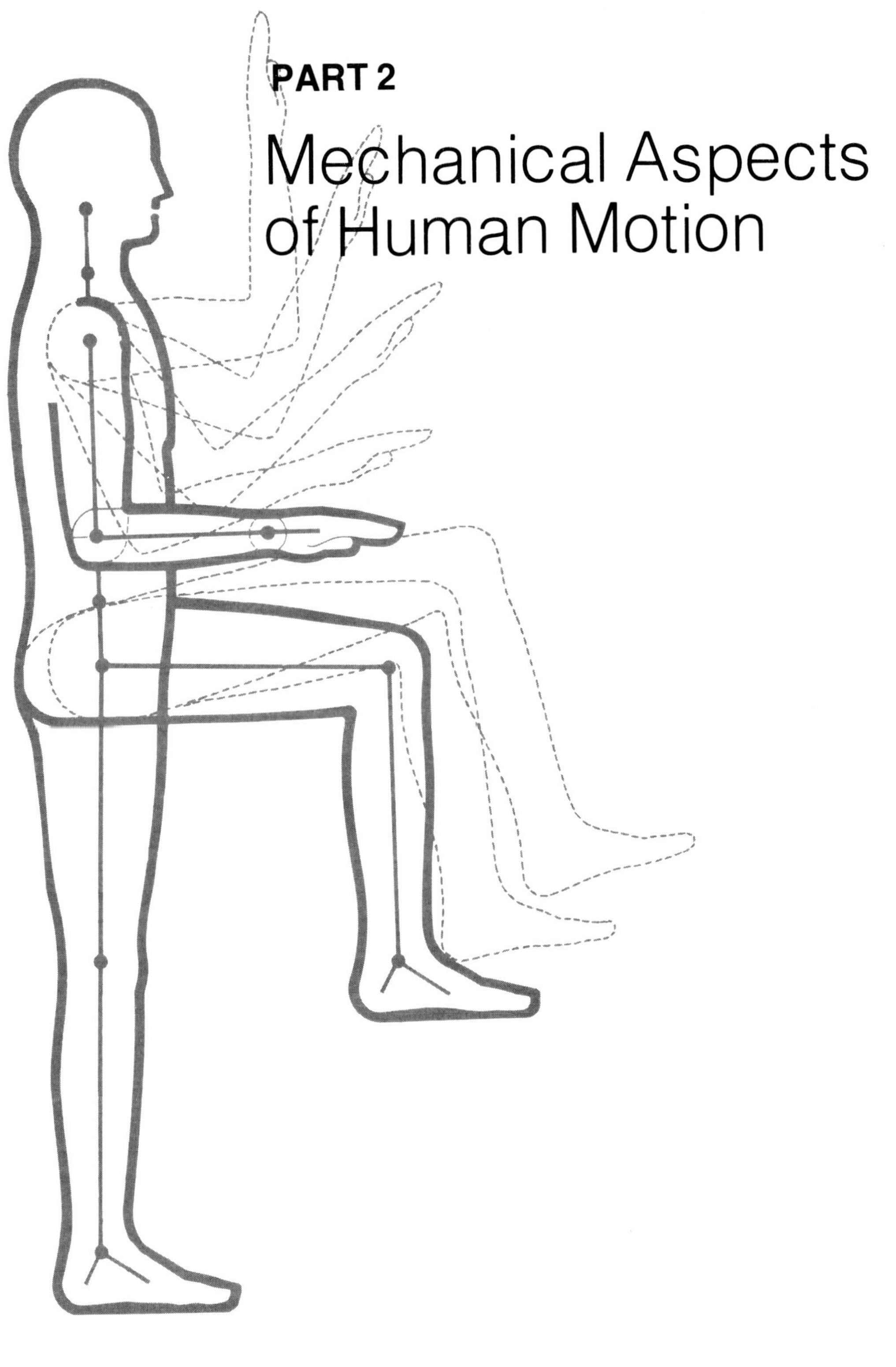

# 11

# Terminology and Basic Concepts

The mechanics of movement deal with motion which results from the application of a force; no regard is given to the nature of the muscular involvement which produced the force. A projectile is studied as it travels the curvilinear path it selects according to its angle and velocity of projection. It does not matter that the projectile is a shot, a football, or a basketball; nor does it matter how the object was pushed, kicked, or thrown into space. By the same token, the efficiency with which it was propelled is of no interest. The effect of spin on a ball is investigated similarly. No regard is given either to the type of ball involved or to the technique used in imparting the spin.

The topics of mechanics to be discussed in the following pages are those which are believed to be most important to coaches, teachers, and performers alike. They include stability, motion, Newton's Laws, projection, spin and rebound, and fluids. Discussions have been kept as free of the mathematics of mechanics as possible. However, where included for use in the verification of the concepts presented, the mathematics have been simplified.

Most of the terminology required to understand the following discussions is included, with definitions and examples, in the chapters devoted to the topics. There are, however, a few terms which are considered basic to all of the mechanical concepts; they appear below.

## Leverage Systems

The mechanics of the three leverage systems were discussed fully in chapter 2; however, the major applications of these systems pertained to the anatomical aspects of movement. For that reason, the principles of leverage will only be reviewed here, but will be applied more specifically to the mechanical aspects of human movement.

First, second, and third class leverage systems comprise a rigid bar (the lever) and the components of force *(F)*, resistance *(R)*, and an axis of rotation *(A)*. Leverage systems are differentiated by the placement of the components along the rigid bar. The first class lever presents the axis between the force and resistance; second and third class levers present the resistance and force, respectively, between the remaining two components. A child's seesaw is an example of a first class lever; a wheelbarrow exemplifies the second class system; and a shovel is a third class lever. Numerous other examples can be found among implements of common use—pliers, scissors, and pry bars are all first class systems; fireplace bellows and nutcrackers are second class systems; tennis rackets, golf clubs, baseball bats, and other such sports implements provide third class leverage.

A lever is considered to includes two arms; the moment arm *(MA)* is the perpendicular distance between the line of force application and axis of the lever; and the resistance arm *(RA)* is the perpendicular distance between the line of resistance and the lever's axis. Figures 11.1, 11.2, and 11.3 illustrate the three leverage classes in both horizontal and off-horizontal positions. It will be seen that it is only when the

Figure 11.1. First class lever

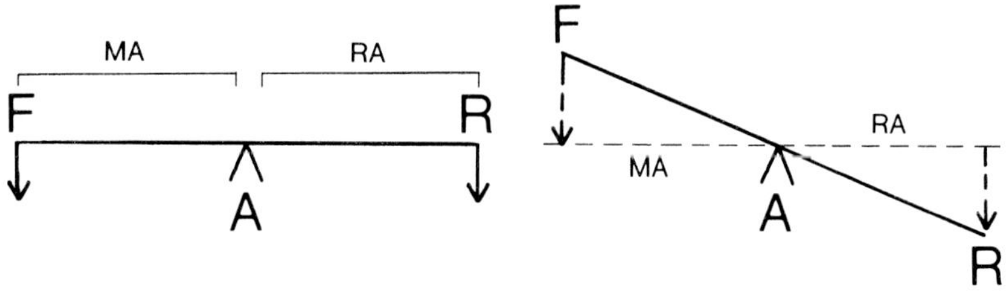

Figure 11.2. Second class lever

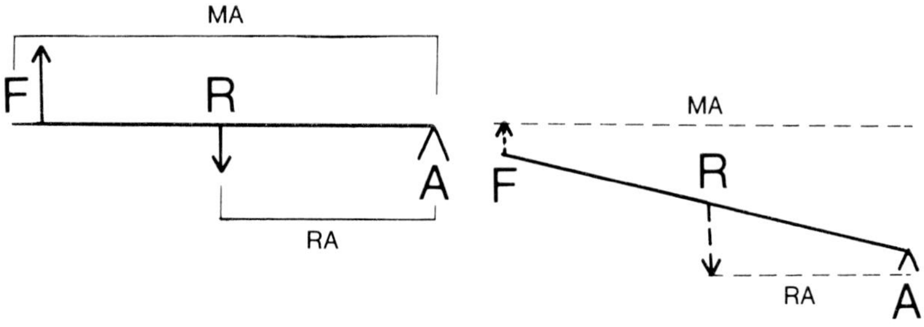

Figure 11.3. Third class lever

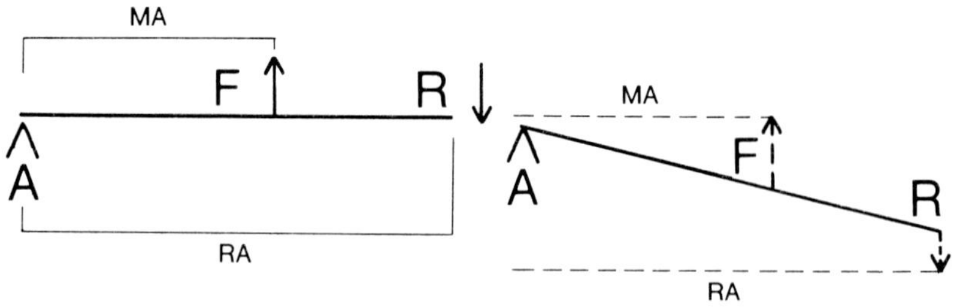

lines of force and resistance are applied at right angles to the lever that the length of the two arms coincide with the actual lever length.

Leverage calculations can be made easily by the use of the formula:

$$F \cdot MA = R \cdot RA$$

If any three of the terms in the formula are known, the fourth can be calculated; thus, if it is known that a weight of 10 kg *(R)* is located perpendicularly 20 cm from the axis *(RA)* and a force is to be applied 40 cm from that axis, it can be found that the force required to balance the lever will be 5 kg. The formula holds true for all classes of levers.

The ratio of moment arm to resistance arm *(MA/RA)* is known as the mechanical advantage of the lever and indicates the number of units of resistance that will be balanced by one unit of force. If a lever comprises a moment arm of two meters and a resistance arm of one meter, its mechanical advantage is 2/1 or 2; for every unit of force applied, two units of resistance can be balanced. If the reverse were true, that is, if the moment arm were one meter in length and the resistance arm measured two meters, the mechanical advantage would be ½. For every unit of force applied, only ½ of a unit of resistance would be balanced.

The product of force and moment arm ($F \times MA$) is termed the *moment of force* or the *torque* of the lever. Increases either in the amount of force applied or the length of the moment arm will increase the moment of force or torque of the lever and enable it to balance a greater resistance or the same resistance at a longer resistance arm. A statement such as, "slide backward slightly on the seesaw to improve the moment," is simply a different way of saying that leverage can be improved by increasing the length of the moment arm.

Study of the configuration of the three levers will indicate that second class levers will always yield mechanical advantages greater than one, since regardless of the placement of the resistance along the lever, the moment arm will be longer than the resistance arm. Conversely, the mechanical advantage of a third class lever will always be less than one, for regardless of the point of force application, the moment arm will be shorter than the resistance arm. First class levers can provide mechanical advantages of either less than one or greater than one depending upon the location of the axis.

Second class levers are known, because of their mechanical advantage, as forceful levers, third class levers forsake force for speed. The human body, with its predominance of third class levers, is capable of generating great speeds during movement but is relatively weak when force is required.

A final look at the four terms comprising the leverage formula will show that if a lever is unable to complete a task, one or more of four adjustments must be made. Force can be increased, resistance can be decreased, and the moment arm can be elongated, or the resistance arm can be shortened. To the athlete, some of these adjustments are more feasible than others. Since resistances encountered in sports and dance are frequently prescribed by official rule, it is fallacious to consider lessening resistance by decreasing their weights. A shot, discus, football, baseball must all conform to standards or they cannot be used. Consideration should be given, however, to appropriate selection of equipment which does afford a range of weight. Tennis rackets, bowling balls, bats, golf clubs should all be chosen carefully so that their respective weights will match the abilities of the athletes (see chapter 13, The Second Law, for additional discussion).

Manipulation of the length of the resistance arm is, for some performers, a possibility for gaining success. A tennis player is instructed, when volleying, to "choke up" on the racket by moving the hand toward the top of the grip. The resistance arm is thus shortened and the force of the opponent's stroke can be better controlled. Baseball and softball batters are instructed similarly when they swing late because of overly heavy bats.

It is perhaps the two components, *force* and *moment arm,* that are adjusted most frequently by performers who wish to increase leverage. Increments of force can be made by increasing muscular strength, lengthening the distance over which the force is applied, decreasing the time of muscular contraction, and patterning the movement so it becomes sequential. Each of these is discussed in following paragraphs and is applied to selected sport or dance movements.

*Increasing Muscular Strength* Whereas a review of the various methods for gaining strength is beyond the scope of this text, a principle common to all programs should be mentioned. The principle is that of "overload" and states that a muscle, if it is to gain strength must contract to its maximum capacity. The contraction may be dynamic or static, and if it is dynamic, it may be concentric or eccentric; regardless, the muscle must be tensed, and tensed maximally. Where maximal contractions are of the concentric, or shortening type, tension of the muscle is developed by attempting to approximate its attachments (origin and insertion); thus, the muscle to be strengthened must be the agonist or mover. Where maximal contractions are static the muscle to be strengthened is still the agonist and attempts to approximate its attachments; however, its resistance is so great that the muscle cannot overcome it. To strengthen the brachialis, for example, the muscle must be made to attempt to pull its insertion closer to its origin, or vice versa, with the greatest tension of which it is capable. The result will be an attempt at flexion of the elbow joint. If the applied resistance can be overcome, a dynamic contraction occurs. If the resistance cannot be overcome a static or isometric contraction occurs. When either of these contractions is performed under appropriate programs strength will be gained.

Muscular strength is said to be specific to the requirements of the task to be performed. The male dancer who is capable of elevating his body to great heights during a leap is not necessarily capable of elevating his partner's body in lifts. Similarly, the ability to execute heavier and heavier bench presses in the weight room does not ensure that a shot-putter will throw farther and farther. It appears logical to employ the same movement patterns in strength-gaining programs as those for which the strength is being gained.

*Decreasing the Time of Muscular Contraction* Quick muscular contractions require more energy than do slow ones; however, it is only through such rapid contractions that our bony levers can be made to generate high rates of speed. The successful place kick in soccer or football is dependent, in part, on the ability of the kicker to move the levers of the leg quickly through the kicking pattern. Similarly, the contribution of the hips to the forcefulness of a golf swing can be greatly enhanced if they are pivoted forward quickly.

*Sequential Movement.* When relatively light sports implements are thrown, kicked, or hurled into space, the force of their projection can be increased if the body parts involved are made to move in the proper sequence. Since the force applied by an object or body depends upon both its mass and acceleration, it can be seen that heavier body parts can generate great forces even though they cannot be moved rapidly. Lighter body parts, however, must be moved very rapidly to make up for their lack of mass. The structure of the human body is such that its heavy portions (hips and shoulders) are centrally located and its lighter portions are located progressively more distal to the center; yet it is with the least heavy portions, the hand and foot, that final forces are delivered to sports objects. Proper sequence of body action must necessitate, then, the movement of the heaviest portion first, followed in turn by the next heaviest portion, in order that each can atone for its loss of mass by sharing the speed of the portions preceding it. The hips will move first, followed in order by the shoulders, upper arm, lower arm, and wrist as the overhand throw is executed. The same sequence prevails during the golf swing, discus throw, shot put, and tennis drive, and is seen to generalize to kicking patterns in that, again, the heavier segments contribute initially to the generation of force with the lighter segments being the last and the fastest of the moving segments.

## Scalar and Vector Quantities

A scalar quantity is one which is characterized by magnitude only. A vector quantity has both magnitude and direction, and can, therefore, be represented graphically as explained in chapter 2. Examples of scalar quantities are mass, distance, speed, and volume; their vector counterparts are weight, displacement, velocity, and pressure. Mass is used to refer to the size or bulk of an object and is equal to weight divided by the acceleration of gravity.*

$$\text{Mass} = \frac{\text{weight (kg)}}{\text{gravity (meters per sec}^2\text{)}}$$

$$= \frac{\text{weight (kg)}}{9.8 \text{ m/sec}^2}$$

The resulting unit is called a *slug*, and can be thought of as that unit of mass which will be accelerated positively at 9.8 meters per second$^2$ when a force of one kilogram is applied.

Weight, on the other hand, comprises magnitude (kilograms, pounds) and direction (toward the center of the earth) to fulfill the prerequisites of a vector quantity. Whereas it is incorrect semantically and mathematically to interchange the words *mass* and *weight*, the two can be conceptualized as equivalents. Since, to calculate mass, weight is divided by the constant representing gravity's pull, weight and mass are proportional to each other; i.e., as weight increases, so will mass. When *mass* is seen in a formula, then, it can be thought of as a representative of weight, and conceptualized thusly.

Distance, another example of a scalar quantity, has magnitude only with no assumption of direction. Distance can be reported simply as a number of units—5 meters—with no reference made to whether the distance lies to the north, south, east, or west. Displacement, on the other hand, is a vector quantity and is, therefore, accompanied by both magnitude and direction. Because of this, displacement can be represented by vectors that can be composed or resolved according to the same procedures that pertain to force vectors.

*The law of gravity is discussed in chapter 13.

As mentioned above, speed (80 kilometers per hour) and volume (a liter of gasoline) are scalar quantities, while velocity (10 meters per second moving from point A to point B) and pressure (300 Newtons per square meter acting in a downward direction) are vector quantities. The latter two may also be represented by arrows that can be composed or resolved.

At this point, it will be helpful for the reader to refer to chapter 2 for a brief review of composition of vectors. It will be noted that the discussion there is limited to the linear case. This was done because knowledge of linear vectors, particularly force vectors, is sufficient for exploring anatomical kinesiology. It is possible, however, to represent angular vector quantities by arrows also. The method for doing so is known as the *right-hand thumb* rule.

Consider the movement of the minute hand on your wristwatch, and, after curling the fingers of your right hand, place them over the dial of the watch. Notice that the direction of the curled fingers is in the opposite direction to movement of the minute hand. Now place the fingers on the back of the watch. The direction of the finger curl is the same as that of the minute hand. Extension of the thumb will serve to represent the direction of a vector scaled to the angular velocity (360° per hour) of the minute hand. It will also denote the direction of a velocity vector for the second hand of your watch. The length of the vector will be longer, of course (60 times longer), since the second hand has a velocity of 360° per minute.

Spiraling footballs can easily be depicted by angular vectors if the right-hand thumb rule is applied. A ball spinning in a counterclockwise direction (when viewed from behind) is accompanied by a vector perpendicular to its long axis and directed through the rear of the ball; clockwise spin velocity is denoted by a vector directed through the nose of the ball.

Angular vectors can be composed and resolved for all quantities except angular displacement. Composition and resolution of displacement vectors will yield results exactly opposite to true direction.

It is unfortunate (or fortunate?) that angular vectors are used so infrequently by kinesiologists and biomechanists. A much more common means of describing angular motion is in terms of degrees, radians, or revolutions per time unit. Further discussion of these descriptors may be found in chapter 14.

Volume, another example of a scalar quantity, is seen to have magnitude only with no assumption made as to direction. Pressure, however, has both magnitude and a direction of application.

## Friction

Friction refers to the ease with which one surface moves on another. Athletes and dancers find themselves attempting to reduce or increase friction to meet the demands of the activity. Footwear is chosen according to its properties of friction; spikes and cleats are worn to increase ground friction, but ice skates are chosen for their ability to reduce friction.

Smoother surfaces generate less friction than do rough surfaces; however, microscopic examination of even the smoothest of surfaces will reveal surprising roughness that can inhibit successful performance. Bowlers, gymnasts, and dancers often revert to use of chalk or powder to fill in rough depressions of balls, bars, and floors in order to decrease friction of contact. Conversely, baseball pitchers and basketball players use a sticky resin to increase friction between the hand and ball.

It is, perhaps, surprising that friction between dry surfaces is independent of the size of the contacting areas. Small and large shoes, and small and large hands apply the same amounts of friction provided the force of application is the same. It is much more profitable to change the type of surface rather than the size of surface when dealing with dry friction.

Amounts of friction can be quantified by a number known as the coefficient of friction. The coefficient is actually the tangent of the angle of lean an object can take before its base slips on the supporting surface. If the object is an athlete and the supporting surface is the ground, the angle of possible lean will attest to the amount of friction provided by his or her footwear.

Coefficients of friction can range, theoretically, between zero and infinity. Practically, however, there is no such thing as zero friction nor is there great possibility of infinite friction. Since the coefficient is proportional to friction (that is, the greater the coefficient, the greater the friction), it is not reasonable to expect a situation in which even the smallest lean would cause slipping. It is equally unreasonable to expect that a performer could lean to as far as a 90° angle without slipping. More realistic lean angles are between 10 degrees (coefficient of .18) and 50 degrees (coefficient of 1.2). The former are characteristic of the forward leans of short-distance runners and the latter represent the precarious leans of basketball players making sharp and quick direction changes.

It is clear that appropriate selection of footwear is requisite to success in performing sport and dance techniques. The dancer, however, is more limited in this respect than is the sports performer. Whereas a track runner, basketball player, etc. is able to choose shoes that will meet the demands of the sport, the dancer is limited to a relatively constant type of footwear—or lack of it. When the ballet shoe or the bare foot cannot offer required amounts of friction, it is the activity that must be altered rather than the type of shoe.

Friction, as it is related to centripetal force, is discussed in chapter 14.

# 12 Stability

A body is stable only when its center of mass is over its base of support. In a position of stability the line of gravity, a perpendicular line dropped from the center of mass, must intersect the supportive base (fig. 12.1). If the body is tilted sufficiently to cause the line of gravity to fall outside the base of support, the body will seek another base (fig. 12.2).

The statements above describe, in the manner of a definition, the concept of stability or static equilibrium. The importance of this concept is far reaching in sports and dance both because of the frequent necessity to maintain stability and also to destroy it for the sake of mobility. The ballerina on pointe is faced with a difficult problem as she seeks to control her center so that the line of gravity continues to pass through the exceedingly small base of support afforded by the toe of her shoe. Conversely, the sprinter in track, who must take a position of stability for the start, aligns body parts to assure that the line of gravity intersects his base of support but falls precariously close to its front edge. The slightest forward lean will cause the line to fall ahead of the base and stability is sacrificed for mobility to begin the race.

The sprinter affords us also with a third condition; that is, the maintenance of instability. Here, the criterion of success is not to regain stability but rather to control the running lean of the body so that each successive step is an attempt to "catch up" with the center of mass. The more the lean, the faster must be the steps taken; similarly, the slower one wishes to run—or walk— the less the lean required to keep the line of gravity moving ahead of the supporting foot. But lean we must, even though in slow locomotion it may be imperceptible.

Stability is perhaps most complicated for those who must begin a skill in the stable posture, then lose it in order to cover space, and finally regain it for the conclusion of the skill. Such would be the case for the vaulter in gymnastics. Having begun the vault in an erect posture, the approach run is initiated by the lean. Instability then becomes the condition and is maintained until the vault is completed and the ending pose is to be taken. At this point, the body alignment must be adjusted to a backward lean which allows the feet to pass under and ahead of the center. The center must then play "catch up" with the

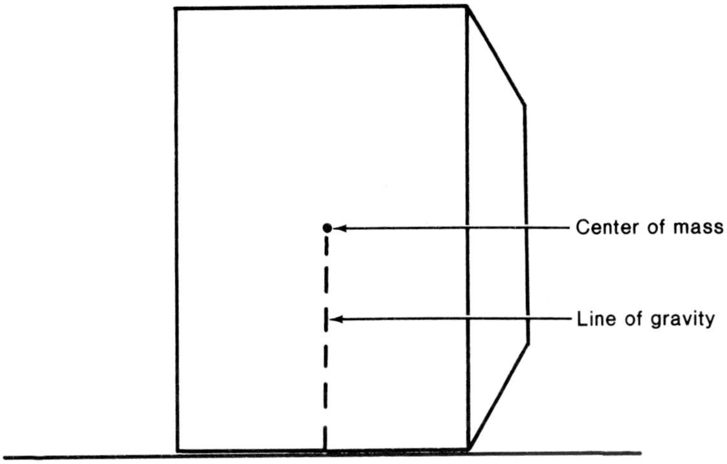

Figure 12.1. An object with stability

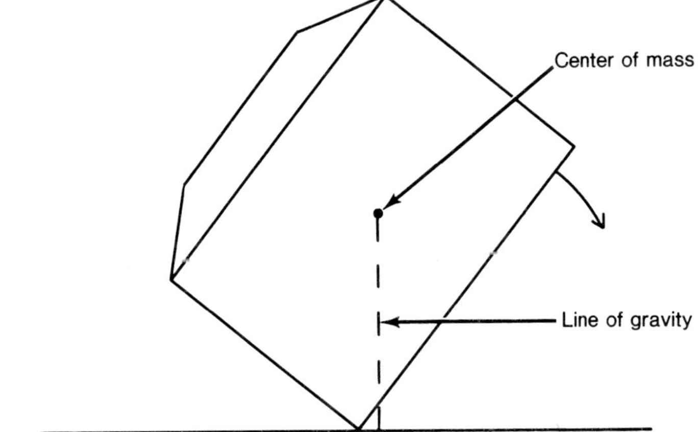


Figure 12.2. An unstable object

base of support and when it does, stability is regained. It is obvious that the timing required must be precise; it is small wonder that so often an additional side or forward step must be taken to gain control of the center's momentum.

Several principles present themselves in the study of stability. One of these can be identified through the examination of the various bases of support employed in sports and dance activities. When the stances of the archer, golfer, and baseball batter are considered, two points of commonality will be noted. In each case the feet are spread, and they are placed side-to-side. Comparison of the stances, at the moment of ball release, of the bowler, softball pitcher, and the basketball player performing a chest pass illustrates again that the feet are spread, but in a front-to-back direction. In all of these activities, the base of support has been enlarged to provide additional stability to the performer in that the line of gravity must travel farther before it falls outside the base. A principle emerges: the larger the base of support of an object, the more stable it is. Effective use can be made of this principle regardless of whether the criterion of success in a skill is stability or instability. The beginning tumbler can more easily achieve the balanced position of a headstand when he is reminded to form a triangle with the head and two hands rather than to place the head between and in line with the hands. The badminton player can profit also from the knowledge of this principle which instructs him, conversely, to maintain a small base of support so he can react quickly to the flight of the shuttlecock.

Mention has been made of the sprinter in track who must be stable during the starting position but who must be able, in the shortest amount of time possible, to become mobile. His position of stability dictates that the line of gravity will intersect his base, but near the edge over which the line will subsequently be directed to achieve mobility. Identical problems of stance are met by competitive swimmers who affect their starts from blocks and by football players just before the ball is snapped. The opposite problem confronts the anchor man in a gymnastic pyramid. He seeks to maintain the stability of his starting position and thus centers the line of gravity over the base so he can make necessary adjustments before the line can fall outside the edge. This second principle of stability states that the more nearly the line of gravity falls at the center of the base, the more stable the body.

A brief look at a fencer, a backpacker, and a dancer will afford insight to a third principle (fig. 12.3). When on guard, the classical stance of the fencer provides that the foil is held in front of and well away from the body in the preferred hand. The nonpreferred arm is held to the rear with the shoulder in abduction and the elbow and wrist in flexion. The position of the nonpreferred arm is one of compensation for the weight of the foil. Were it not for this compensation, the center of mass and its line would be "pulled" by the foil to a point close to the forward edge of the base, and the fencer would find difficulty in controlling his advance as well as in initiating a retreat. So it is with the backpacker who must lean forward at the hips to compensate for the backward shift of his center caused by the weight of the pack. The dancer, though not usually encumbered by external weights, yields further evidence of the validity of compensation. During such techniques as the arabesque and grand battement, the arms are positioned to compensate for the weight of the elevated leg.

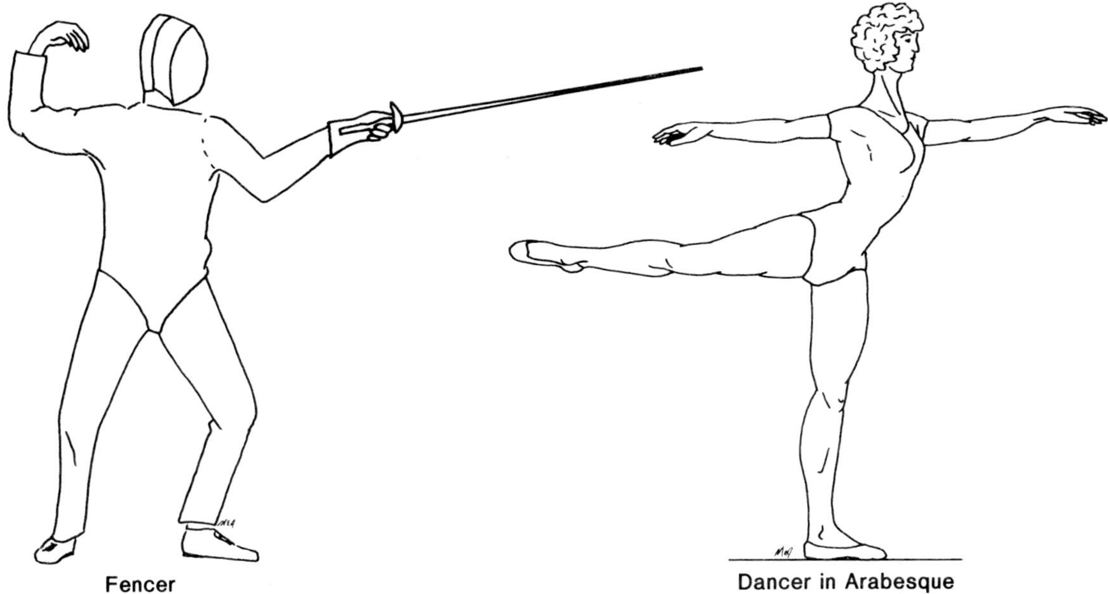


The third principle becomes: when an external weight is added anywhere to the body, except directly above or below the center of mass, the line of gravity shifts toward the weight, and compensatory movements are required to re-establish its alignment over the center of the base. Movement of a body part away from the midline causes the same effect as the addition of an external weight. This principle is important also to therapists and to physical educators in adapted and developmental areas of specialization when they work with amputees. Amputation of a limb causes the center to migrate to the opposite or "heavier" side. The amputee is unaccustomed to the new position of the center and must relearn the feeling of stability. Those who sustain the loss of both legs present a center of gravity at about the xiphoid process, and when they are placed in wheelchairs, must exercise caution when reaching for or picking up items so that they do not overlean the chair's base of support.

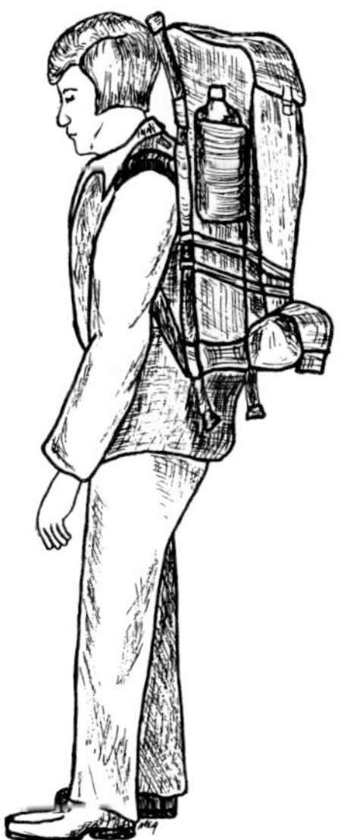


Figure 12.3. A fencer, dancer, and backpacker illustrating compensatory actions to improve stability

Returning to the archer, golfer, baseball batter, bowler, softball pitcher, and basketball player with whom this discussion originated; the question of the shape of the supportive base can now be explored. These performers select a base in accordance with the direction in which they must apply force. The center of mass fluctuates in a direction parallel to that of force application; the base is widened, therefore, in that direction to prevent the line of gravity from falling outside and causing a loss of balance. A fourth principle of stability instructs, then, that the base of support should be widened in the direction of force application. This principle can be broadened to include, also, force absorption. If one is expecting to be pushed from the side, the feet are placed in a side-to-side stance; expectation of a shove from the front or rear leads to a front-to-back stance. In each case, the base is broadened to make it more difficult for the line of gravity to fall outside the base.

A fifth principle of stability concerns the height of the center of mass. Figure 12.4 illustrates two objects, *A* and *B*, which are identical except for the heights of their centers of mass. Object *A* must be tilted farther than object *B* in order to move its line of gravity outside its base; thus, the lower the center of mass, the more stable the object. The short gymnast will tend to excel in balance beam; women, by virtue of their broad pelvic girdles and comparatively narrow shoulder girdles, will be more stable than men; a young child is quite unstable since his relatively heavy head causes an upward displacement of his center. Acrobats who balance two, three, or even four performers with each one standing on the shoulders of the other perform a difficult feat indeed, for as each additional performer is balanced, their collective center moves higher. Badminton, tennis, and softball players make use of this principle as they leave the ready position to intercept the flight of the shuttlecock or ball. The badminton and softball players elevate their centers by extending the knees and hips slightly just before the opponent makes contact with the implement. The tennis player elevates the center by actually jumping slightly from the ground before the opponent hits the ball. In each case, the performer becomes less stable and more able to become mobile quickly without committing himself to any direction of progress which may either place him in an unfavorable position to affect the interception, or "tip" the opponent.

Discussion of stability or static equilibrium often comprises the statement, "the sum of the moments is equal to zero." The terminology may seem confusing at first glance; however, when it is remembered that a moment of force is equal to a moment arm multiplied by the force applied (F $\times$ MA), a glimmer of clarification may be seen. Return, briefly, to consideration of the first class lever known as a seesaw. If the seesaw is balanced, the sum of its moments must be equal to zero; i.e., the product of its moment arm and their respective forces are equivalent. Two forces of 10 kg each applied at 5 meters on either side of the axis will cause the seesaw to balance.

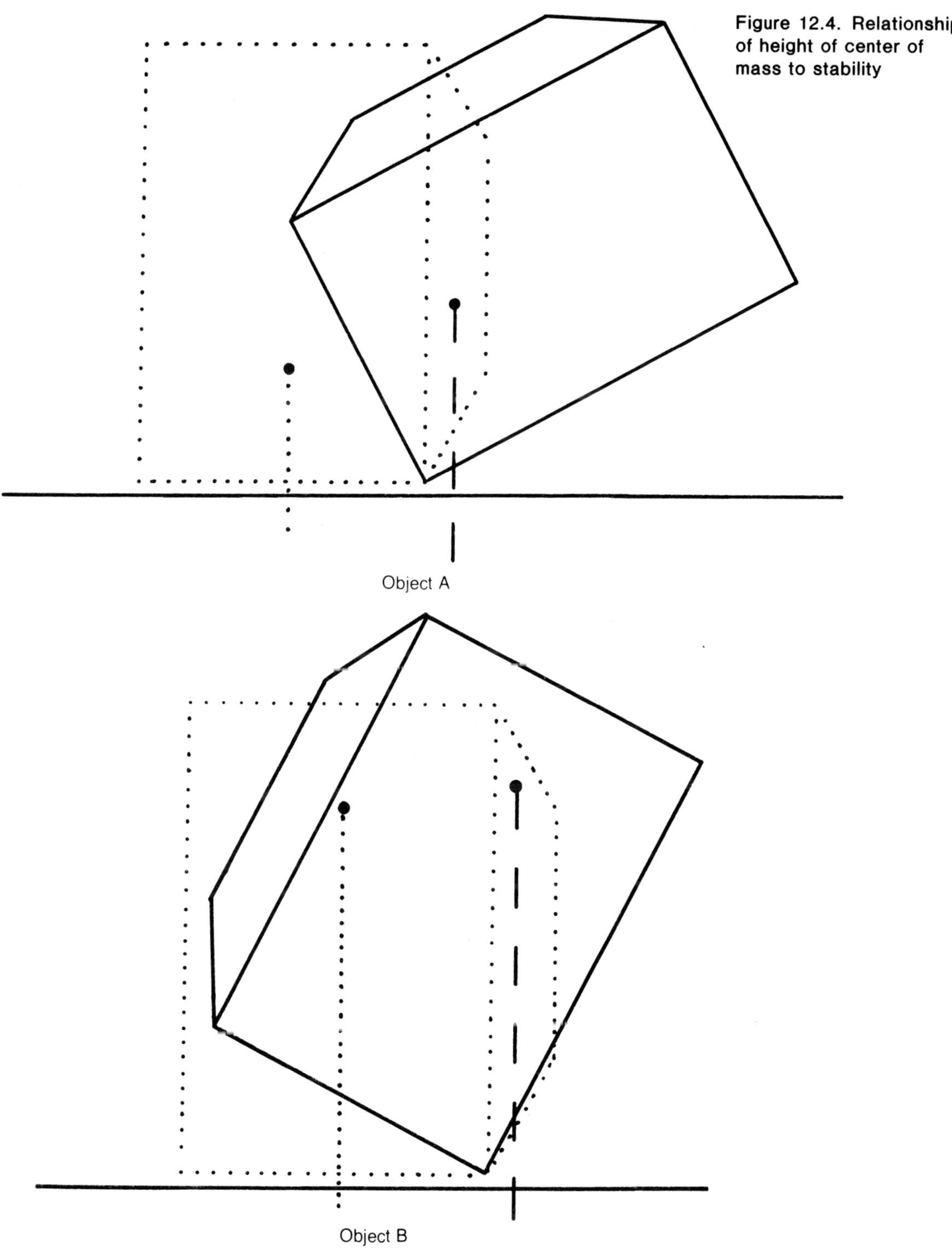


Figure 12.4. Relationship of height of center of mass to stability

$$F \times MA = R \times RA; \text{ or}$$

$$F_1 \times MA_1 = F_2 \times MA_2$$

$$10\text{kg} \times 5\text{M} = 10\text{kg} \times 5\text{M}$$

and

$$\text{moment}_1 = \text{moment}_2$$

therefore

$$\text{moment}_1 - \text{moment}_2 = 0$$

In other words, the sum of the moments equals zero.

Use of the concept of sums of moments is frequent in static equilibrium, for it entails the very basis of stability. Only when all moments on one side of the body equal those on the other will the body be stable with its line of gravity passing through the center of its base of support. To hold an arm at shoulder level rather than at the side increases its moment because the moment arm is increased. The increased moment must be neutralized by the other side of the body if stability is to be retained. Perhaps the other arm could be abducted, also, or the head could be tilted sufficiently so its weight multiplied by its moment arm could equal the moment of the extended arm on the opposite side.

All of this is by way of reinforcing, mathematically, principles set forth above. To retain static equilibrium requires that compensation be made above and below, on either side of, and forward and back of the center of mass to ensure that the sum of the moments is equal to zero.

## Determination of the Center of Mass

The center of mass of the body is probably the parameter most frequently used to describe movement of the body through space. Because position of the center of mass is so influential to stability or mobility of the body, and because it is also a prime factor in the calculation of the amount of work done by an individual, the procedures for its location can be of utmost importance to the teacher and coach.

The mathematical determination of the location of the center of mass is not a complex calculation, but it is somewhat laborious if done by hand. The data needed for making the calculation include total body weight, individual body segment weight, location of the center of mass of each segment, and horizontal and vertical coordinates of these centers. The coordinates can be obtained by projecting film of the subject on graph paper that has been labeled in arbitrary linear units. The origin of the graphic system is placed so the projected image is in the first quadrant; i.e., the coordinates X=0, Y=0 (0, 0) are placed in the lower left-hand corner of the graph paper. A stick figure of the subject's position is then completed (fig. 12.5). A millimeter ruler can be used to locate the centers of mass of the various segments by using the segmental data presented in figure 12.6. Having marked all segments, their respective X and Y coordinates are found on the graph paper. The procedure is illustrated in figure 12.7 for the left upper leg, which measures 35 millimeters in length. From figure 12.6, it is found that the center of mass of the upper leg is located 37.2 percent of the segment length from the hip axis. Thus, 35 millimeters $\times$ .372 = 13.02 millimeters. When that distance is measured to the nearest millimeter from the hip, a mark is made on the segment and

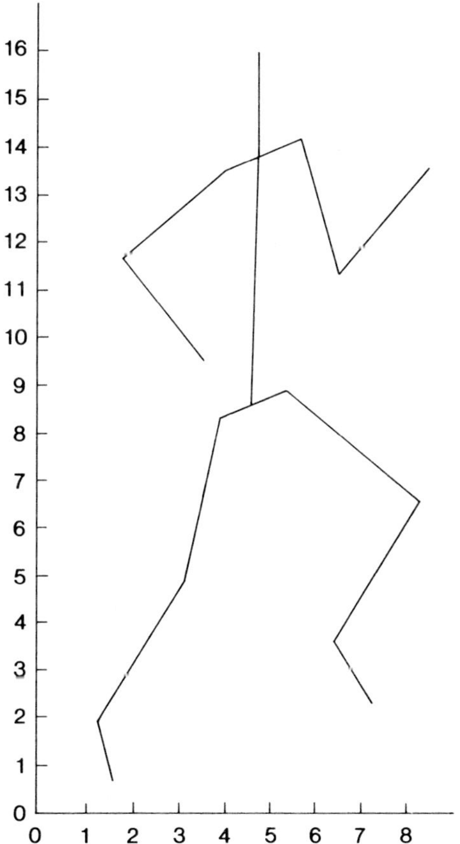


Figure 12.5. Stick figure on graph paper

Figure 12.6. Location of centers of gravity (mass) of body segments*

| Segment | Center-of-Gravity Location Expressed as Percentage of Total Distance between Reference Points |
|---|---|
| Head | 46.4% to vertex; 53.6% to chin-neck intersect |
| Trunk | 38.0% to suprasternal notch; 62.0% to hip axis |
| Upper arm | 51.3% to shoulder axis; 48.7% to elbow axis |
| Forearm | 39.0% to elbow axis; 61.0% to wrist axis |
| Hand | 82.0% to wrist axis; 18.0% to knuckle III |
| Thigh | 37.2% to hip axis; 62.8% to knee axis |
| Calf | 37.1% to knee axis; 62.9% to ankle axis |
| Foot | 44.9% to heel; 55.1% to tip of longest toe |

*AMRL Technical Report 69-70, Wright Patterson Air Force Base, Ohio, 1969.

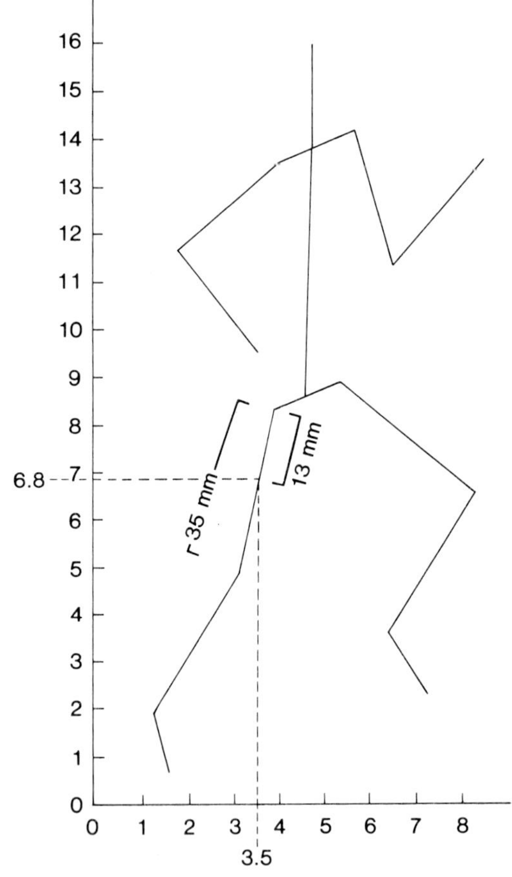


Figure 12.7. Location of center of mass of right upper leg

| Segment | Percent Body Weight |
|---|---|
| Head | 0.073 |
| Trunk | 0.507 |
| Upper arm | 0.026 |
| Forearm | 0.016 |
| Hand | 0.007 |
| Thigh | 0.103 |
| Calf | 0.043 |
| Foot | 0.015 |

*AMRL Technical Report 69-70, Wright Patterson Air Force Base, Ohio, 1969.

Figure 12.8. Weights of body segments relative to total body weight*

perpendiculars are dropped to the two axes. Their points of axis intersection (3.5, 6.8), are the coordinates of the center of gravity of the upper leg. The only remaining step is to multiply both the X and Y coordinates by the weight of that body segment. These data are found in figure 12.8. Results of multiplication are added to those of all other segments, with X coordinates kept separate from Y coordinates. The two sums are then divided by the body weight. The divisions provide X and Y coordinates of the total body center of mass for the position analyzed.

$$X_{cg} = \frac{(X_1 \cdot Wt._1) + (X_2 \cdot Wt._2) + \ldots + (X_{16} \cdot Wt._{16})}{\text{Body Weight}}$$

$$Y_{cg} = \frac{(Y_1 \cdot Wt._1) + (Y_2 \cdot Wt._2) + \ldots + (Y_{16} \cdot Wt._{16})}{\text{Body Weight}}$$

Subscripts indicate segment number; i.e., if segment number one is the foot, its coordinates should each be multiplied by the weight of the foot, etc. It must be remembered that both the right and left arms and legs are to be considered in the calculation; however, if only one side of the body can be seen, and if bilateral symmetry of the limbs can be assumed, the calculations from the observed limb can simply be doubled.

A less mathematical solution to determining the location of the center of mass lies in the use of a board, two "knife-edges," and a weight scale. One end of the board is placed on the scale and the other on a block of sufficient height to level the board. The "knife-edges" (two lengths of angle iron will do quite nicely) are placed between the ends of the board and the scale and block, respectively. Length of the board between the edges is recorded, and the scale is set to zero.

A subject whose weight is known can now lie on the board with feet toward the scale. The scale reading is recorded and the following calculation is performed.

$$\text{Center of Mass} = \frac{\text{Scale reading} \times \text{length of board between edges}}{\text{Weight of subject}}$$

Suppose our subject weighs 60 kilograms and the length of the board between knife-edges is 180 centimeters. If the scale reading is 30 kilograms, we can solve for the location of the center of mass as follows:

$$\text{Center of Mass} = \frac{30 \text{ kg} \times 180 \text{ cm}}{60 \text{ kg}}$$

$$= 90 \text{ cm}$$

The center of mass is located 90 centimeters from the knife-edge that is on the block.

The process can be repeated if locations of the center are desired in the sagittal and frontal planes. The subject would stand on the board with his or her side to the scale and then facing the scale. Results of the calculations will yield the desired locations. It is also possible to place the subject in some sports posture on the board and determine, in the same fashion, the location of the center of mass.

## Summary

Stability is the condition of a body in which its center of mass is aligned perpendicularly to its base of support. Five major principles relating to stability are:

1. The size of the base of support is proportional to stability; that is, the larger the base, the more stable the body; the smaller the base, the less stable the body but the more easily mobility can be achieved.
2. Intersection of the line of gravity at the center of the base of support yields greatest stability for that base; intersection of the line near the edge of the base lessens stability but makes mobility easier to achieve.
3. The addition of weights to the body anywhere but directly above or below the center of mass causes the center to move in a sideward direction toward the weight. Realignment of the center is achieved through compensatory movements in the opposite direction. Movement of a body part away from the midline has the same effect as the addition of a weight.

4. To maintain stability as force is being applied or absorbed, widen the base of support in the direction of the force.
5. The lower the center of mass of a given base of support the more stable the body; the more the center is raised, the less stable the body becomes.

The location of the center of mass can be calculated mathematically through the use of a stick figure on graph paper, or a board, "knife-edges," and a weight scale.

## Laboratory and Field Experiences

1. Stand with your arms at your sides as you raise one foot from the ground and notice that it is relatively difficult to remain stable. Now, abduct your arms to shoulder level and use them to help stabilize your position. Explain why the arms contribute to your ability to maintain stability while standing on one foot. Extend your explanation to include the tightwire walker and his use of the long balancing pole.
2. What foot stance (side-to-side, front-and-back, and so on) would you use when performing the following activities?
   a. "ready" position in tennis
   b. removing a heavy object from an overhead closet shelf
   c. standing, facing forward, in a moving vehicle
   d. standing, facing sideward, in a moving vehicle
   e. catching a forceful chest pass in basketball
3. Perform a reaching rescue on a partner who is simulating a swimmer in trouble. What position should you take to prevent the swimmer from pulling you into the water?
4. Watch a softball or baseball pitcher deliver a pitch and notice any tendency he might have to lose his balance to one side after the ball is released. If you were signaled to bunt to the pitcher, to which side of him would you direct the bunt?
5. While watching a dancer perform an arabesque, locate her center of mass, using the principles of stability.
6. Relate the principles of stability to your success (or lack of success) when climbing a Bachman Ladder.
7. From a sports magazine, trace on graph paper the outline of an athlete performing some activity. Within the outline, draw a stick figure that joins the several joint centers and the head/neck segment. Determine the location of the center of mass of the athlete.

# 13 Newton's Laws

Sir Isaac Newton is the discoverer of three laws, or truths, which form the basis for the mechanical analysis of all motion. Many of the motion situations encountered in sports and dance bear a clear and straightforward relationship to the laws; other situations are more difficult to relate, and for that reason, are usually excerpted by textbook authors to be discussed in separate chapters. The chapters on stability, projection, spin and rebound, and so on, that follow all encompass principles which are based upon the laws, but which have been treated separately in the interest of simplicity. Nevertheless, all motion is based on the laws; as motion is analyzed, therefore, the laws must present the front line of defense, and when the questions "why?" or "why not?" perplex the coach and performer, those questions should be examined initially from the viewpoint of the laws. More often than not, the answer will be found thereby.

## The First Law: Inertia

An object will remain in its state of motion until it is acted upon by an external force sufficiently large to disturb that state.

It must be remembered, when exploring the ramifications of the first law, that objects which are at rest are in a state of motion—that of no motion. The law addresses itself, therefore, both to objects which are moving and to objects which are still. In the varied techniques of sports and dance activities, examples can be found in which either the condition of rest or of movement is prevalent over the other; frequent examples can be found also which illustrate the blending of both aspects of motion.

Application of the law of inertia to situations in which the object of concern is at rest can be made by recalling the often-heard statement, "the hardest part of lifting a weight is getting it off the floor." Certainly the statement is true, for the barbell will tend to exercise its inertia by remaining on the floor—a good thing for those who frequent the weight room! Similarly, it can be said that the most fatiguing part of partner work in pas de deux is the overcoming of inertia of the female dancer by the male dancer who must lift her into space. To aid him in his task, the female partner is taught to help overcome her own inertia by extending the joints of the legs at the moment of his lift. Other examples of the effect of inertia on the resting body can be found in the standing long jump in track, back dives from the springboard, and in the starting position on the still rings. In all of these activities, the athlete must expend energy simply to overcome his own inertia.

It would be remiss not to point out that the law of inertia can place excessive demands on the muscular systems of the body. Consideration must be given to the choice of muscles to be used when lifting, pushing, and pulling. Heavy, difficult tasks must be matched with large, powerful muscles if injury is to be avoided. This is particularly important during lifting, when the tendency is to lift with the small muscles of the back rather than the large muscles of the hip and thigh.

Application of Newton's first law to situations in which inertia of movement predominates is seen particularly well in bowling. It is typical to teach beginning bowlers to deliver a "straight" ball—one that has no sidespin. Once the ball has been released, it will tend to continue its state of motion by rolling in a straight line down the alley. There is no external force being applied, except the friction of the ball against the wood, and friction will not cause the ball to veer to the side. The bowler has only to concentrate on directing the ball toward the pocket. As the bowler becomes more skilled, however, he may change from the straight ball delivery to that of a hook in which he imparts a counterclockwise spin (or clockwise, if he is lefthanded) to the ball. Upon release, the ball will again yield to its inertia and travel in a straight line down the alley. As friction slows the ball, the external force of the spin imparted is allowed to manifest itself and when it exceeds the inertia of the ball, will cause the ball to veer, or hook, into the pocket. Obviously, the timing must be quite precise; if the ball is rolled with a great deal of force, the spin will not be able to overcome the inertia and the hook will not occur. If the ball is rolled with too little force, the hook will be premature.

Inertia of the moving body has no doubt been appreciated also by the beginning snow skier who often complains that although lessons are quite adequate in their treatment of initiating movement on skis, they are dismally lacking in methods of stopping. Unless friction between the skis and snow can be increased by proper edging or waxing techniques, the skier is likely to become an inertia casualty.

Probably the greatest relationship of the law of inertia to sports and dance occurs within those techniques in which an implement is thrown or swung. One key to success lies in the ability to overcome the resting inertia of the implement and then to maintain its moving inertia. Both the starting and stopping of motion requires energy; in the interest of efficiency, extraneous starts and stops should be avoided. Once the windup has begun in baseball or softball pitching, the ball should never come to rest; the swimmer should time each successive stroke to maintain his moving inertia; the golfer must establish a looping swing pattern to ensure that the head of the club will remain in motion from the beginning of the backswing through the hit of the ball.

At this point, a second look at the law of inertia is indicated. A body will remain in its state of motion until some force causes a change. Description of the state of motion of an object must necessarily include both its rate and direction of movement. Objects at rest have zero rate of motion and thus have no direction; however, moving objects display both a rate and a direction. That these two conditions remain the same is stated implicitly by the law, but is not easily observable. Friction, gravity, air and water resistance all function as external forces to change the rate of motion. Equally important are forces which change direction—and under the law that direction can be linear, angular, or curvilinear. The amount of force necessary to change direction is dependent upon the amount of change desired. In the case of the hook ball in bowling, the comparatively small force of the spin is sufficient to deflect the ball from its inertial straight line of direction. A great deal more force would be required to stop the ball completely.

The angular aspect of Newton's first law is demonstrated by the diver and gymnast who initiate rotation of their bodies to perform somersaults. Actually, the rotation is initiated as the supporting surface is left by directing the force of the projecting thrust through the body along a path which does not pass through the center of mass. Once the athlete is airborne, the velocity of that rotation is controlled by manipulating his radius of rotation. During the takeoff phase, the body is held extended to elongate the radius and ensure a slow rate of rotation so that height can be attained. The body is then tucked or piked to shorten the radius and increase the rate of spin. Having completed the somersault, the body is again extended to slow the rotation and prepare for landing or entry to the water. That rate of rotation can be controlled by altering the radius is a function of the fact that, under the first law, the body has been made to achieve a certain angular inertia (or angular momentum) which will remain constant until some external force acts to change it.

## The Second Law: Acceleration

The acceleration of a body is proportional to the force imparted to it and inversely proportional to its mass. In symbols,

$$A = \frac{F}{M}\text{, or Acceleration} = \frac{\text{Force}}{\text{Mass}}$$

By rearranging the terms of the formula the law can be stated differently; for example: the force which can be generated by a body is directly proportional both to its acceleration and to its mass.

$$F = MA\text{, or Force} = \text{Mass} \times \text{Acceleration}$$

Conceptualization of the second law is simplified by examining it through both of its forms. The first form instructs us, for instance, that application of the same amount of force to a golf ball and a twelve-pound shot will cause the golf ball to accelerate more than the shot because of its smaller mass. The second form indicates, however, that if these two objects are made to accelerate equally, the shot, because of its greater mass, will make the larger dent when they land. Certainly neither of these two statements is surprising, but when the forms of the law are extended to other events, they become of great importance to the analysis of technique.

When the human body is considered as the object of acceleration in such situations as jumping or leaping, the force applied is that which results from the strength of the contracting muscles, and the mass is that of the body itself. If increased acceleration is demanded for success in jumping to rebound in basketball, to spike in volleyball, or to increase the height of jump to perform the entrechat, the performer must either apply more force by strengthening the muscles and/or he must reduce his mass. Accordingly, the typical body build of such athletes incorporates a well-muscled but lean body. Successful sprinters in track also display these body characteristics as do long jumpers, high jumpers, and pole-vaulters for whom the ability to accelerate is a key to success.

When force is to be applied to implements or other human beings, attention must be given to the elevation of both acceleration and mass. Football linemen are large (mass) and powerful (acceleration), and thus can apply a great deal of force in blocking and tackling. An archery arrow is a more lethal projectile over short distances than a bullet because, even though its acceleration is less than that of the bullet, its mass is considerably greater. At long distances, the bullet can be more damaging since air resistance so slows the arrow that even its greater mass cannot compensate.

The second law is of particular importance in the selection of sports implements. Certainly it is true that the large baseball bat in the hands of a powerful hitter deserves respect, for if the ball is contacted, it will react with great force. The large bat in the hands of a weak hitter causes no concern whatsoever since the ball probably will not be hit. Unless the hitter is strong enough to accelerate the bat properly, he will swing late. Even if contact is made, it will probably result in a slow foul ball. So it is with the tennis player who consistently swings late—the fault may not lie in technique at all, but rather with a "too heavy" racket. Young girls and boys learning golf will have difficulty controlling their swings if they must use their mothers' or fathers' "hand-me-down" clubs. Bowlers often fall into this trap by theorizing that the heavier the ball, the easier the strike. Unfortunately, loss of control and incomplete pin action is, more often than not, the result of improper ball selection.

## The Third Law: Action-Reaction

When one body exerts a force on a second, there is an equal and opposite force exerted by the second body on the first. To clarify the application of Newton's third law to sports and dance, two conditions will be discussed: (1) when the body is supported directly or indirectly by the earth; and (2) when the body is in space without such support. Under the first condition will fall almost all of the techniques in which an implement (ball, shot, discus) is thrown or struck. Throwing a ball overarm, for example, involves a forceful forward action of the arm. The accompanying reaction tends to rotate the rest of the body backward. If the feet are contacting the ground securely, however, the body cannot comply and the reaction is transmitted to the ground. There are countless examples of ground transmission of reaction since so many sports involve throwing and hitting, and thus, the law of action-reaction, because it is frequently not observable, is difficult to conceptualize. Verification of the presence of the law can be found, however, if one imagines the outcome of such activities if they were performed on a slippery surface such as ice. Without firm foot contact, reactions of the body can manifest themselves and the feet will slip from under the body in the direction of the reaction (or in the opposite direction to the action).

When the body is in space the law of action-reaction is usually more observable. The diver tucks the head forcefully causing the hips to elevate to perform a somersault. A hurdler clears the trailing leg by elevating the opposite shoulder or dipping the head. The high jumper who employs the Fosberry Flop technique drops the hips sharply after they have crossed the bar to cause the legs to rise and clear the height.

When applying Newton's third law to movement, the relative masses of the acting and reacting bodies must be considered. Since the law states that the two forces must equal each other, it follows that the product of mass and acceleration of the acting body must equal that of the reacting body. Thus, the hand or forearm, even though it may be accelerated rapidly, is hardly of sufficient mass to cause a clearly observable reaction of the larger and heavier legs or trunk. The basketball player executing a jump shot will testify to the fractional forward movement of the legs as they react to the force of the shooting hand and forearm. The reaction is not large enough to cause any problem to the shooter—in fact, it can be used to good advantage if it is localized in the lower legs and paired with an action of snapping the knees into extension. The resulting reaction will be a slight raising of the rest of the body mass and the shooter will stay in the air longer. This technique can also be employed by the volleyball spiker.

At the other extreme of action-reaction in the air is the long jumper who employs the hitch kick to prevent the body from rotating in a forward direction after takeoff. Since the action of the arms and legs in the hitch kick involves forward rotation, the reaction will seek to rotate the body in the opposite direction and thus neutralize the athlete's tendency to land head first. A strong reaction is required; therefore, the action must involve heavy, accelerated body parts.

An outgrowth of the law of action-reaction is the principle referred to as transfer of momentum and relates to the redistribution of angular momentum generated by the movement of body parts. For example, when one wishes to execute a vertical jump, the arms will be forcefully elevated to above the head just as the feet leave the ground. The momentum established by the arms will be transferred to the body when the arms reach the overhead position and become still. The competitive swimmer displays a similar transfer as he executes a racing dive; he generates angular momentum with the arms, and when that momentum is reduced to zero by virtue of the arms having been positioned over head, it will manifest itself by increasing the angular momentum of the body. The swing of the forward leg by high jumpers and dancers performing leaps and tour jetés are other examples of the transfer of momentum.

## Force Absorption

The ability to absorb force is frequently as important to athletes as is the ability to impart it. Two major principles, both of which are derived from Newton's laws, instruct us in successful force absorption and are: (1) the velocity of a moving object should be slowed gradually, and (2) the area of force absorption should be as large as possible under the confines of proper performance.

Illustrative of the first principle are those techniques in which an implement must be caught or during which the body must affect a landing after having been airborne. The baseball player knows well the sting of a ball which was caught in the palm of the glove rather than in the absorbent webbing; similarly, a pass receiver in football must "give" with the ball to prevent it from bouncing off of the hands or shoulder pads. In these instances, force is being absorbed by elongating the time over which the velocity of the implement is slowed. If sports objects are moving excessively fast, it may be necessary to lengthen the absorption time even more by allowing the arms to swing backwardly after the initial "give" or even by taking a backward step. Such force absorbing movements can often be used to place the caught object in a position from which a subsequent throw can be made. A baseball shortstop frequently employs this technique to speed his throw to first base after having fielded a ground ball.

When the body is airborne, landings must be made in such a way that either the body or the surface upon which the landing is made absorbs the force. Dancers, gymnasts, and volleyball players gradually slow the force of descent from leaps, vaults, and spikes by flexing the joints of the lower limb upon ground contact. Trampolinists, high jumpers, and pole-vaulters allow the landing surface to absorb the force and can, therefore, land in positions which would otherwise be injurious.

To further illustrate the first principle of force absorption, consider the shoulder roll technique taught to tumblers, sky divers, and football players. For these athletes, the absorption provided by the gradually flexing joints may not be sufficient; continued absorption is made possible by the execution of a shoulder roll.

The second principle of force absorption, to the effect that the area of absorption should be enlarged as permitted by the situation, may best be discussed from the viewpoint of winter sports. Skis and snowshoes are both pieces of equipment that have been developed in deference to this principle, for without the enlarged area over which the body weight is spread, locomotion through deep snow would be virtually impossible. It will be recalled also that the rescuing of individuals who have fallen through thin ice should be performed in a prone position so that the rescuer's weight will be dispersed over the surface of his body, thus lessening his tendency to break through also.

The second principle applies, in addition, to falls in dance. The front fall is seldom performed, either by men or women, because the force of the fall must be taken on the hands and then transmitted to the body as the chest is lowered to the floor. Without precise timing of the flexing joints, the force will be localized at the wrist joint with disastrous results. A more popular, and safe, fall is the sliding fall during which the force is spread over the lower rib cage, abdomen and hips.

## Summary

Newton's three laws form the basis of all mechanical principles of human movement. The laws are those of inertia, acceleration, and action-reaction.

*First Law: Inertia* An object will remain in its state of motion until it is acted upon by an external force sufficiently large to disturb that state.

*Second Law: Acceleration* The acceleration of a body is proportional to the force imparted to it and inversely proportional to its mass.

$$\text{Acceleration} = \frac{\text{Force}}{\text{Mass}}$$

$$\text{Force} = \text{Acceleration} \times \text{Mass}$$

*Third Law: Action-Reaction* When one body exerts a force on a second, there is an equal and opposite force exerted by the second body on the first. In accordance with the third law a principle referred to as transfer of momentum has been derived. When a body part reduces its momentum to zero or near-zero, that momentum will be conserved and transferred to another body part.

Force absorption is characterized by two major principles, (1) the time of absorption should be lengthened, and (2) the area of absorption should be enlarged. The ability to absorb force successfully is highly related to the avoidance of injury.

## Laboratory and Field Experiences

1. Observe a swimmer executing one of the glide strokes. Does the swimmer's technique represent agreement with the law of inertia?
2. A professional track athlete who specializes in the long jump is experimenting with the use of a forward tuck somersault during his flight between takeoff and landing. In terms of the law of acceleration as it applies to angular motion, do you find his experiment a valid one?
3. You are told that a certain tennis professional uses a heavyweight racket when he is the server in a singles match but substitutes a medium-weight racket for it when he is the receiver. Explain his action through the application of Newton's second law.
4. Explain why the times for four-man bobsledding are faster than those for two-man teams.
5. Stand on a piano stool or similar piece of apparatus and swing the arms forcefully to the left in the transverse plane. What is the reaction of the hips? Which of Newton's laws does this illustrate?
6. Explain why it is more difficult to walk in sand than on a hard surface such as concrete.
7. Drop a golf ball on a hard surface and then on a pillow or tumbling mat. Describe the difference between the two reactions of the ball in terms of the principles of force absorption.
8. Hold a discus at shoulder height so it is aligned vertically and drop it onto soft ground. Now hold the discus horizontally and drop it as you did before and notice the difference in the two marks made in the ground. Explain your observation by applying the principles of force absorption.

# Motion

# 14

Motion of the human body and of objects propelled by the human body is subject to the same mechanical laws that govern all motion on earth. The two types of motion, linear and angular, were discussed in chapter 2 and will only be reviewed here.

## Linear Motion

Linear motion is characterized by the movement of all parts of a body in the same direction and at the same velocity. The sports of bobsledding and luge entail linear motion of the vehicles and their occupants.

## Angular Motion

Angular motion is characterized by the circular rotation of an object around an axis. A wheel exhibits angular motion as does the forearm when the elbow joint is flexed or extended.

Linear and angular motion are frequently performed simultaneously. Walking and running allow for linear progression of the trunk because of the angular motion of the limbs. A bowling ball, while rolling down the alley, shows linear motion of its axis of rotation as the parts of the ball rotate angularly.

## Curvilinear Motion

While description of motion as either linear or angular is sufficient for the discussion of anatomical considerations, it is necessary to explore a subcategory of linear motion when mechanics are discussed. The subcategory is that of curvilinear motion and is characterized by the progress of a body along a curved, but not circular, path. A javelin traveling through the air is undergoing curvilinear motion. All of its parts are moving in the same direction at the same velocity but its path is curved rather than straight.

It is possible to combine angular and curvilinear motion just as angular and linear motion can be performed simultaneously. Dancers and long jumpers exhibit the combination during leaps from the ground which move them from one point in space to another. Their centers of mass progress curvilinearly by virtue of the explosive angular motion of the limbs. A discus is released with spin—angular motion—but its axis of rotation follows a curvilinear path.

Curvilinear motion, whether occurring alone or in combination with its angular counterpart, is specific to the mechanics of projection. For this reason, further discussion of curvilinear motion is reserved for chapter 15, which deals with projection.

## Linear Velocity vs. Speed

Velocity can be defined simply as *displacement* (S) covered per unit of time. When the action transpires along a straight line, linear velocity occurs; if the action takes place through a full or partial circle, angular velocity occurs.

To illustrate the linear case, consider an athlete who runs directly from Point *A* to Point *B*, a displacement of 100 meters, in ten seconds. His linear velocity is equal to 100 meters divided by ten seconds, or ten meters per second.

$$\text{velocity} = \frac{\text{displacement}}{\text{time}} = \frac{\text{S}}{\text{t}}$$

$$= \frac{\text{100 meters}}{\text{10 sec.}} = \text{10 meters per second}$$

Implicit in the definition of linear velocity are the requirements that the distance between Point *A* and Point *B* has both magnitude (100 meters) and direction (straight line beginning at Point *A* and ending at Point *B*). These two conditions categorize linear velocity as a vector quantity which can be described diagrammatically as discussed in chapter 2.

That velocity is a vector quantity differentiates it from speed, which is a scalar quantity. Scalar quantities have magnitude only, with no assumption regarding direction. A simplified distinction between velocity and speed can be made by considering the 440-yard dash event in American track. On those tracks which are 440 yards around, the sprinter begins and ends at the same point. The straight line displacement between the start, Point *A*, and the finish, Point *B*, is zero feet. The sprinter's velocity is zero feet per second; his speed, on the other hand, is equal to 440 yards of *distance* (D) divided by the time required to complete the sprint, say 60 seconds.

$$\text{speed} = \frac{\text{distance}}{\text{time}} = \frac{D}{t}$$

$$= \frac{440 \text{ yds.}}{60 \text{ sec.}} = 7.33 \text{ yds. per second}$$

It will be noted that the calculations of both speed and velocity are essentially the same. The difference lies only in the manner in which the measurement is made. It is correct, then, to refer to the velocity of a sprinter performing the 100-meter dash if the dash takes place on the straightaway; however, one must speak in terms of speed when discussing a 200-meter dash if the 200 meters are measured along the curve of the track.

The examples given above entail a total displacement or distance and the total time required to cover the ground. Resulting calculations would, therefore, yield *average* linear velocity and *average* speed, respectively. Whereas these calculations may be of interest to those who monitor the record books, they are often of little help to the teacher or coach. Of more interest is the knowledge of what transpired during the race to produce the overall elapsed time. Answers to such questions as, "What was the velocity over the first 10 meters of the race?" or "What was the velocity/speed over each 10 meters of the race?" or "Over which 10 meters of the race was velocity/speed the greatest?" are of great interest. Even these calculations would yield averages, however, but over shorter displacements/distances. Knowledge of these facts can be further enhanced by determining, for a given segment of a race, the frequency of stride (stride rate) and the ground covered by each stride (stride length). It is clear that the product of stride rate and stride length is equal to velocity/speed. As rate and length vary, so will the velocity/speed of the runner. Which of these two should be emphasized at the start, middle, or end of the race? There does not seem to be consensus on the answer to that question; however, it is known that "overstriding" can cause a slowing of progression because the center of mass is behind the base of support rather than over or in front of it. Equivalently, fast stride rates are not physiologically economical, whereas comparatively slow stride rates coupled with long stride lengths do not allow the runner time to apply the needed force to the ground (the "airborne" effect).

It has been mentioned that calculations of speed or velocity thus far considered were averages over a period of time. One might well question the point at which averages of velocity/speed no longer pertain. The answer is somewhat difficult to envisage, but is stated as "when the time period of concern approaches zero." In other words, when a displacement or distance has been covered in little more than zero time, calculations are no longer averages but rather are termed *instantaneous.* Instantaneous velocity will be discussed in more detail under angular velocity.

### Linear Momentum

Momentum is defined as the product of mass and velocity. Linear momentum is, therefore, the product of mass and linear velocity. Heavy objects moving at great velocities display tremendous momentum, a quality that makes them difficult to stop or deflect. Light objects must move rapidly to generate momentum, just as slow-moving objects must possess a large mass if they are to achieve momentum. Contrast the momentum potential of a shuttlecock with that of a medicine ball and a bowling ball. The shuttlecock is handicapped by its small mass; the medicine ball must be tossed at a slow velocity; but the bowling ball, with its mass moving at velocities typical of the skilled bowler is capable of attaining great momentum.

Examination of the formula for linear momentum will serve to initiate a discussion of conservation of linear momentum.

$$\text{linear momentum} = \text{mass} \times \text{linear velocity}$$

$$M = mv$$

Once a quantity of momentum has been established, it will be conserved either within the object or within the system within which the object reacts. A cue ball reaches a certain magnitude of momentum when it is struck by the cue. If the cue ball strikes a counter ball, it will lose some of its momentum, not because its mass is changed by the contact but rather because its velocity is slowed. The loss of momentum of the cue ball will be observed as an increase in momentum by the counter ball. The momentum of the cue ball after contact added to the momentum of the counter ball after contact will equal (within the confines of friction and air resistance) the momentum generated initially by the cue.

### Angular Velocity

When objects display angular rather than linear motion, their velocities or speeds are said to be *angular,* and are commonly referred to as *revolutions, degrees,* or *radians* traveled per unit of time. If a basketball rotates four complete times between release and the hoop, and two seconds are required for flight time, its angular velocity may be calculated as:

$$\text{angular velocity} = \frac{\text{revolutions}}{\text{time}} = \frac{4}{2 \text{ sec.}}$$

$$= 2 \text{ revolutions per second}$$

When objects travel through only a portion of a circular path, it is more convenient to report their angular velocities or speeds in terms of degrees or radians per second. Figure 14.1 illustrates a softball pitcher performing the windmill pitch. Suppose it is of interest to calculate the angular velocity of the humerus as it flexes through an arc

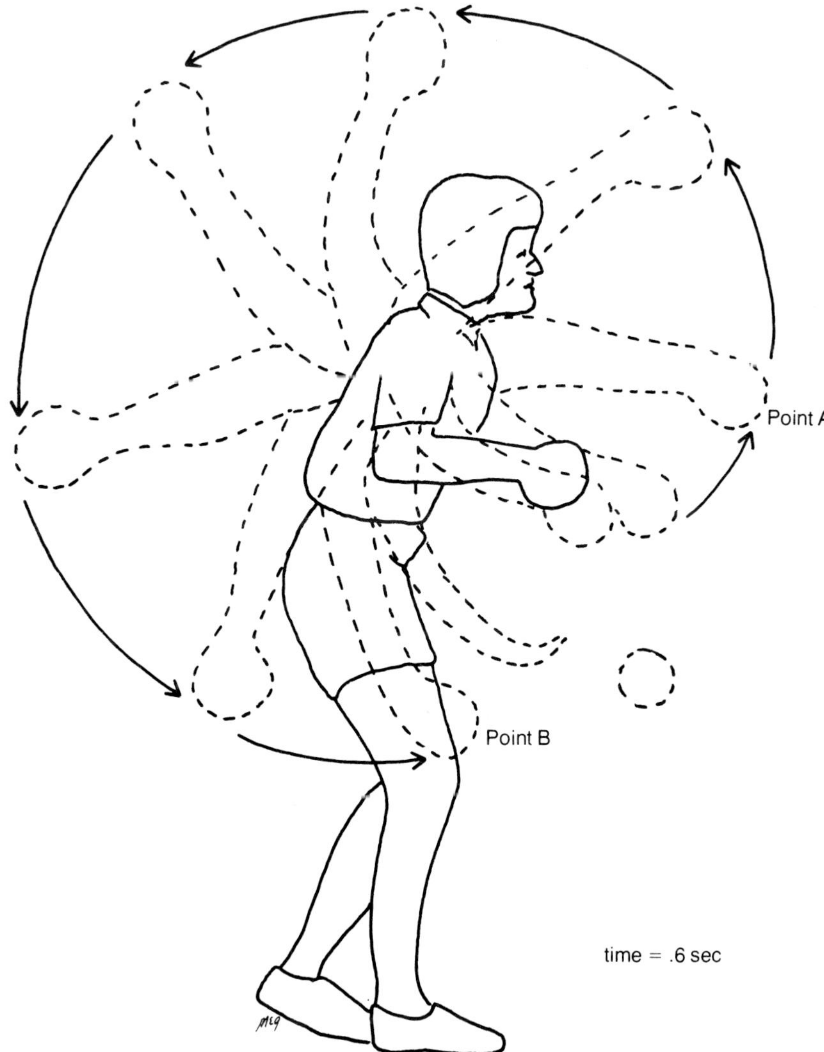


**Figure 14.1. Angular motion of the humerus during the windmill pitch in softball**

around the shoulder joint. From Point *A*, the beginning arm position of the pitch, to Point *B*, the release, a total of 275 degrees are negotiated. The time required for the movement is .6 seconds.

It is at this point that the difference between angular velocity and angular speed becomes critical. The actual *distance* traveled by the humerus is 275 degrees; division of distance by time (.6 seconds) yields as its result *angular speed* or, more properly, *average* angular speed.

$$\text{average angular speed} = \frac{\text{angular distance}}{\text{time}}$$

$$= \frac{275 \text{ degrees}}{.6 \text{ sec.}}$$

$$= 458.3 \text{ degrees per second}$$

*Average angular velocity,* on the other hand, would be calculated by dividing the shortest *displacement* between point A and B (360° — 275° = 85°) by the elapsed time (.6 seconds) or

$$\text{average angular velocity} = \frac{85 \text{ degrees}}{.6 \text{ seconds}} = 141.67 \text{ degrees per second}$$

It will be seen that angular speed will equal angular velocity when angular motion is performed between 0 degrees and 180 degrees. Beyond that point, the two calculations will differ. It is important to note this difference when reading the literature or when analyzing movement, lest the wrong interpretation be made. Fortunately, there are few instances in which a segment of the human body is rotated through displacements exceeding 180 degrees.

Conversion of angular displacements or distances from degrees per second to radians* per second is a simple matter. Since a radian subtends 57.3 degrees, it is only necessary to divide the degrees traveled per second by 57.3. For the softball pitcher in figure 14.1,

$$\text{Radian/sec} = \frac{275°/\text{sec}}{57.3} = 4.8 \text{ radians per second}$$

Mention was made before of the concept of instantaneous velocity or speed as opposed to average velocity or speed. The difference between the two will be related to the angular case of motion, but can be generalized easily to the linear case.

*A radian is that portion of a circle which results when the length of its radius is measured along its circumference. The degrees subtended by one radian are 57.3.

The movement to be analyzed will be that of the hand as it is moved through its full range of motion between flexion and extension. The subject has placed the left forearm on a tabletop and, with the thumb up and wrist held stable, moves the hand as rapidly as possible from flexion to extension. A camera placed above the hand will supply film data of the action. Camera speed is set at 100 frames per second.

Upon viewing the film, it is noted that 10 frames or .1 seconds (10 milliseconds) elapsed while the movement was performed. Also noted were the beginning and ending positions of the hand. We will assume these were 6° and 129°, respectively. Angular distance is equal, therefore, to angular displacement, since the total excursion was less than 180 degrees. For the sake of brevity, then, only the word *velocity* will be used in further discussion.

Based on the foregoing facts, we know that the hand was displaced 123 degrees (129° minus 6°) in 10 milliseconds (one-tenth of a second).

$$\text{Average angular velocity} = \frac{123 \text{ degrees}}{10 \text{ milliseconds } (.10 \text{ second})}$$

$$= 1230° \text{ per second}$$

Now we shall address instantaneous velocity. The first step is to determine the angular position of the hand in each of the ten frames of film. The starting position will be referred to as $P_0$ and each subsequent position will be $P_1$, $P_2$, etc. The ending position will then be $P_{10}$. Suppose the following position data were found.

| Time (milliseconds) | Position (degrees) |
|---|---|
| 0 | 6 |
| 1 | 9 |
| 2 | 13 |
| 3 | 20 |
| 4 | 32 |
| 5 | 47 |
| 6 | 66 |
| 7 | 87 |
| 8 | 107 |
| 9 | 122 |
| 10 | 129 |

The column of time data arises from the camera speed of 100 frames per second. Elapsed time between frames is easily determined to be .01 seconds (1 millisecond).

From the position data, displacements are calculated by subtracting the initial angular position (6 degrees) from each of the other positions. In other words, we will determine how far the hand moved from its starting point during time increments of one millisecond.

| Time (milliseconds) | Position (degrees) | Displacement (degrees) |
|---|---|---|
| 0 | 6 | |
| 1 | 9 | 3 |
| 2 | 13 | 7 |
| 3 | 20 | 14 |
| 4 | 32 | 26 |
| 5 | 47 | 41 |
| 6 | 66 | 60 |
| 7 | 87 | 81 |
| 8 | 107 | 101 |
| 9 | 122 | 116 |
| 10 | 129 | 123 |

It is recommended that displacement data be converted from degrees to radians for this example. The graphing of the data will be greatly facilitated because the range of radian calculations will be much smaller than the range of degree calculations.

| Time (milliseconds) | Displacement (radians) |
|---|---|
| 0 | |
| 1 | .05 |
| 2 | .12 |
| 3 | .24 |
| 4 | .45 |
| 5 | .72 |
| 6 | 1.05 |
| 7 | 1.41 |
| 8 | 1.87 |
| 9 | 2.02 |
| 10 | 2.15 |

The next step in the procedure is to graph the displacement data on the Y axis against the time increments on the X axis (fig. 14.2).

Viewing the completed graph will confirm that there are portions of the curve that are steep, while other portions are less steep or even have no steepness at all; i.e., the curve is horizontal. This can be

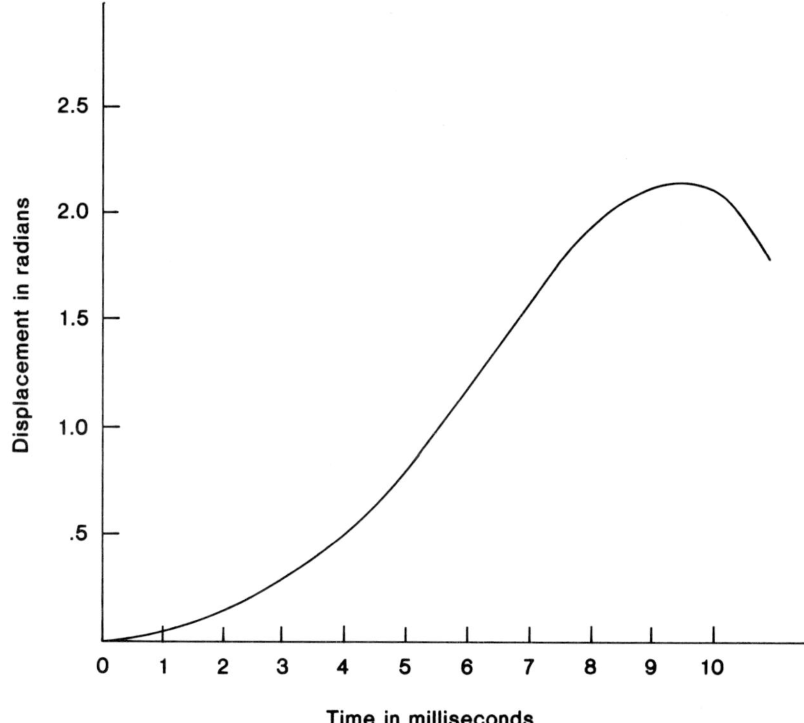


**Figure 14.2. A curve of displacements**

verified by drawing tangents (straight lines that touch the curve at some point) as several time points (fig. 14.3).

The steepness of a tangent is referred to as its slope and slopes are proportional to instantaneous velocity. The steeper the slope, the greater the instantaneous velocity; when slope is zero, instantaneous velocity is also zero.

It is interesting to graph the slopes at their time periods in order to get a picture of instantaneous velocity. This will be done initially in qualitative fashion by labeling the Y axis simply from zero slope to greatest slope. Time periods remain on the baseline.

The resulting graph indicates that instantaneous velocity is greatest at or about the midpoint of the action and is lowest at beginning and end of the movement. This is logical, since we know that the hand was still at the start and finish. Time is needed to accelerate to a high instantaneous velocity and when it is reached, time is needed to slow gradually to a final stop.

It is, of course, possible to quantify graphs of instantaneous velocity. The process is cumbersome when done by hand; however, one example will be given.

Figure 14.3. A displacement curve with selected tangents

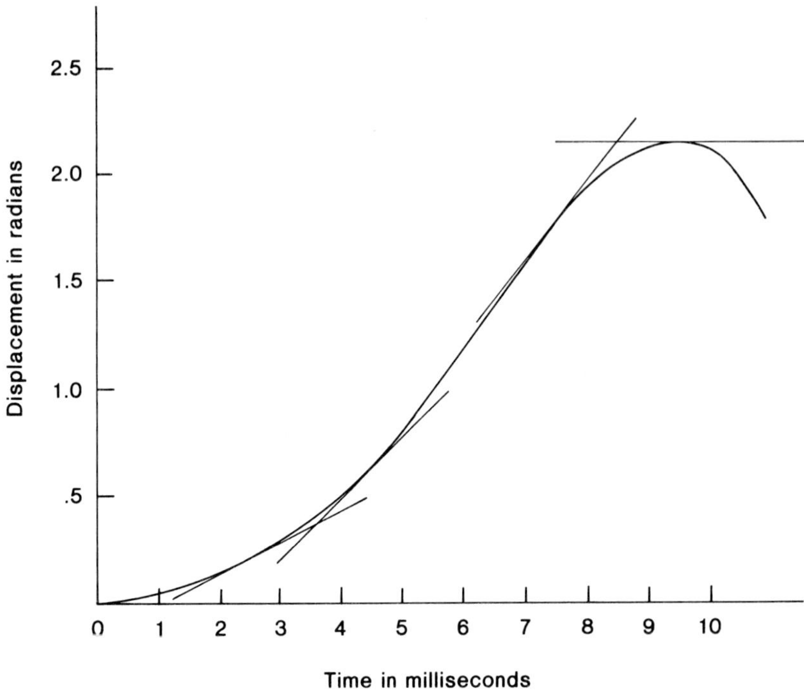


Figure 14.4. Qualitative graph of instantaneous velocity

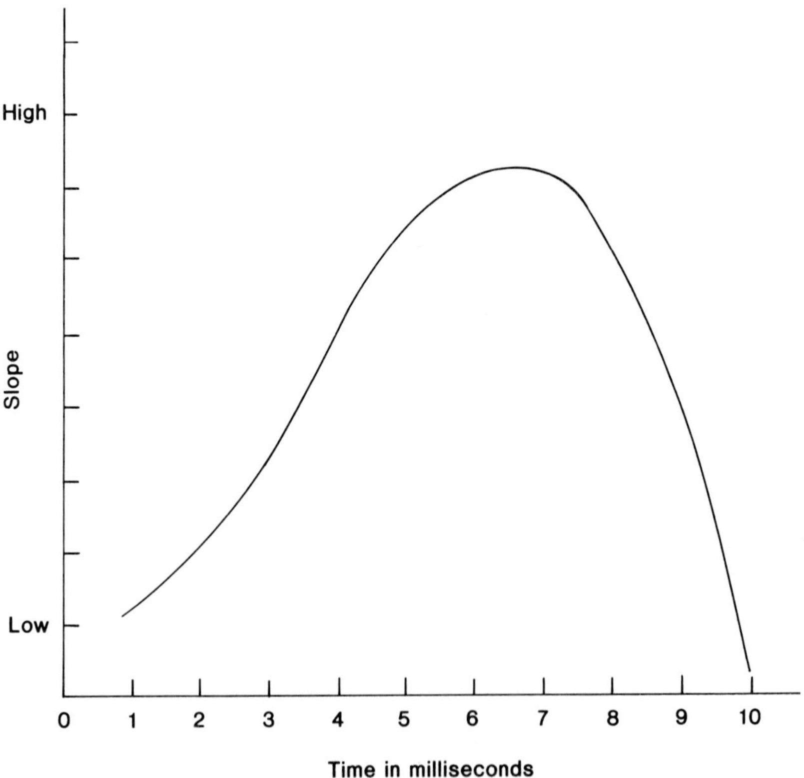

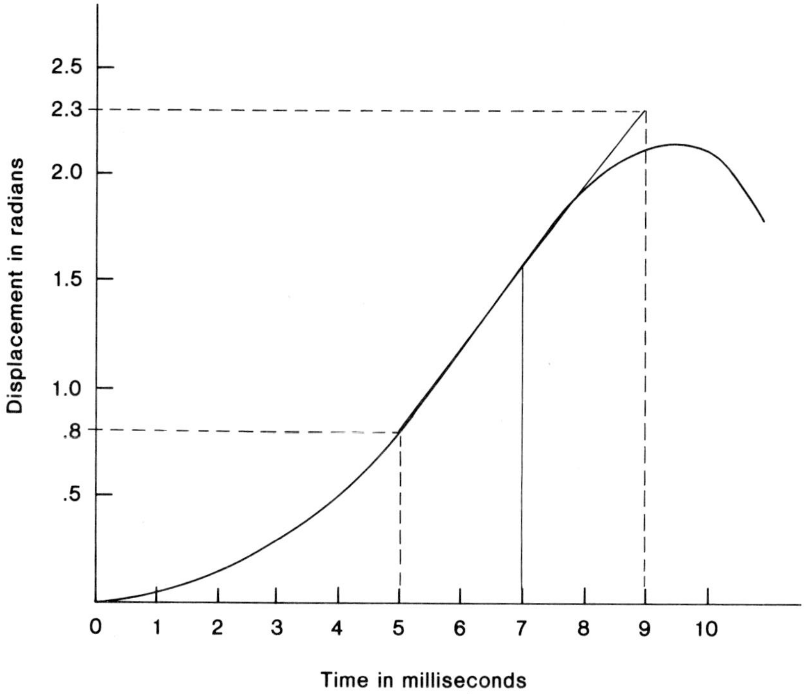

Displacement in radians
2.5
2.3
2.0
1.5
1.0
.8
.5
0 1 2 3 4 5 6 7 8 9 10
Time in milliseconds

Figure 14.5. Instantaneous velocity at 7 milliseconds

We must return to the displacement graph and select a time point at which we wish to know instantaneous velocity; for example, 7 milliseconds. A tangent to the curve is drawn at that time and extended forward or backward to cover several time periods. We shall extend ours both forward and backward so that it covers the time period between 6 and 8 milliseconds.

Now, determine the number of radians covered by the horizontal extension from each end of the tangent to the Y axis. The tangent has "risen" from .8 to 2.3 radians as it "ran" from 5 to 9 milliseconds. Displacement was, therefore, 1.5 radians (2.3 minus .8 radians) in 4 milliseconds. Instantaneous velocity becomes:

$$\text{Instantaneous velocity} = \frac{1.5 \text{ radians}}{4 \text{ milliseconds}}$$

$$= 37.5 \text{ radians per second}$$

When the process has been completed for the entire curve, the calculated velocities can be plotted. The shape of the resulting graph will be similar to the qualitative graph shown in figure 14.7.

## Angular Momentum

Angular momentum is defined as the product of angular velocity and mass. Conceptually, angular momentum and linear momentum are the same; they are both quantities that speak to the resistance of a moving body to a change in its movement—to its inertia.

In the linear case, increases in mass or in velocity will increase the momentum of an object and, therefore, increase the amount of force necessary to change its state and direction of motion. In the angular case, an increase in mass or in velocity will similarly increase momentum; however, a third factor must be recognized and that is the location of the mass relative to the axis of rotation.

Consider a slingshot with thongs 50 centimeters long hurling a missile weighing 30 grams. It is true that if the angular velocity of rotating the slingshot is increased, or if the weight of the missile is increased, the inertia of the system—its angular momentum—will be increased. It is also true that given the same rotational velocity and missile weight with thongs that are 75 rather than 50 centimeters long, the angular momentum will increase. The radius of rotation must be taken into account when dealing with angular momentum.

The formula for angular momentum is:

$$\text{Angular momentum} = \text{moment of inertia} \times \text{angular velocity}$$

Let us compare that formula to the one for linear momentum.

$$\text{Linear momentum} = \text{mass} \times \text{linear velocity}$$

It is seen that the term *moment of inertia* appears in the angular formula rather than the term *mass*. It can be said, then, that mass is the single determinant of moment of inertia in linear momentum. As mass is increased or decreased, the linear moment of inertia is increased or decreased. In the angular case, however, moment of inertia is defined in formula form as

$$\text{Angular moment of inertia} = \text{mass} \times \text{radius}^2$$

Substituting for terms, we can write

$$\text{Angular momentum} = (\text{mass} \times \text{radius}^2) \times \text{angular velocity}$$

The three quantities that influence angular momentum are clearly set forth and will be seen to have relevance to centripetal force.

**Centrifugal and Centripetal Forces** When an object achieves velocity along a curved path, centrifugal and centripetal forces are exerted simultaneously. Because a large portion of the movements involved in sports and dance are angular, it is necessary to examine the nature of these forces, and the methods by which adjustments can be made for their presence.

Centrifugal force is that force which is said to act away from the axis of rotation, whereas centripetal force acts toward the axis of rotation. The forceful swinging of a baseball bat is accompanied by a tendency of the bat and the arms to pull away from the vertical axis around which they are being rotated. Centrifugal force is thus being manifested. The musculature of the back, shoulders, and arms, as well as those muscles involved in gripping the bat, contract simultaneously to exert a force toward the vertical axis—centripetal force—in an effort to neutralize the outward pull. If neutralization is realized, in other words, if the two forces equal each other, the bat and arms will swing, undisturbed, through their arc. Should the centrifugal force overcome its centripetal counterpart, however, the angular path will be disturbed, most probably resulting in loss of hand contract with the bat. Accordingly, the bat will depart from the arc of the swing and travel, instead, along a path tangential to that arc. We are all familiar with the devastating potential of such implements when they slip from the hands.

To prevent such occurrences, grips of leather, tape and other materials are placed on the handles to increase friction and thereby contribute to the total centripetal force. Athletes are well-advised to change the grips on sports implements when they become worn and slippery.

Study of the formula by which amounts of centripetal force is calculated will clarify the concept.

$$\text{Centrifugal Force} = \frac{\text{mass} \times \text{velocity}^2}{\text{radius of rotation}}$$

As mass and velocity (actually its square) are increased, centripetal force must also be increased if angular rotation is to be continued. If the radius of rotation is increased, centripetal force requirements are decreased, and vice versa. Let us examine each of these quantities as they relate to sport and dance.

*Mass* The selection of an "overheavy" tennis racket, baseball bat, etc., will increase centripetal force requirements to prevent the implement from pulling away from the grip.

Heavy gymnasts will require greater grip strength than lighter gymnasts during performance of the giant swing.

*Velocity* The faster the rate of body rotation in the discus throw, the greater will be the need to apply centripetal force to prevent premature release of the discus. When the discus has been released, however, the greater will be its resulting linear velocity.

The greater the speed of a track runner around an unbanked curve, the greater must be the friction between shoes and ground (centripetal force) to prevent slipping as the body leans inwardly.

*Radius* Sharp turns in dance, basketball, softball, etc., are made in a path that has a short radius from the center of the arc of the turn. Centripetal force is, accordingly, very great. High levels of friction between the foot and the turning surface are demanded if the turn is to be made safely. If there is insufficient friction, velocity of the turn must be sacrificed to avoid falling.

The presence of centripetal force will be noted in all activities in which an implement—racket, golf club, bat—is swung forcefully, through space. Equally dramatic in the exhibition of the two forces are those sports techniques which require, for success, that an object be hurled into space. The discus throw, bowling delivery, overarm throw, and softball pitch are examples, and have in common a windup action intended to build centrifugal and centripetal forces to an optimum peak, at which time release occurs. Angular velocity is converted to linear velocity and directs the object along a path tangent to the arc at the point of release. These activities have in common also the demand for some degree of accuracy. Figure 14.6 presents sequence tracings of a softball pitcher executing the windup and release. Points *A* and *B* mark the approximate locations at which the earliest and latest releases can occur to ensure that the ball will enter the strike zone. The distance between the two points is surprisingly short—probably no more than four or five centimeters—and represents a challenge of timing that an athlete, even with the sophisticated nervous and muscular structure comprising the human body, cannot meet with any consistency. Yet, it is not rare to observe a high degree of accuracy in pitching and other such sports. How is this accomplished in the face of such odds? The answer lies in the use of a technique called *flattening the arc*. Figure 14.7 shows the actual pattern executed by the pitcher, and the flattening of the arc traveled by the softball that results from a forward linear movement of the shoulder joint. Points *A* and *B* are used, again, to show the approximate locations of the earliest and latest successful release points, and include a distance considerably longer than that pictured in figure 14.6. It is obvious that the athlete's timing need not be as precise if the arc is flattened.

The influence of centrifugal and centripetal forces is not limited to only those sports in which implements are swung or objects are thrown or kicked into space. Tumblers, gymnasts, skaters, dancers, and divers must adjust constantly to the two forces anytime rotation is initiated around a frontal, sagittal, or vertical axis. These athletes are concerned primarily with conserving and controlling the angular momentum they have at their disposal.

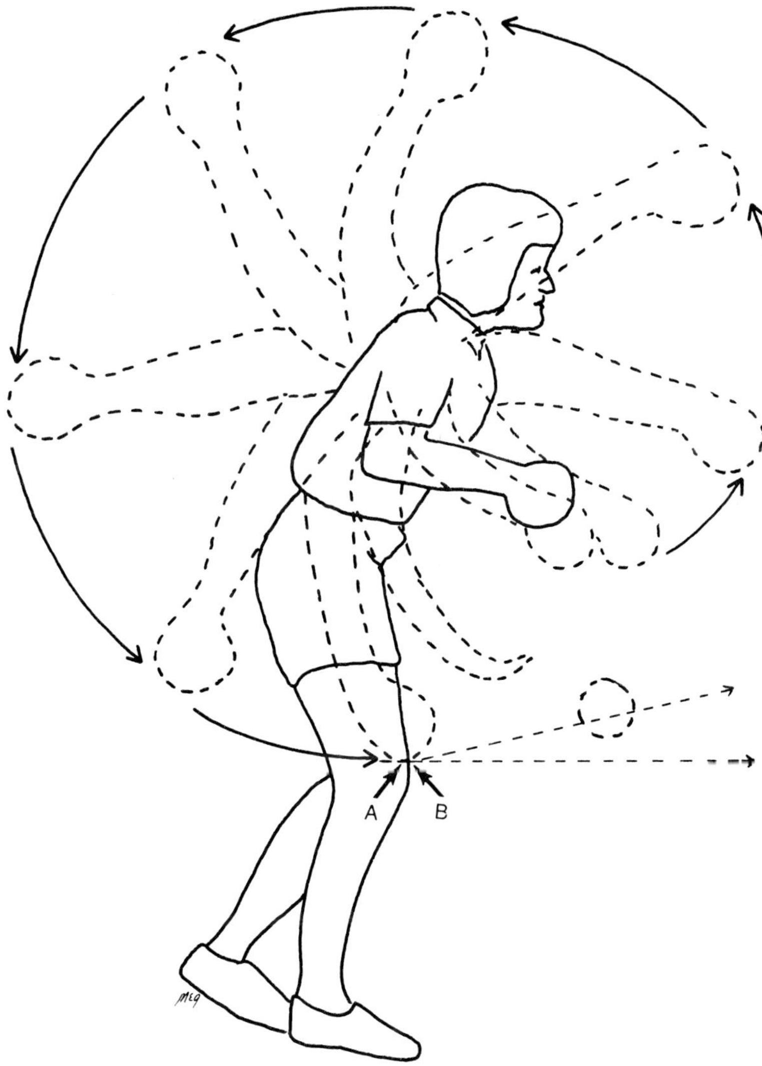

Figure 14.6. Sequence tracings of a softball pitcher executing the windmill pitch in place

A restatement of the formula for angular momentum will clarify the concept of conservation of angular momentum.

Angular momentum = (mass × radius$^2$) × angular velocity

The term *mass* in the formula refers to the mass of the rotating object; in the discussion here, the rotating object is the athlete and since his mass will not fluctuate appreciably in the course of a given rotational pattern, it can be viewed as a constant and is, therefore,

Figure 14.7. Actual sequence tracings of a softball pitcher executing the windmill pitch

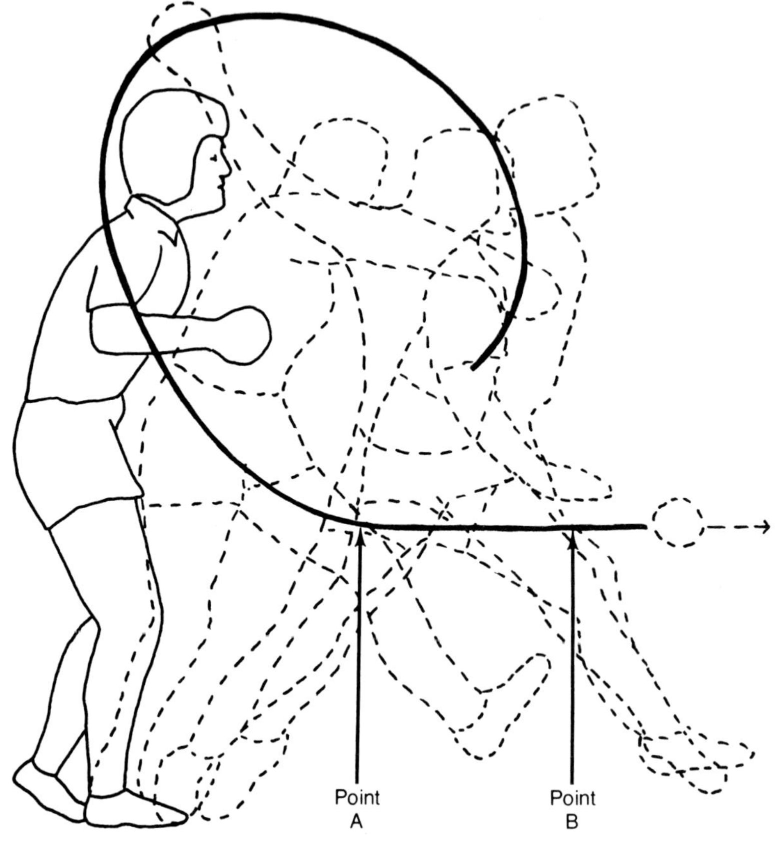


disregarded. The remaining terms of velocity and radius are the ones which can be manipulated to conserve angular momentum.

It will be noted that velocity is proportional to angular momentum as is the radius of rotation; hence, an athlete with a given amount of momentum can increase or decrease his velocity of rotation by shortening or lengthening his radius of rotation. Consider the skater who enters a vertical spin with a certain force. The arms are gathered to the body to increase the velocity of the spin, but when the spin is to end, the arms are spread into space to increase the radius and slow the velocity. The dancer performing the tour jeté (fig. 14.8) swings the arms upward to gain vertical lift, then pulls them close to the body to increase the velocity of rotation, and finally extends them to regain control for the landing. Tumblers and divers can control their rotations by shortening their radii if they are short of completing somersaults or by lengthening their radii if they are "over-rotating" their stunts.

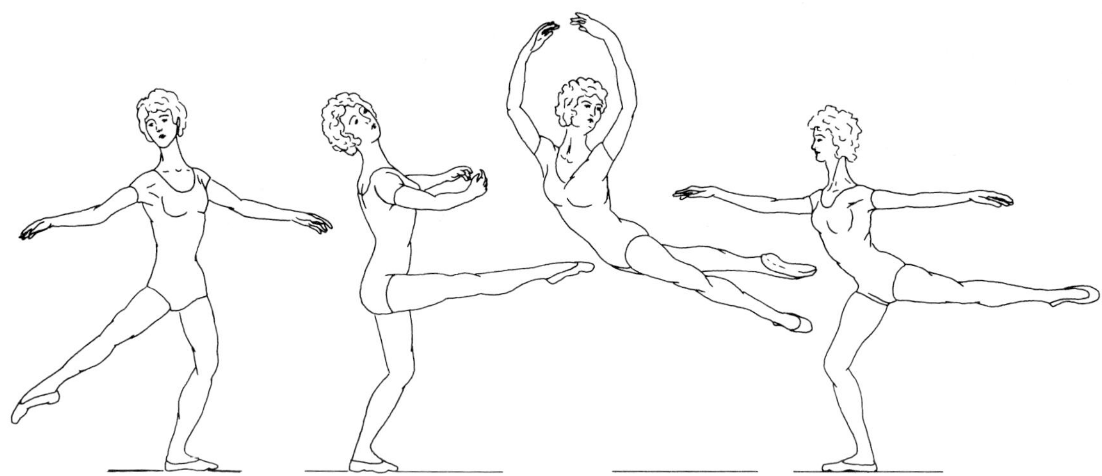

Figure 14.8. Dancer performing the tour jeté

The concept of conservation of angular momentum can occasionally benefit those in racket sports, and even the football quarterback. When the foreswing of a forehand drive has been miscalculated and will result in a late hit, the elbow can be flexed somewhat and, with the shortened radius of swing, the racket can be brought to contact more quickly. If a quarterback must pivot quickly to hand the ball off to a running back, he can speed his pivot by holding the ball close to the body, thus shortening the radius of rotation.

## Acceleration

Acceleration is the rate with which an object changes its velocity. If the rate of change yields greater velocity, the object is undergoing positive acceleration; if lesser velocity results, that is, if the object slows its velocity, negative acceleration is being experienced.

The word *deceleration* was long considered a slang term in kinesiology and was omitted from the terminology in deference to the phrase *negative acceleration*. Deceleration is being more frequently used, however. Its increased usage is probably an attempt to clear confusion regarding the use of the word *negative* to indicate both a slowing of velocity and a direction of movement. To illustrate, assume a ball is being tossed into the air. It is tossed with a certain velocity and is gradually slowed by the pull of gravity until it reaches its peak. The ball will then enjoy a gradual increase in velocity as it drops back toward earth. It would appear to be clear that the ball undergoes negative acceleration until it reaches its peak; it then is positively accelerated until it is caught. The confusion arises from the use of the words *positive* and *negative* to indicate direction. Upward movement is in a positive direction whereas downward movement is in a negative direction. Movement to the right is positive; leftward movement is negative; and so on. Thus, the tossing of a ball could be described as undergoing negative acceleration while moving in a positive direction to its peak and then accelerating positively in a negative direction. Need more be said? Terminology, in this case, creates rather than clarifies confusion. In deference to the situation, the word *deceleration* has been revived. The tossed ball can now be described as experiencing positive deceleration to its peak and negative acceleration as it approachs the ground.

Acceleration can pertain to objects moving in either linear or angular paths. As was the case with velocity, accelerations can be calculated as average or instantaneous values.

Average linear acceleration can be seen easily when one watches a runner. At the start, the runner has zero velocity; on the sound of the gun, the runner positively accelerates to reach peak velocity; the runner then undergoes either constant acceleration or positive deceleration until the finish line is crossed. The difference between the runner's final velocity and initial velocity divided by elapsed time is equal to the average linear acceleration.

$$\text{Average linear acceleration} = \frac{\text{Final velocity} - \text{initial velocity}}{\text{elapsed time}}$$

Average angular acceleration is calculated in a similar fashion. Reference to the displacement data shown on page 284 will indicate that the hand segment used in the example was displaced 3° in the first millisecond of movement and 7° during the last millisecond. Average angular velocities for those two time periods were:

First millisecond

$$\text{Average angular velocity} = \frac{3^\circ}{.01 \text{ sec.}} = 300^\circ \text{ per second}$$

Last millisecond

$$\text{Average angular velocity} = \frac{7^\circ}{.01 \text{ sec.}} = 700^\circ \text{ per second}$$

Average angular acceleration is, then equal to 4000° per second squared since

$$\text{Average angular acceleration} = \frac{700^\circ \text{ per sec.} - 300^\circ \text{ per sec.}}{.10 \text{ sec.}}$$

$$= 4000^\circ \text{ per sec}^2$$

Instantaneous acceleration, like instantaneous velocity, occurs over time periods so short that they approach zero seconds. Calculation of instantaneous accelerations, whether they are linear or angular, follows the same procedure as that outlined previously for instantaneous velocity. One begins by drawing tangents to the instantaneous velocity curve. Consider, for example, the curve shown in figure 14.9. It is repeated below in quantitative form with selected tangents drawn in place.

The slope or steepness of each tangent is indicative of the magnitude of instantaneous acceleration. The greater the slope, the higher the instantaneous acceleration. A qualitative graph of the slopes of the tangents appears in figure 14.10.

A quantitative expression of instantaneous acceleration may be found by drawing a tangent at some time period, such as 5 milliseconds (fig. 14.11). Extension of the tangent over four time periods and then intersecting its two ends with the Y axis shows that within 4 milliseconds change in velocity, the tangent rose from 20 to 42.5 radians per second.

$$\text{Instantaneous acceleration} = \frac{42.5 \text{ rad} - 20 \text{ rad}}{.04 \text{ sec}}$$

$$= 562 \text{ rads per sec}^2$$

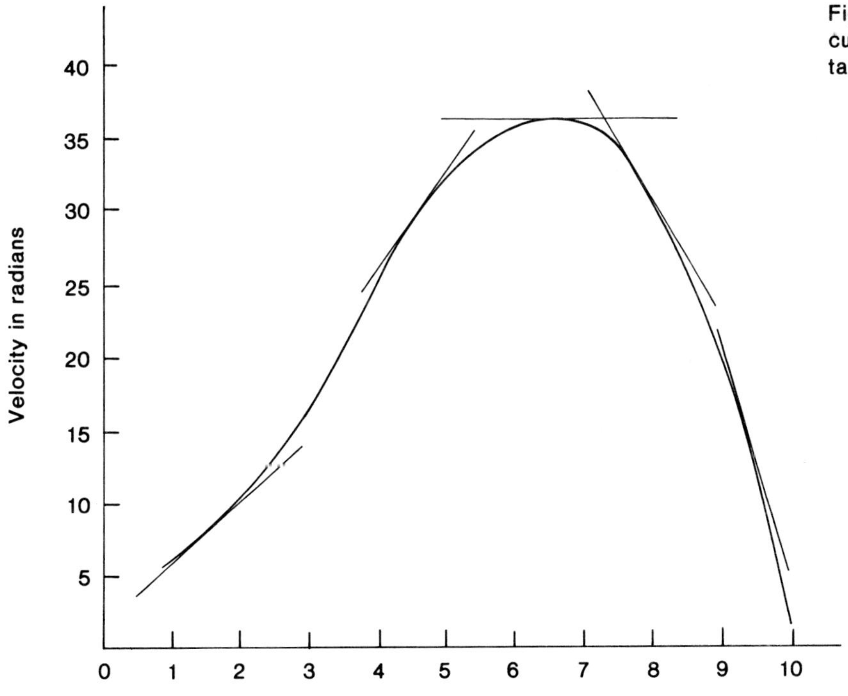


Figure 14.9. A velocity curve with selected tangents

Figure 14.10. Qualitative graph of instantaneous acceleration

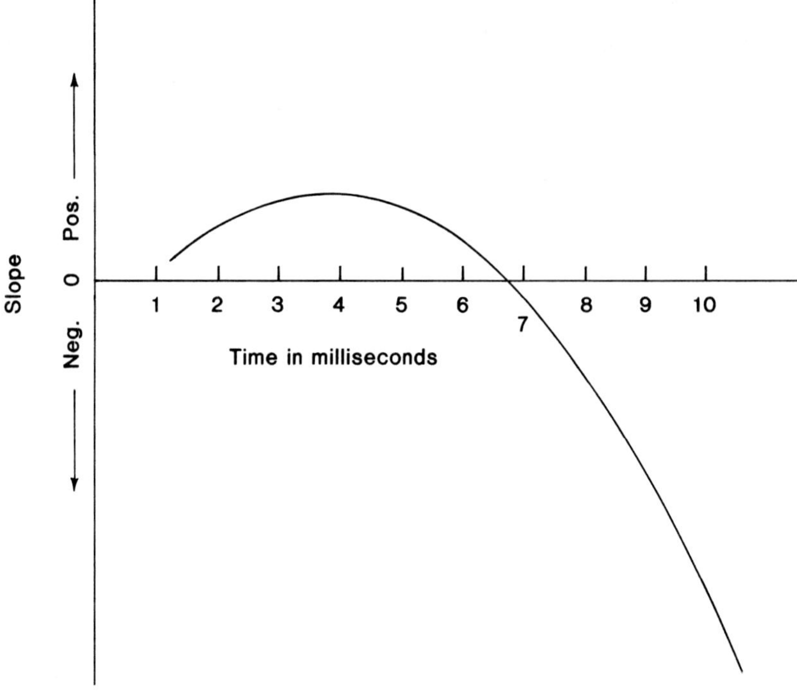


Figure 14.11. Instantaneous acceleration at 5 milliseconds

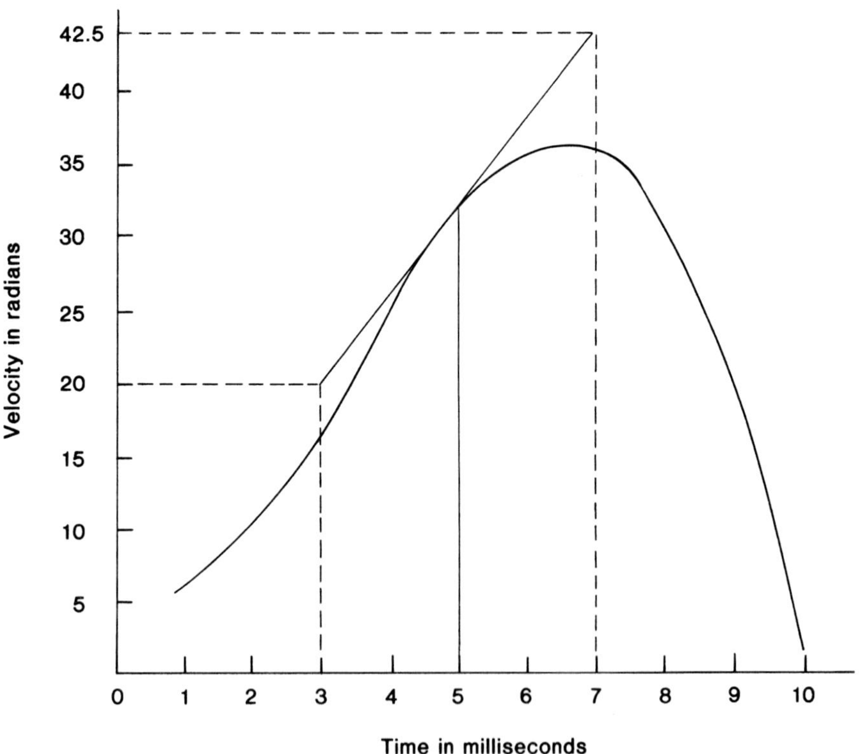

One form of acceleration with which we live every day is that described as the law of gravity. The influence of gravity's pull, with its property of acceleration, is pertinent to several sports and dance techniques. The law of gravity stipulates that an object falling toward earth will accelerate at the approximate rate of 9.8 meters per second squared; that is for every second an object falls, it will accelerate an additional 9.8 meters. During the first second of fall, the object accelerates from zero velocity to 9.8 meters per second. During the second second, the object will undergo another 9.8 meters per second of positive acceleration in addition to that of the first second, and so on. The distance and time of fall bear a simple relationship to the pull of gravity as in the following equations.

$$\text{Distance of fall} = \frac{\text{Pull of gravity}}{2} \times \text{time}^2 \text{ (seconds)}$$

or

$$s = \tfrac{1}{2}\, gt^2$$

rearranged,

$$\text{time of fall} = \sqrt{\frac{\text{distance of fall}}{\tfrac{1}{2}\text{ pull of gravity}}}$$

or

$$t = \sqrt{\frac{s}{.5g}}$$

Suppose a foul tip in baseball has risen to a point twenty meters above the ground. How long will it take the ball to fall to earth? By replacing terms in the formula, it is found that:

$$t = \sqrt{\frac{s}{.5g}} = \sqrt{\frac{20 \text{ meters}}{4.9}}$$

$$= \sqrt{4.08} = 2.02 \text{ sec}$$

The catcher has approximately two seconds in which to position himself to catch the ball after the ball reaches its peak.

Examination of the formula relating to gravitational pull will show that the use of the symbol $g$ carries no reference to whether the acceleration for which it stands is positive or negative. The foul tip which requires two seconds to fall to earth required two seconds to rise to its peak. Implicit in this concept is the fact that the velocity of the ball at the moment it is caught is equal to the velociy with which it left the bat (provided the ball was hit and caught at the same height from the ground). It is small wonder that catchers frequently drop the ball, for, at such high velocities, a momentary blink of the eyes is all that is required to lose eye contact completely and commit the error. Similarly, it is understandable that the tennis smash is so difficult a shot to execute—especially so if the opponent's lob was hit high into the air.

## Summary

Linear motion is characterized by the movement of all body parts in the same direction and at the same velocity. Angular motion provides for the circular rotation of an object around an axis, and curvilinear motion, a subcategory of linear motion, is characterized by movement of an object along a curved, but not circular, path.

Linear and angular velocity are defined as the displacement in a given direction that is covered in a unit of time and is differentiated from speed because speed carries no requirement of direction. When velocity is multiplied by mass, the product is known as momentum and can either be linear or angular in nature.

Acceleration is the rate at which an object changes velocity and can be used to describe both linear and angular motion. An object undergoing the pull of gravity, with its constant acceleration of 9.8 meters per second$^2$, is an example of linear acceleration.

Angular momentum is the product of mass, radius of rotation$^2$, and angular velocity. Angular momentum is relevant to conservation of momentum and centripetal force in activities that involve swinging and hurling of sports implements, and body rotations in diving and tumbling. When centripetal force is eliminated, objects will leave their circular paths along a tangent to the point of release.

## Laboratory and Field Experiences

1. Categorize each of the following activities according to whether it is linear, curvilinear, angular, or a combination motion.
   a. Free throw in basketball
   b. Bicycling
   c. Long jump in track
   d. Glide in the sidestroke
   e. Action of the leg during the football punt
   f. Free fall of a sky diver
   g. Movement of a pool cue during the break
2. Determine whether the following are examples of speed or velocity.
   a. Cross-country ski racing
   b. Throw from shortstop to first base
   c. Motocross
   d. Fifty-meter freestyle race in swimming

3. Sketch a water skier being pulled along the surface of water. Draw vectors to represent all of the forces being applied to the skier.
4. Assume you are point-after-touchdown kicker in football and are faced with a wind blowing toward you from your left. Where will you direct your kick? To the right or left of the goal?
5. Run the bases in softball or baseball as rapidly as you can. Can you continue your straightaway velocity as you round a base? What does centrifugal force have to do with the rate at which you can round a base?
6. What are the degrees of difficulty of a forward somersault dive in (1) tuck position, (2) pike position, and (3) lay-out position? Do these degrees of difficulty agree with what you know about angular momentum? Explain.
7. Explain why the curves of a bicycle track are banked.
8. Using the following data, calculate and graph displacements, velocities, and accelerations.

| Time (sec.) | Position (meters) |
|---|---|
| 0 | 0 |
| .1 | 5 |
| .2 | 10 |
| .3 | 15 |
| .4 | 22 |
| .5 | 32 |
| .6 | 43 |
| .7 | 55 |
| .8 | 58 |

# 15 Projection

The principles which relate to projection depend upon the reason for the projection. If an object is to reach its destination in the shortest possible time, the angle at which it is projected will be selected specifically and will differ from the angle chosen if the technique demands that time of flight be as long as possible. If distance or accuracy rather than time of flight is the critical factor, still other angles may be selected. As all of these situations are examined below, air resistance is disregarded.

Any projectile follows a curvilinear path through space and is governed by two conditions: (1) the angle at which it is projected will equal the angle at which it hits the ground (angle of incidence), and (2) the pull of gravity influences it in a constant manner regardless of its angle of projection. Figure 15.1 illustrates the first of these conditions and depicts, as examples, four angles of projection at equivalent velocities, from ground level. In each case, the angles of projection and incidence are equal; the distances covered by the object vary, however, but in a predictable manner. When the projection angle is 90 degrees, the object rises higher than it does at any other angle, requiring maximum flight time, but it covers no distance. As the projection angle decreases from 90 degrees to 0 degrees, the height of projection gradually lessens, and less time will be used between projection time and impact time. Distance covered by the projectile is seen to increase as the angle approaches 45 degrees where it is greatest, and then to decrease as the angle nears 0 degrees. It will be noted that the angles of 30 and 60 degrees result in equal distances covered by the projectile. This will be the case, also, for angles of 20 and 70 degrees, 40 and 50 degrees, and any other pairs of angles which sum to 90 degrees, for these angles involve complementary components of vertical and horizontal force.

From the discussion to this point, it follows that if distance of projection is the criterion of success, and if projection is to occur from ground level, the 45-degree angle should be selected. Kickoff specialists in football, as well as golfers, long jumpers and dancers performing distance leaps, can benefit from this knowledge as they select appropriate projection angles. Golfers must consider, however, that the

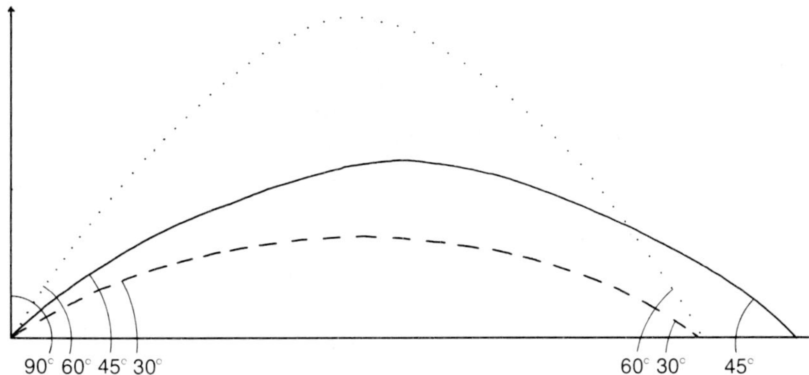


Figure 15.1. Four angles of projection at a constant velocity and their relationships to distance covered

slant of the face of the club imparts backspin to the ball, and this coupled with the complicated aerodynamics of the dimpled surface of the ball, causes it to rise. A lower projection angle is chosen, therefore, in order that the ball can rise into its optimum path. Long jumpers and dancers must recall that their respective projection velocities are built up through an approach run. Their horizontal component is thus far greater than their vertical component as takeoff is approached. To convert this horizontal force to a vertical one would require more muscular force than the human body can generate, and even if it were possible, the conversion would necessitate such a level of energy that there would scarcely be enough remaining to allow the athlete to leave the ground. For greatest distance of body projection, the projection angle of choice is somewhat less than 30 degrees.

In those techniques which depend upon the element of flight time as well as distance, the selection of projection is more involved. The football quarterback knows, through practice, where in the pattern his pass is to be caught. If he chooses a low projective angle, his teammate will not have sufficient time to run to the predetermined point. On the other hand, the choice of projection which is too high may require more strength of his throwing arm than he is capable of giving. The same problems face the baseball outfielder who must project the ball at an angle which allows it to reach a specific point in the shortest time possible. The basketball player faces other problems of projection as he shoots. To him, the selection of projection angle must be quite precise to ensure accuracy, and yet he is always at the mercy of varying distances to be covered by the ball, as well as his own inconsistent velocities of projection.

Athletes participating in field events such as the discus throw and shot put must make yet another adjustment in the selection of optimum angles of projection. Whereas the angle of 45 degrees yields optimum distance from ground level projection, it is not optimum for

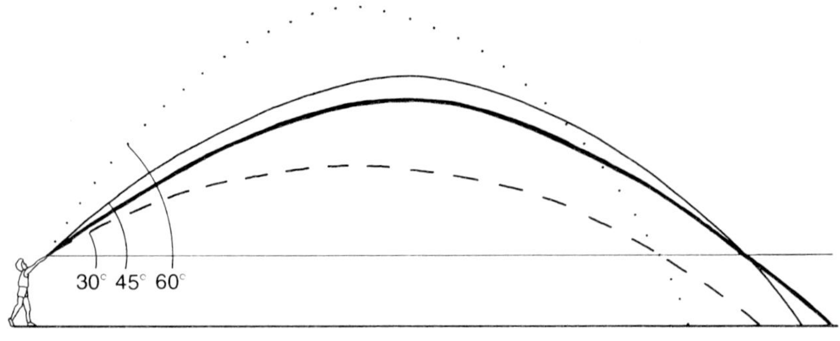


Figure 15.2. Effect of height of projection on distance when angle and velocity of projection are held constant. The projection angle represented by the heavy line is less than 45 degrees, but provides for greatest ground distance

above ground projection. Figure 15.2 illustrates the effect of height of projection on distance when angle and velocity are held constant. It is seen that as height of release increases, the projection angle should decrease if all possible ground distance is to be covered. In the actual situation, velocity of projection must also be considered since no two athletes, regardless of their height difference, will be able to generate equal velocities. In general, the tall athlete who is able to project at high velocities (and thus throw for long distances) should choose angles which are from 5 to 10 degrees less than 45 degrees. The shorter and weaker individual will find more success if he projects at angles closer to but never equaling or exceeding 45 degrees.

In order to further clarify the principles of projection, two formulas will be introduced. The first is used for calculating horizontal displacement (range) of a projectile when projected from ground level and states that:

$$\text{Range} = \frac{\text{velocity}^2 \times \text{sin of } (2 \times \text{ angle of release})}{\text{acceleration of gravity}}$$

$$= \frac{v^2 \sin 2\,\theta}{g}$$

Since the acceleration of gravity (9.8 meters per sec$^2$) is constant, it can be ignored as a factor that will increase or decrease range. Range of a projectile depends, then, on its velocity ($v^2$) and its projection angle.

It is no surprise that range is dependent on velocity of projection; we commonly accept the fact that if two objects are projected at the same angle, the one projected at the greater velocity will go farther than the one with lesser velocity. The relationship of projection angle to range may not appear so logical, since it is not actually the projection angle with which we are dealing but rather the sine of twice that angle. The trigonometric function sine varies between zero (0°) to one (90°). The largest value that can be assigned to the term sine $2\ \theta$ is, therefore, one. It follows that $2\ \theta$ must equal 90° and $\theta$ will be 45°. This confirms the statement made above that 45° is the optimum angle for ground-level projection.

Let us now substitute some arbitrary values for the terms in the numerator and then vary them to determine which has the greater influence on range. Assume a projection velocity of 10 meters per second at a projection angle of 30°.

$$R = \frac{10^2 \times \sin 2(30^\circ)}{9.8}$$

$$= \frac{100 \times \sin 60^\circ}{9.8}$$

$$\sin 60^\circ = .866$$

$$= 8.84 \text{ meters}$$

Now, each of the values arbitrarily selected will be increased, in turn, by one unit; i.e., velocity will be increased to 11 kilometers per second and range will be calculated. Following that, velocity will be returned to 10 meters per second and $\theta$ will be increased to 31°. The calculation will be repeated. Thus,

$$R = \frac{11^2 \times \sin 2(30^\circ)}{9.8}$$

$$= 10.69 \text{ meters}$$

and

$$R = \frac{10^2 \times \sin 2(31^\circ)}{9.8}$$

$$\sin 62^\circ = .883$$

$$= 9.01 \text{ meters}$$

It is obvious that increasing either of the two values improves the range. Equally obvious is the greater increase per unit that is achieved by varying velocity.

The formula for calculating range if an object is projected from some height (h) above the ground can now be introduced.

$$R = \frac{V^2 \sin\theta \cos\theta + V \cos\theta \sqrt{(V \sin\theta)^2 + 2\ hg}}{g}$$

Using the same values selected for the previous calculations and setting height at 2 meters, we see that

$$R = \frac{10^2\,(.5)\,(.866) + 10\text{km/sec}\,(.866)\,\sqrt{(10 \cdot .5)^2 + 2 \cdot 2 \cdot 9.8}}{9.8}$$

$$\sin 30^\circ = .5$$

$$\cos 30^\circ = .866$$

$$= 11.5 \text{ meters}$$

Each of the values will now be increased, one at a time, by one unit as the other values are kept the same.

1. $V = 11\text{M/sec} \qquad \theta = 30^\circ \qquad h = 2\text{M}$

$$R = \frac{11^2\,(.5)\,(.866) + 11(.866)\,\sqrt{(11 \cdot .5)^2 + 2 \cdot 2 \cdot 9.8}}{9.8}$$

$$R = 13.45 \text{ meters}$$

2. $V = 10\text{M/sec} \qquad \theta = 31^\circ \qquad h = 2\text{M}$

$$R = \frac{10^2\,(.515)\,(.857) + 10(.857)\,\sqrt{(10 \cdot .515)^2 + 2 \cdot 2 \cdot 9.8}}{9.8}$$

$$R = 11.59 \text{ meters}$$

3. $V = 10\text{M/sec} \qquad \theta = 30^\circ \qquad h = 3\text{M}$

$$R = \frac{10^2\,(.5)\,(.866) + 10(.866)\,\sqrt{(10 \cdot .5)^2 + 2 \cdot 3 \cdot 9.8}}{9.8}$$

$$R = 12.51 \text{ meters}$$

Comparison of the results of the calculations again shows that a one-unit increment in velocity increases range more than similar increments in either projection angle or height. It would be more beneficial for the coach of distance throwers to emphasize the development of velocity of projection rather than searching for optimum projection angles and heights. On the other hand, projection angle is probably the easiest factor to change in a short period of time. Since velocity is a function of strength and projection height is a function of the athlete's height, it is likely that neither of these can be changed appreciably from week to week. It is for this reason that many athletes keep on file a film record of their top performances. Should their performances suddenly fall off, they can determine their errors by comparison. It is not unusual to find that the cause of their problem is improper selection of projection angle.

It was pointed out earlier that all projectiles are influenced in like manner by the pull of gravity. If two projectiles reach the same height, they will fall to the ground in the same interval of time. Their respective angles of projection make no difference to time lapse; distances covered will, of course, vary. This principle holds true, likewise, for objects which are projected horizontally from above ground level. If an object is projected horizontally from a height of 4.9 meters, it will strike the ground one second later regardless of the velocity with which it was projected. The time interval can be calculated by using the formula already introduced:

$$t = \sqrt{\frac{S}{.5g}}$$

$$t = \sqrt{\frac{4.9}{.5(9.8)}} = \sqrt{1}$$

$$\text{time} = 1 \text{ second}$$

It is seen, then, that the projectile will strike the ground at the same time whether it is projected horizontally or whether it is simply dropped. Application of this principle to ballistics yields surprising—almost unbelievable—results. If a bullet is fired from a gun trained along the horizontal, it will strike the ground at the same time as will a second bullet which was dropped from the muzzle height at the moment of firing.

## Summary

Projectiles follow a curved path through space which is governed by velocity and angle of projection, and height of release. The projection angle of 90 degrees provides height but no distance, and the projection angle of 0 degrees, from ground level, provides for distance but no height.

Greatest distance of an object projected at ground level will be reached when the angle of projection is 45 degrees. As the height of release is elevated, the optimum angle decreases.

Three factors govern the range that will be covered by a projectile: (1) velocity of projection, (2) projection angle, and (3) projection height. Increments in velocity will produce the greatest increases in range. Given constant projection velocity and zero height (ground level), greatest range will be attained at a 45° projection angle. As height of projection is increased, however, projection angles should be decreased slightly from 45°.

Flight time of an object projected horizontally from above ground level is governed by the influence of gravity just as all projectiles are. The longer flight times must be accompanied by high projection angles; if short flight times are required, the projecting angle should be lessened.

## Laboratory and Field Experiences

1. Attach a hose to a water faucet and open the valve for full pressure. Hold the end of the hose next to the ground and train the water stream upwardly until it covers maximum distance. Have a partner use a protractor to determine the angle at which you are projecting the water. Now, hold the hose at shoulder level and adjust the angle for maximum distance. Is your second projection angle lower or higher than your first? Do your findings agree with the principles of projection?
2. Sketch a gymnast at three or four time-points as he performs the forward giant swing on the horizontal bar. Mark the approximate location of his center of gravity on each figure and connect them to form a circle. If the gymnast were to release the bar just before he reaches the bottom of his arc, where would he be projected? If he releases just past the bottom of the arc, where would he be projected? Considering his acceleration during the downswing, at what point do you think he will develop his greatest angular momentum? If his grip strength is not sufficient to provide the necessary centripetal force at the point of greatest angular momentum, he will be pulled from the bar. Where would he be projected if this were the case? Does this indicate appropriate positioning of spotters?
3. Explain why a football punter frequently chooses the higher of the two complementary angles at which to project the ball. How do the two "hang times" differ?
4. Assume that a baseball shortstop has approximately three seconds to field a batted ball and throw it to first base. What projection angle should he choose to ensure that the ball will arrive in time to make the out? What does this mean with regard to the velocity of his throw?
5. Why is it possible to shoot an arrow at zero degrees of projection when shooting at 18 to 20 meters and hit the target? Why must the arrow be shot at greater than zero degrees from 60 meters?

# Spin and Rebound

# 16

The mechanics of spin and its effect upon ball flight and rebound reflect combinations of aerodynamics, force composition, and principles of action-reaction. Aerodynamics explain the behavior of the ball in flight; force composition and related basics of action-reaction explain departures from normal paths of rebound.

For purposes of the discussion that follows, friction of rebound will not be considered. It should be noted, however, that friction between the ball and the rebounding surface will always dampen, to some degree, the rebound response.

## Spin and the Ball in Flight

When a ball moves through space, the air which it encounters is forced to part and, as the ball passes through, exerts a certain amount of resistance on its cover (fig. 16.1). When the ball is not spinning the resistance applied at each point is neutralized by that applied on the opposite side and no deviation will be noted. If spin has been imparted, however, air resistance over a portion of the ball acts with the spin, while on the other side the resistance is against the spin (fig. 16.2). Where air resistance acts with the spin, air is allowed to pass quickly over the ball and a low-pressure area develops. The portion of the ball 180 degrees removed is spinning against air flow and develops

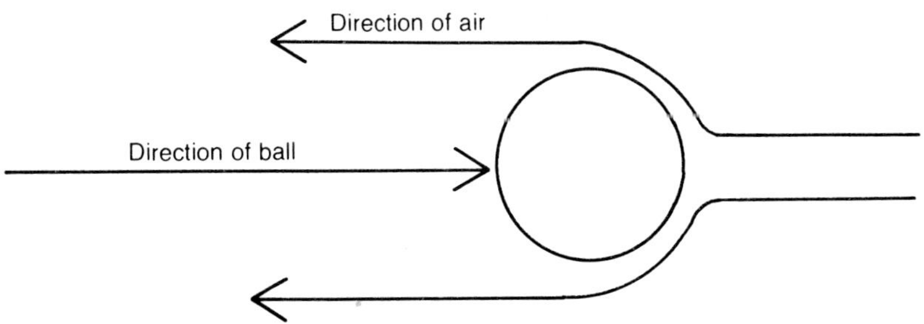


**Figure 16.1. A ball with no spin encountering air flow**

Figure 16.2. High and low pressure areas developed by a ball with spin

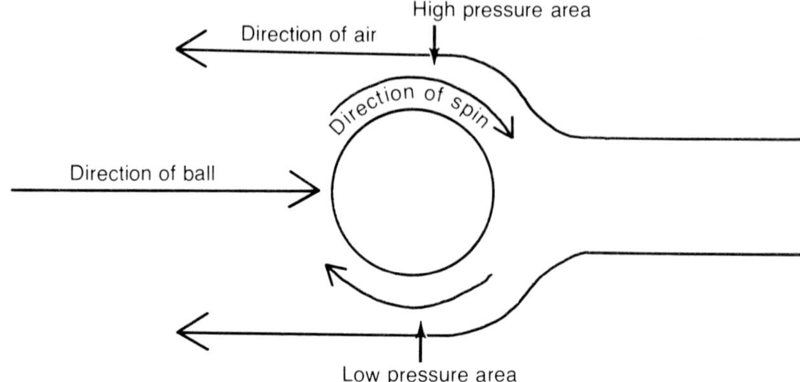


a high-pressure area. As a result the ball is pushed by the high-pressure area into the low pressure area, and will rise, drop, or curve, accordingly.

There are an infinite number of spin directions that can be imparted to a ball and all of these cause it to behave uniquely. Only the three common spins will be discussed here for any other spin will be a combination of at least two of these; if the mechanics of the three major spins are mastered, any combination can also be deciphered.

### Spin around the Frontal Axis—Top Spin and Backspin

Figure 16.3 is presented to show, from the side view, the effect of top spin and backspin on balls in flight. The top spin ball is seen to drop into the low pressure area created by the faster moving air as it passes below the ball. With backspin, however, the ball will rise into the low pressure area created above it. Top spins and backspins are seen commonly in the tennis drive and basketball shot, respectively.

### Spin around the Sagittal Axis—Clockwise and Counterclockwise Spin

In figure 16.4, two balls are pictured from the back as though the reader has thrown them. The spins illustrated are characteristic of a bullet, archery arrow, or a passed football. It will be seen that as the balls come into contact with the surrounding air, they meet it throughout their circumferences with a spin direction of 90 degrees to air flow. The effect at any single point on the cover of the ball is neutralized by the effect 180 degrees removed. The ball will not, therefore, depart from its normal curvilinear path, and will even enjoy a certain stabilizing effect in that path.

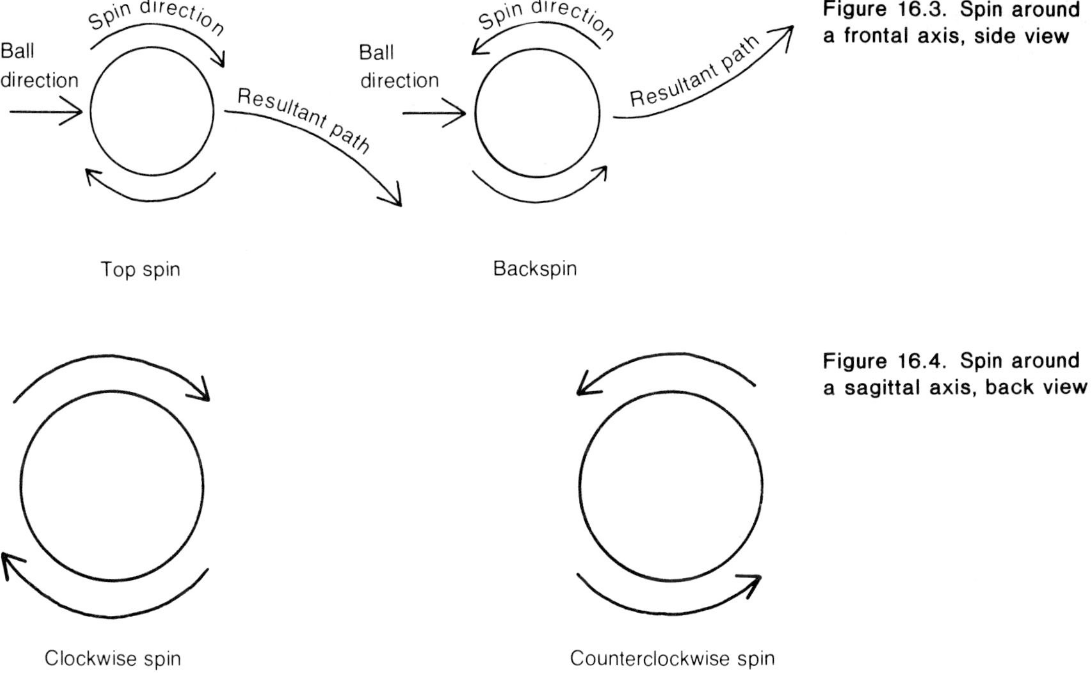


**Figure 16.3. Spin around a frontal axis, side view**

**Figure 16.4. Spin around a sagittal axis, back view**

### Spin around the Vertical Axis—Right-to-Left and Left-to-Right Spin

The balls shown in figure 16.5 are seen to be spinning around the vertical axis. They are pictured from the back as though they had been thrown by the reader. The labeling of right-to-left and left-to-right is, accordingly, made from that vantage point. Study of balls rotating in these two directions will demonstrate that low-pressure areas are made to occur along that side of each ball which moves in the same direction as the passage of air. Right-to-left spin will result in a curve to the right; left-to-right spin will cause the ball to curve left. Such spins frequently accompany golf drives and result in a sliced or hooked shot.

## Rebound

The ability to predict the path of a rebounding ball is important to success in several of the sports. If all balls had equal ability to rebound, bounced with equal velocity, had no spin, prediction of the rebound path would be a simple matter. Such is not the case, however,

Figure 16.5. Spin around the vertical axis, back view

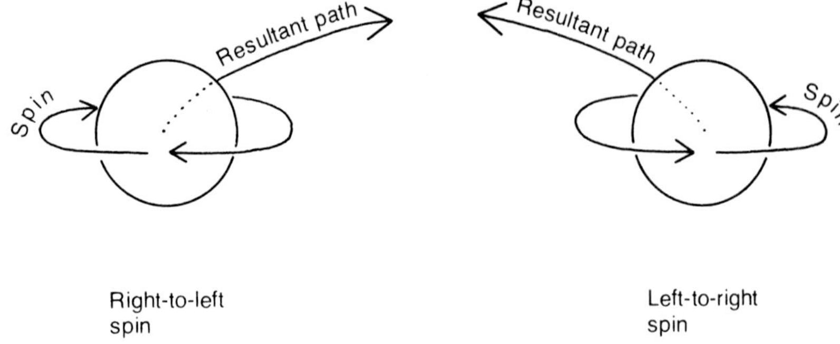


for almost every sport involving rebounding objects incorporates balls of different elasticities which can be hit or thrown with or without spin at different velocities onto surfaces of varying hardness.

## Coefficient of Restitution

The amount of bounce possessed by a ball, or any object, can be quantified by calculating its coefficient of restitution (e) as follows:

$$\text{coefficient of restitution} = \sqrt{\frac{\text{height of bounce}}{\text{height of drop}}}$$

If a ball is dropped from a height of 150 centimeters and achieves a height of 121.5 centimeters from the bounce, its coefficient of rebound is equal to the square root of 121.5 centimeters divided by 150 centimeters, or:

$$e = \sqrt{\frac{121.5}{150}} = \sqrt{.81}$$

$$e = .9$$

Proper coefficients of restitution of the objects used in sports are ensured by various means. Basketball rule books include the regulation that when a basketball is dropped from a height of 1.83 meters, measured from the bottom of the ball, it must bounce to a height of from 1.24 to 1.37 meters, measured to the top of the ball. The coefficient of a volley ball is the responsibility of the manufacturer who provides a ball that will have proper bounce when it is inflated according to specifications. Tennis balls retain their coefficients through vacuum packing. Old and worn balls have a decreased coefficient and are said to be "dead." Golf balls, squash balls, even "superballs" have their own coefficients of restitution, and they will range between greater than zero and less than one. Objects which have coefficients of zero do not rebound; objects which possess coefficients of one exist only in the imagination, since some energy is always lost to the action of the object against the rebounding surface. The energy remaining in the bounce is, therefore, always less than that built up during the drop.

### Angles of Incidence and Rebound

With no spin, the ball will rebound from the striking surface at the same angle as that with which it approached the surface. The angle of approach is referred to as the angle of incidence; the angle at which it leaves the striking surface is the angle of rebound (fig. 16.6). When spin has been imparted to the ball, however, the angle of rebound will not equal the angle of incidence, and rebound will no longer be as predictable.

In the preceding pages, the three major types of spin were discussed with regard to ball behavior in flight. Here, the effect of those spins will be examined as they relate to ball behavior from the rebound. The three spins are those resulting from rotation of the ball around the frontal, sagittal, and vertical axes.

### Rotation around the Frontal Axis: Top Spin and Backspin

When a ball strikes a rebounding surface with top spin, the bottom of the ball—its rebounding surface—is moving backward (fig. 16.7). The reaction to the spin direction will be forward, in much the same way that one's body will move forward as a result of a backward push

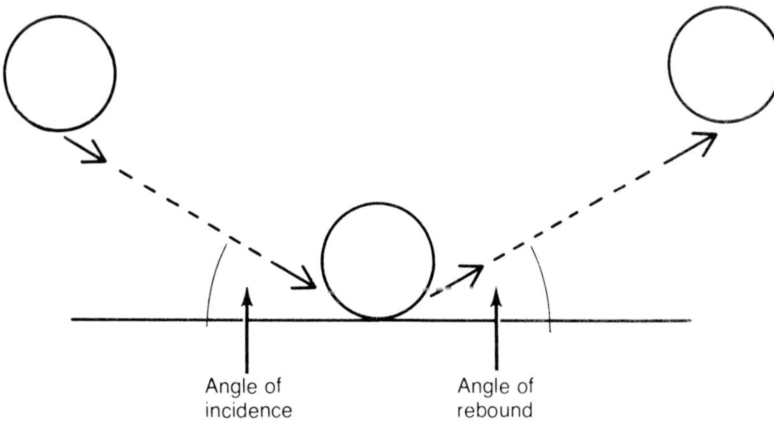


**Figure 16.6. Angles of incidence and rebound, side view**

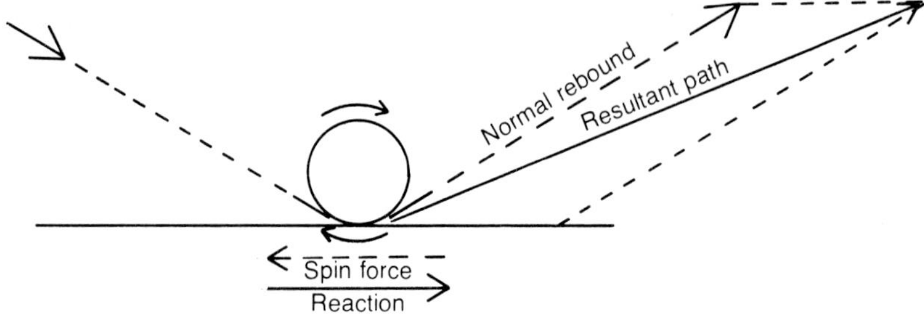


Figure 16.7. Rebound of a ball with top spin, side view

with the foot against the ground. This forward reaction, when coupled with the force vector of the ball as it rebounds, yields, through composition, a vector longer than either the reaction vector or the normal rebound vector. The result will be a ball which travels faster after the rebound that before it. In addition, the ball will rebound lower than normal. The greater the spin, the longer will be the spin reaction vector, and the more the ball will display the fast, low rebound of the top spin ball.

The rebounding ball which has backspin will react in exactly the opposite fashion (fig. 16.8). The portion of the ball which strikes the surface is moving forward; the reaction will be backward, and again, through composition of the two vectors representing spin reaction and rebound force, it can be seen that the ball will bounce at a greater angle than normal but with less forward velocity. If a great deal of backspin is applied with a soft hit, the ball can even be made to rebound backwardly.

### Spin around the Sagittal Axis—Clockwise and Counterclockwise Spin

The rebounding portion of the ball with clockwise spin (as viewed from the thrower's or hitter's vantage point) will be moving to the left (fig. 16.9). The ball's reaction will be a "kick" to the right. When paired with the ball's directional vector, the reaction vector will indicate a rebound which is to the right of normal. Figure 16.9 illustrates the rebound of a ball with counterclockwise spin. The ball is seen to bound to the left of normal.

### Spin around the Vertical Axis—Right-to-Left and Left-to-Right Spin (Sidespin)

In figure 16.10, a ball with sidespin is illustrated from the top view as it rebounds. Every point of the rebounding surface is moving in some direction and is causing an opposite reaction; but, for every reaction

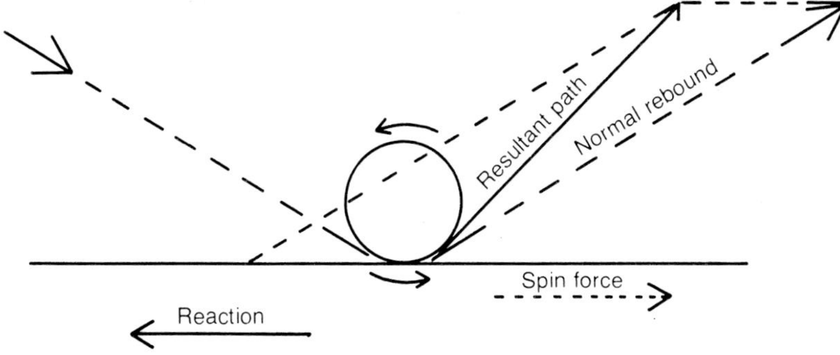


Figure 16.8. Rebound of a ball with backspin, side view

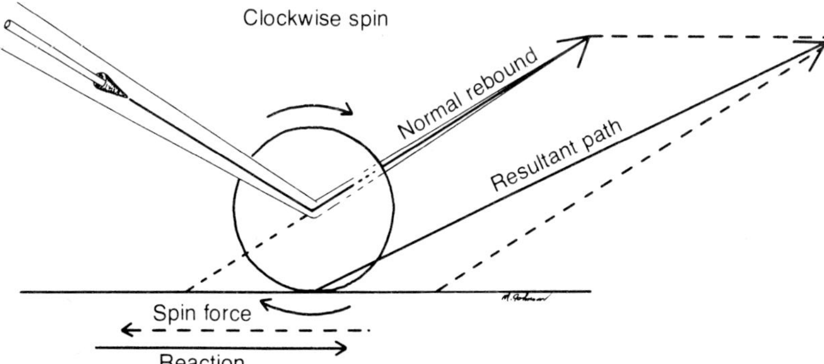


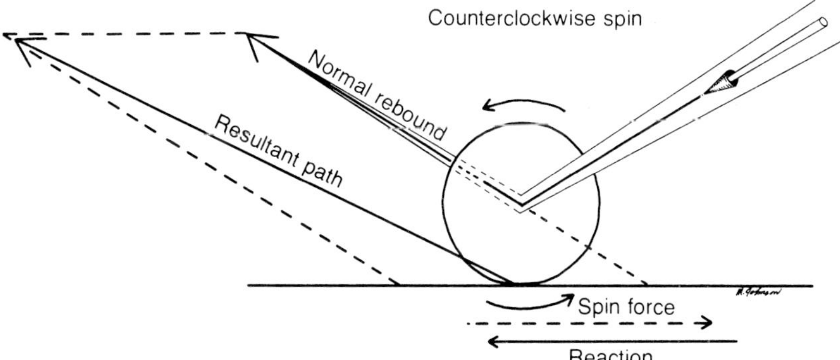


Figure 16.9. Rebound of a ball with clockwise or counterclockwise spin, back view

forward there is an equal one backward. For every reaction to the right, there is an equal one to the left. The net result of all of the reactions is zero; hence, the ball will not deviate from its normal directional path after the rebound. It may bounce a little lower than normal because of the energy-consuming friction it creates as it bounces.

Figure 16.10. Rebound of a ball with right-to-left or left-to-right spin, back view

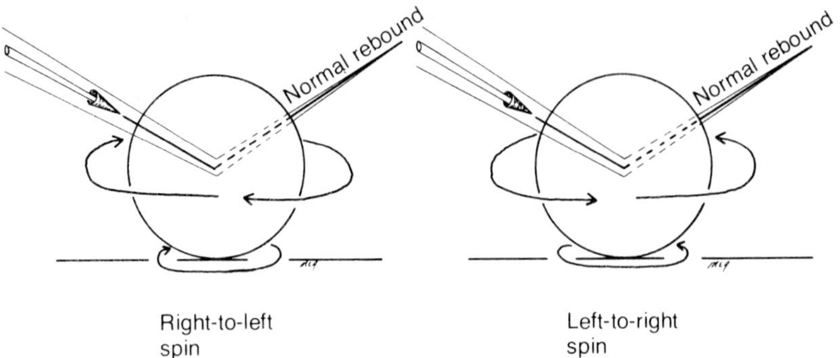


## Impact between Two Moving Bodies

To this point, discussion has been limited to the type of impact in which a moving body collides with a stationary one. It is often of equal interest to examine the factors involved when a moving object (a ball) collides with another moving object (a bat or racket). The common coefficient of restitution of the objects must be considered as must their masses, velocities, and the angle at which they meet.

For our example, let us consider the impact between ball and stick in field hockey. For the sake of simplicity, friction between the ground and rolling ball will be disregarded, as will be the friction between the two objects when they collide.

To determine the velocity of the ball after impact with the stick, the following formula must be used:

$$v = \sqrt{\left[\frac{m_2 v_2 (1 + e) + v_1 \cos \alpha \, (em_2 - m_1)}{m_1 + m_2}\right]^2 + (v_1 \sin \alpha)^2}$$

where $m_1$ = mass of ball
$m_2$ = mas of stick
$v_1$ = velocity of ball at impact
$v_2$ = velocity of stick at impact
$e$ = common coefficient of restitution between ball and stick
$\alpha$ = angle of impact between ball and stick

To determine the angle of rebound ($\beta$) the ball will take after impact:

$$\beta = \arctan\left[\frac{(v_1 \sin \alpha)(m_1 + m_2)}{m_2 v_2 (1 + e) + v_1 \cos \alpha \, (em_2 - m_1)}\right]$$

Both formulas are rather lengthy and are presented mainly for the purpose of showing the factors involved in studying this type of impact. Should the interested student wish to select arbitrary values for use in the formulas and then vary each one in turn, he or she is urged to do so. The findings will indicate that the velocity of the ball after impact can be increased if (1) the mass of the stick is increased, (2) the preimpact velocity of the stick is increased, (3) the preimpact velocity of the ball is increased, and (4) the angle of impact ($\alpha$) is made to approach 90°.

These results can be generalized to tennis, baseball, softball, and many other sports. It must be remembered, however, that one must possess sufficient strength to increase velocity of the swing and/or to control increased mass of the hitting implement. Nonetheless, if a high velocity of return is desired, pick a ball that has been hit hard to you and attempt to contact it as close to 90° as possible.

Such sports as tennis, racquetball, squash rackets, and badminton deserve special consideration in discussion of impact because it is possible to string rackets to varying degrees of tension. The tighter the strings, the higher will be the common coefficient and the greater will be the velocity of the ball after impact. Caution is again advised, however. Strings with high tension can cause loss of control precisely because their coefficients are high and there is little "give" at impact.

## Summary

The table below summarizes ball behavior during flight and rebound when the various spins have been imparted. In all cases the ball is described as it is seen from the rear, as though the reader has hit the ball with the spin indicated. Clockwise spin is designated *CW;* counterclockwise spin is designated *CCW;* right-to-left spin and left-to-right spin appear as *R-L* and *L-R,* respectively.

Numerous examples emphasizing the relevance of spin to athletic success can be pointed out. Only a few of them will be given here, with the expectation that these examples can be applied as needed.

| | Top | Back | CW | CCW | R-L | L-R |
|---|---|---|---|---|---|---|
| Ball in flight will: | drop | rise | not react | not react | curve right | curve left |
| Ball will rebound: | fast, low | slow, high | right | left | not react | not react |

The passing shot in tennis is usually hit with top spin, both because the ball will drop into the court and also because it will rebound with added velocity. Backspin is imparted to a basketball when shooting to insure its downward deflection if it hits the backboard or the back edge of the rim. Clockwise and counterclockwise spins are imparted to footballs when the quarterback passes because stability in flight is desired; however, since right- and left-handed quarterbacks spin the ball in opposite directions, receivers must take care to absorb the spin force by proper positioning of the arms and hands. Spin around the vertical axis is used successfully by pitchers to curve the ball toward or away from the batter.

The principles of rebound are not limited to impact between a moving body and a stationary one. Masses and velocities of two moving objects together with their common coefficient of restitution and their angle of impact all combine to characterize the result of the collision.

## Laboratory and Field Experiences

1. Attach a tape measure to a wall so that it is vertically aligned. Have a partner drop a golf ball, volleyball, tennis ball, squash ball, and superball from the top of the tape as you watch carefully to note the height of rebound. Calculate the coefficients of rebound of these balls by using the formula introduced in this chapter. How do the respective coefficients contribute to the flavor of the games or activities in which they are used?
2. Observe a volleyball player executing the bump and relate the angulation of her arms to the angle at which the ball is approaching her. Generalize this relationship to beginning volleyball players who frequently bump the ball back over their heads or even into their faces. It is interesting to note, with regard to the latter error, that unskilled players commonly close the eyes and turn the head as they make contact with the ball—perhaps a reflex developed from an earlier rebound disaster!
3. With a partner, execute basketball bounce passes and investigate the responses of the ball, when it rebounds, to the various spins you impart. Make any generalizations you can, and then bounce the ball, with spin, against a wall. Do your generalizations hold true? Can you add to them? Repeat the experience while bouncing the ball off of a hard ceiling. Are there differences in rebound directions from those you observed while executing the bounce pass on the floor?

4. What types of spin must a pitcher have imparted to the following pitches?
   a. Drop ball
   b. Rise ball
   c. Curve ball, inside
   d. Curve ball, outside
5. Explain why top spin is commonly imparted to a volleyball by a backline player who has the third hit.
6. Using a tape measure as described in Experience #1, determine the various coefficients of rebound of a golf ball when it rebounds from such surfaces as a concrete, wood, carpet, etc. What is the influence on rebound of surfaces with varied degrees of hardness?

# 17 Fluids

A fluid is a substance which is comprised of easily moveable particles—a substance which is capable of flowing. To the performer in sports and dance, the fluids of import are air and water. Certainly the fluid most typically encountered is air; however, the underwater swimmer must be more cognizant of the fluid properties of water than air, while the competitive swimmer is at the mercy of both environments as he propels himself to reach his goal.

The study of fluids is simplified by sorting athletic activities into two categories. One category pertains to static conditions of performance; the second concerns dynamic or moving aspects of performance.

## Fluids and Statics

When air comprises the fluid environment of an athlete and the athlete as well as the environment are in static conditions, there is no effect on performance. The principles of stability which were discussed in chapter 12 continue to pertain without change. When the environment is water, however, a different set of principles apply and will be discussed below.

**Principle 1—Archimedes' Principle** When an object is placed in water, it is buoyed up by a force equal to the weight of the water it displaces.

Suppose a tank is filled with water to a level even with the bottom of a drain tube which leads to an empty container. Suppose further that an object weighing one kilogram is placed in the water tank (fig. 17.1). The water displaced by the object will flow through the drain tube and into the container. If the container is weighed after water ceases to flow through the drain tube, and corrected for its own weight, a decision can be made as to the condition of the one-kilogram object in the tank. If the displaced water weighs one kilogram the object will be floating; however, none of its parts will be above water. If the displaced water weighs more than one kilogram, the

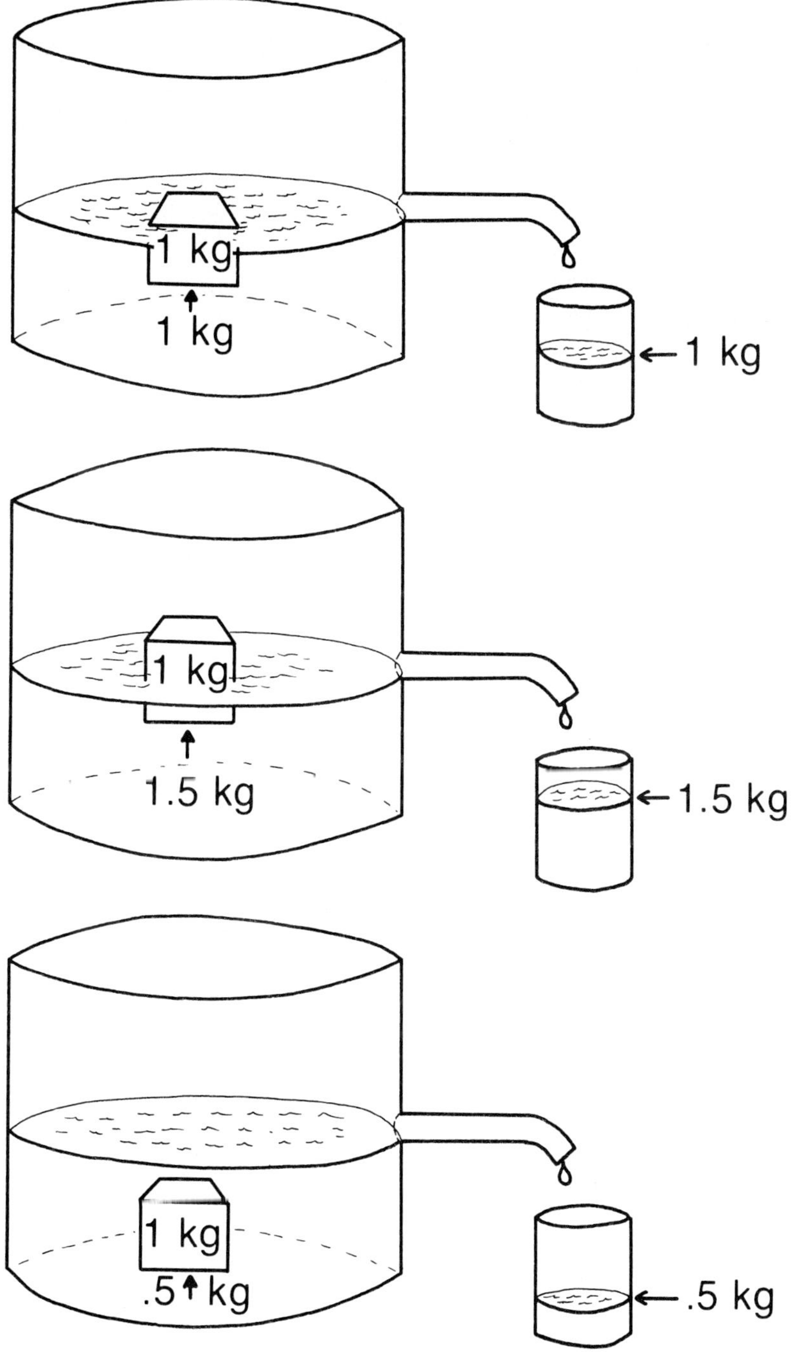


Figure 17.1. Archimedes' principle

object will be floating with some of its parts above water. If the displaced water weighs less than one kilogram, the object will have fallen to the bottom of the tank.

The predominant characteristics of objects which will float are large surface area and light weight. Cork, inflated balls, and most wood all exhibit these characteristics and are, likewise, known to float. Rock, metal, and other such materials are quite heavy in proportion to their surface areas and will not float.

When Archimedes' principle is applied to humans, it can be seen that one's ability to float is a function of body build. Overweight or obese individuals float easily because of the large surface area of their bodies and because, despite the fact that they certainly are not light in weight, they possess great amounts of buoyant fatty tissue. Extremely lean individuals present neither large surface areas nor significant amounts of fatty tissue, and find floating difficult or impossible. Similarly, muscular individuals, although exhibiting large surface area, experience difficulty in floating because they have a low percentage of body fat.

The size and amount of inflation of the lungs must not be overlooked as a factor in the ability of individuals to float. For those who are on the borderline between floating and sinking, the degree of inflation of the lungs may be critical. The advice "take a deep breath and hold it" is not without basis as an aid to the beginning swimmer to float. However, since the life of the float may be limited to the length of time one can hold the breath, a further piece of advice is in order. If the swimmer will exhale and inhale in the shortest time possible between each breath-holding bout, it will be noted that the float can be maintained. The body reacts rather slowly to adverse floating conditions, and if the exhalation-inhalation phase is performed quickly and explosively, the body will not have time to sink.

Only a small percentage of people are actually unable to float, and for these, some type of buoyant garment must be worn if motionless floating is to be performed. Life vests and other such garments are designed to increase significantly the surface area of the body while adding only slightly to its weight. Thus, the displaced water weighs considerably more than the vested swimmer and floating is possible.

The positioning of a body part above water decreases the ability of the body to float because no water is displaced by the protruding part. Attempts to keep the head above water while floating are doomed to failure because of its heaviness; some compensation must be made to support it. These compensatory actions can be sculling of the hands or kicking of the legs or both, as done while treading water. Treading water consumes, of course, much more energy than motionless floating, but if the head is to be held clear of the water, movements must be made by body parts below the water to offset its downward press.

A similar problem confronts the synchronized swimmer who attempts a stunt called the "ballet leg." The swimmer is required to support one or even both legs above water. Tremendous downward force must be generated by the hands and arms to equal the weight of the legs.

Another application of Archimedes' principle is made by those certified to teach swimming for the handicapped. Immersion of the body has the effect of making it weigh less because of its buoyancy. It is possible that muscles too weak to cause movement against gravity can do so within a water environment. Some muscular exercise as well as maintenance of range of joint movement can thus be obtained.

**Principle 2** An object will float motionless only when its center of mass intersects or is perpendicularly aligned with its center of buoyancy. Although the object will float motionless regardless of which of the two centers is uppermost, it will be more stable if the center of mass is below the center of buoyancy (fig. 17.2).

Swimmers frequently misconstrue the meaning of the word *float* to include not only lack of motion but also the requirement of a horizontal position in the water. In view of Principle 2, it is erroneous to

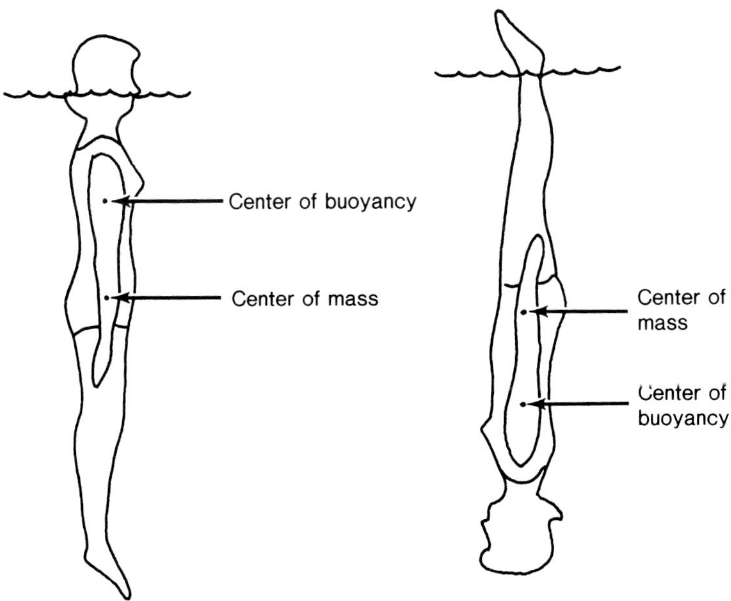


Figure 17.2. Alignment of the center of mass and center of buoyancy

expect that all swimmers will float in the same position and that this common position will be a horizontal one. Figures 17.3, 17.4 and 17.5 illustrate three positions of floating which are representative of the many positions possible. The swimmer in figure 17.3 will assume a vertical floating position since it is only in this position that the center of mass is perpendicularly aligned with that individual's center of buoyancy. The swimmer in figure 17.4 will assume the horizontal position since, again, this is the only position in which the two centers can be aligned. For this individual, the center of buoyancy is noted to be located in the hip region. The downward displacement of the individual's buoyancy center is caused by a high concentration of fatty tissue in the hips and thighs, coupled with relatively small lungs. The swimmer in figure 17.5 will assume a position between the two extremes in deference to a lesser downward migration of the buoyancy center. Floating position can be seen, then, to be a function of lung size, and amounts and locations of fat deposits. It follows that most adult women will approach the horizontal in their floating positions because of their higher body fat percentages which are located particularly around the hip and thigh region. Adult men, on the other hand, must rely on inflated lungs and expanded chests to buoy them up and will float, typically, in a more vertical position.

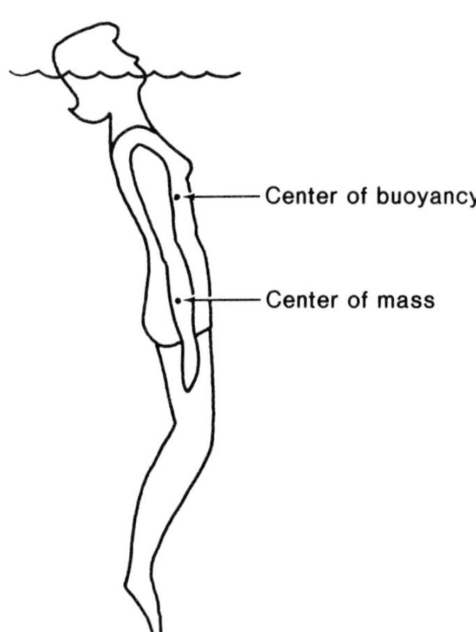


Figure 17.3. Vertical floating position

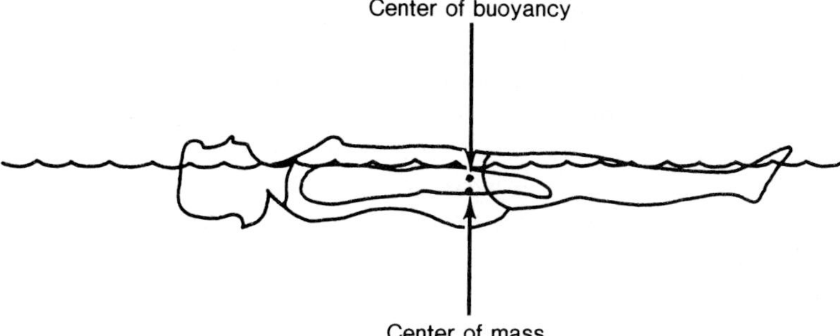


Figure 17.4. Horizontal floating position

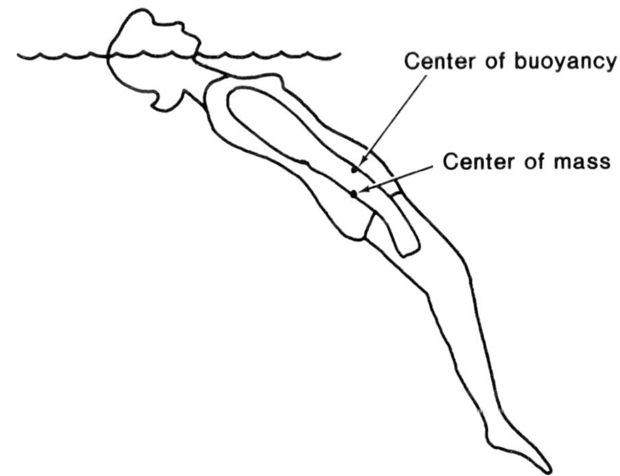


Figure 17.5. Diagonal floating position

This principle is of some import to those teachers of swimming who, without further thought, teach the technique of floating from a horizontal position. Unless the learner happens to be a horizontal floater, the lower limbs must necessarily sink in order that a position of alignment of the two centers be established. Unfortunately, the feet and legs will not stop when the proper position has been reached; rather, they will continue to drop because of their own inertia and will literally pull the swimmer underwater. The result is not only one of some discomfort but also one of miseducation, for the swimmer will undoubtedly conclude that he is a "sinker." The problem is easily solved, however. If the initial floating position is vertical rather than horizontal, the legs and feet are as deep as they can possibly be; the limbs will either maintain their position or they will rise until the centers of mass and buoyancy are aligned. The swimmer's comfort and feeling of success will, thereby, both be enhanced.

Since the body acts as a first class lever while it rotates around its center of buoyancy to find its floating position, it can be treated as such. By adding weight above the center of buoyancy, the feet may be made to elevate; similarly, subtraction of weight from below the center will cause the same response. Figure 17.6 presents a swimmer whose floating position is near vertical when her hands are at her sides. Elevation of the arms to overhead is accompanied by an elevation of the center of mass and a repositioning of the lower limbs. If it is desired that the feet be even higher, the wrists may be flexed so that the hands are out of water. Without the buoying force of the water, the weight of the hands is magnified and causes even greater elevation of the center of gravity with the subsequent realignment. For individuals who find extreme difficulty in floating, a final adjustment may be made and is illustrated in figure 17.6. Since flexion of the knees will cause the center of mass to migrate even farther toward the head, the two centers will be made to approximate each other to the limit. The position of alignment will, it is hoped, be reached and the swimmer will float successfully.

The various adjustments discussed above are relevant also to the synchronized swimmer who is frequently called upon to perform floating patterns. Subtle changes in arm, hand, and head placement, as well as in breath control, can establish the necessary alignment of centers and yield the motionless float.

## Fluids and Dynamics

The study of the dynamics of fluids concerns the environments of air and water under conditions in which either an athlete or a sports implement is moving through the environment; or the environment is moving around an athlete or implement; or both are moving around each other. Fortunately, the principles which pertain to fluid dynamics are common for all of the above conditions, for probably every athlete has been in situations requiring that certain adjustments be made to meet the challenges offered by his fluid environment.

The principles of fluid dynamics are those related to the tendency of the fluid to change the state of motion of an object, and are referred to as the principles of *drag* and *lift*. Drag is that force which is applied by a fluid as it strikes the surface of an object; lift is the force which is generated at right angles to the drag force (fig. 17.7).

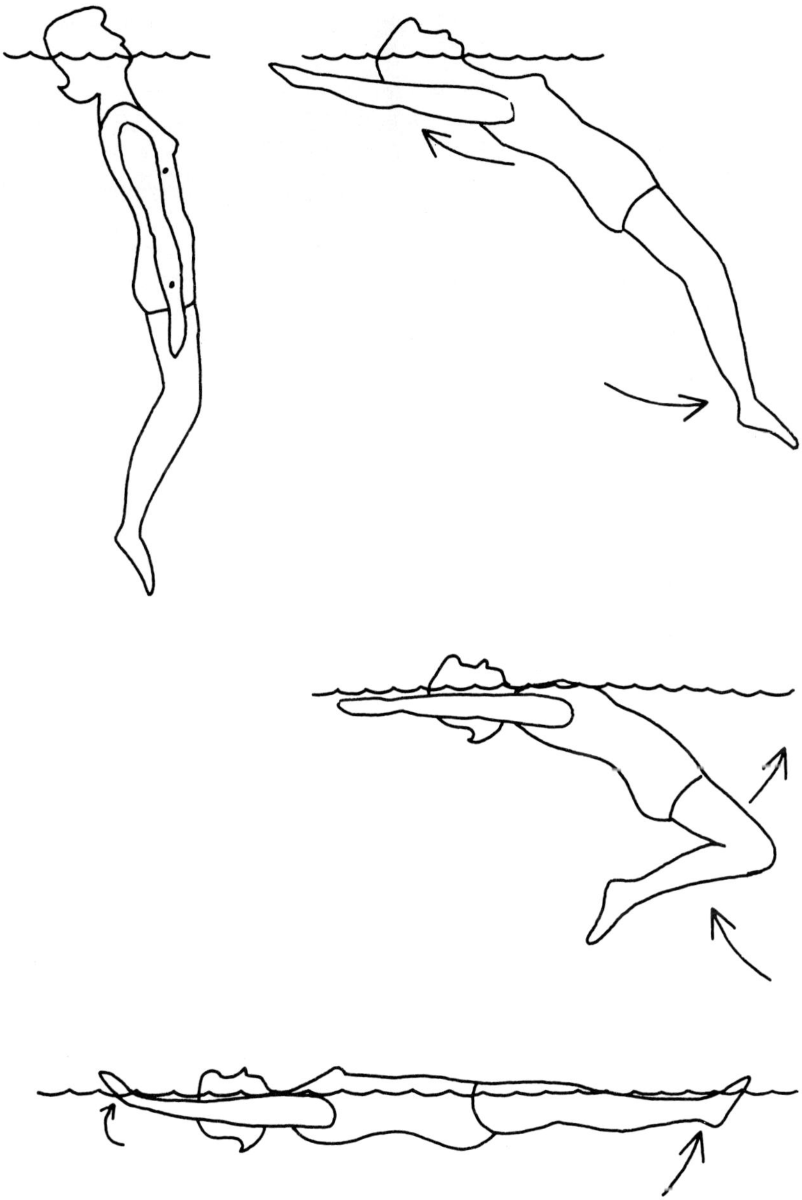

Figure 17.6. Limb positions and floating

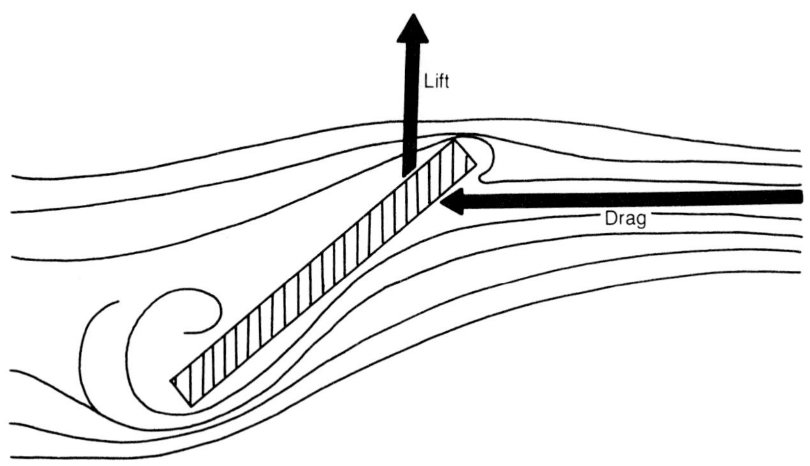


Figure 17.7. Drag and lift forces

As fluid passes over the object shown in figure 17.7, the forces it applies tend to slow the object as well as to elevate its path. If air is the fluid, the drag force is usually the more important of the two forces since the lift force generated at velocities typically encountered is seldom great enough to overcome the weight of the object, whether the object is an athlete or a sports implement. Exceptions can be noted, however. For example, discus and javelin throwers can choose certain angles of inclination to reduce drag while exploiting the lifting force in order to elongate the time and distance of the throw. Nevertheless, the lifting force of airflow is usually so much less effective than the drag force that it is considered to be inconsequential. This is not true when the fluid is water, for, with its higher density, it can generate lifting forces which are indeed large. Contrast the water level of a speedboat before it begins moving with the water level when peak velocity is reached—clear testimony to the effectiveness of the lifting force of water. It might be remembered, also, that the depth of an underwater swimmer's glide can be adjusted simply by changing the inclination of the hands when the arms are held overhead. Further use can be made of this concept by the swimming teacher who is puzzled by the inability of thin or muscular swimmers to execute the gliding strokes with expected form. Since lift is proportional to velocity, these non-buoyant swimmers can maintain the glide phases of the strokes for only short periods of time.

An aspect of the study of lift as a component of fluid dynamics is the Magnus Effect. This relates to the behavior of spinning objects as they pass through their fluid environments. Since the application of the Magnus Effect is so important to the kinesiologist, a special chapter, "Spin and Rebound," has been included to treat behavior of the ball while it is airborne and rebounding (see chap. 16).

The drag provided by fluids as they contact objects is dependent upon the factors of surface area, surface smoothness, shape of the object, and velocity of flow. When flow velocity is considered, it must be remembered that flow can be caused by an object moving through the fluid, or by fluids flowing past the object, or by both. Regardless of the cause, the faster the flow, the greater will be the resistance, or drag. In fact, resistance increases approximately with the square of velocity. For example, if velocity is 4 meters per second, it will be accompanied by some magnitude of resistance, say 12 units. Increasing velocity to 8 meters per second causes the resistance to rise to 48 units. Doubling velocity increases resistance by a factor of 4 or $2^2$. Equivalently, tripling velocity increases resistance by a factor of 9 or $3^3$, and so on.

Mathematically, resistance can be approximated by multiplying the square of velocity by the constant .7.

$$\text{Resistance (drag)} = \text{velocity}^2 \times .7$$

The importance of this relationship to swimming is easily seen in those strokes requiring that recovery be made underwater. Rapid movements should obviously be avoided during the recovery phase.

Surface area is proportional to drag; the greater the area, the greater the drag. Skiers, bicyclists, and bobsledders, to name but a few, must strive to reduce surface area to a minimum if minimum air drag is to be attained. Skintight ski outfits, smaller profiles resulting from dropped handle-bars, and streamlined bobsleds are all designed for this reduction. Even beyond these reductions, which have come about largely as the result of efforts on the part of manufacturers, many reductions can be made by the athlete himself. For example, the bicyclist can clip his water bottle to the frame of the bicycle in such a way as to reduce surface area. Similarly, briefcases, books, and packages can be strapped on the bicycle so as to present their smallest surfaces to the airflow.

Swimmers are no less concerned with the relationship between surface area and drag. Competitive swimmers choose swimming apparel which is tight fitting so as not to "catch" water at the neck, arms, or waist. Further reduction is accomplished by positioning body parts to present the smallest possible surface to the water through which the body is directed. Conversely, the shallow water jump performed by lifeguards is predicated upon exposure of a large surface area to the water in order to use the resulting drag to maintain the head above water.

A final example of the consequences of water drag is offered from the world of the synchronized swimmer whose costumes must be chosen on the basis of aesthetics as well as efficiency. The design and fabric of headwear and costumes must be selected with great care to prevent the generation of overwhelming drag with resulting lack of maneuverability.

Smoothness of surface is inversely proportional to drag; that is, the smoother the surface, the less the drag will be. The sleek and shiny material used in the making of speed-skaters' clothing is intended to reduce drag as is the use of fiberglass by the manufacturers of bobsleds. Woolen swimsuits have given way to those made of a silkier material—swimmers have even explored, with negligible results, the practices of shaving body hair and coating the skin with oil to minimize drag.

Shapes of objects as determinants of drag are particularly important to those involved in activities of high velocity and/or in the design of water craft. Shape is important with respect both to the leading surface of the object and its trailing surface. Consideration of the shape of a football will clarify the shape-drag relationship, for it will be seen in figure 17.8 that the football presents the same cross-sectional area to the air regardless of whether the nose of the ball is tapered or blunt. It is easily seen, however, that the passage of air is enhanced by the taper of the leading surface, and drag is effectively reduced. Figure 17.8 illustrates also the adverse effect of a blunt trailing surface on the ball. A low-pressure area is formed behind the ball because of inability of air to fill the trailing space. A suction force is thus established which will slow the ball. The optimum condition of air passage will again be provided by the tapered shape. An interesting application of the effect of shape on efficient fluid dynamics has been

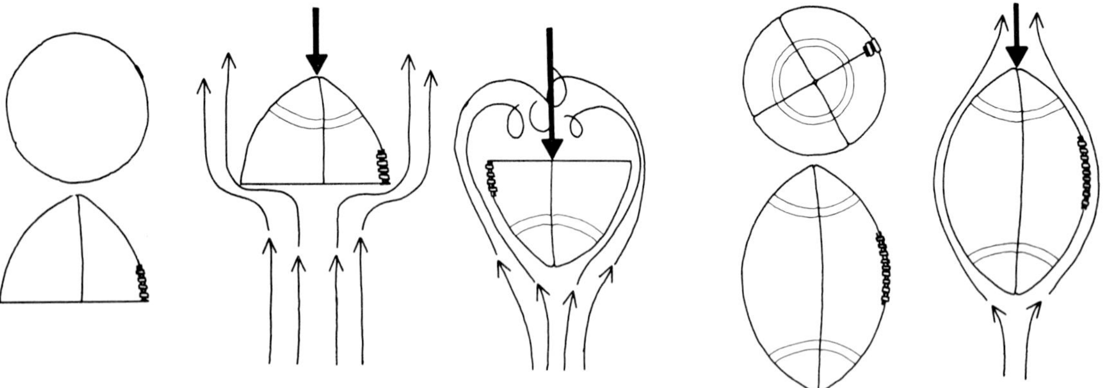

**Figure 17.8. Fluid flow and selected object shapes**

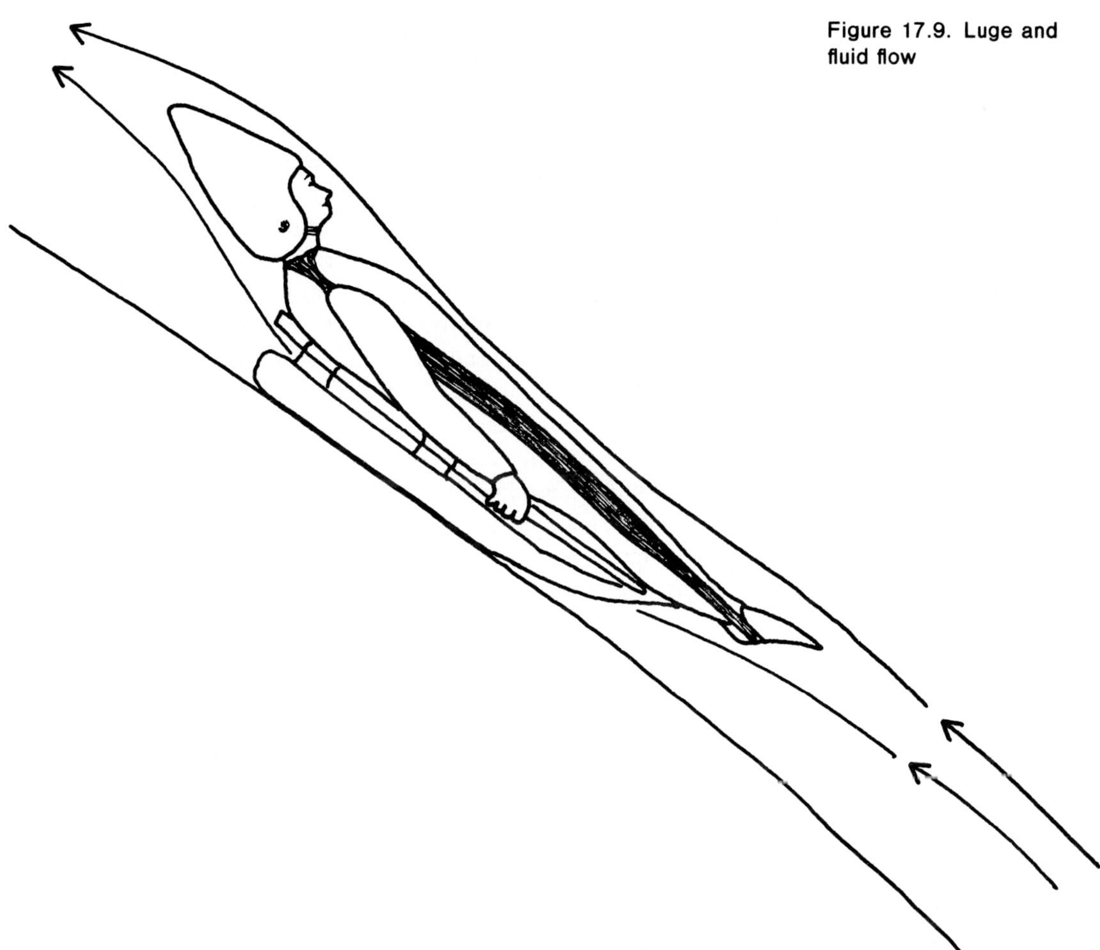

Figure 17.9. Luge and fluid flow

made by competitors in luge. Not only are the ankles plantar-flexed to provide a tapered forward surface, but the headgear has been designed with a bullet shape to facilitate the filling of the trailing space with air (fig. 17.9).

The effect of shape is even more observable in the water environment because of the higher density involved. In addition to noting the tapered shapes of water craft designed for speed, it should be remembered that streamlined positions of the arms and legs are dictated for greatest efficiency while executing swimming strokes.

## Summary

A fluid is comprised of easily moveable particles; to the athlete, the fluids of importance are water and air. Fluids, and their effects on sport and dance, can influence movement in either a static or dynamic fashion.

Under static conditions in a fluid environment of air, the principles of stability pertain to the analysis of movement. When the fluid environment is water, however, two additional principles must be noted; (1) when an object is placed in water, it is buoyed up by a force equal to the weight of the water it displaces (Archimedes' principle), and (2) an object will float motionless only if its centers of mass and buoyancy are perpendicularly aligned.

Under dynamic conditions, the athlete is concerned with his movement through the fluid and/or the fluid's movement around him. The principles of fluid dynamics are referred to as those of *drag* and *lift*. Drag is the force applied by the fluid as it strikes the surface of an object, and its magnitude is dependent upon the object's surface area, surface smoothness, and shape. Lift is the force which is generated at right angles to drag force and gives rise to the behavior of spinning objects as they pass through their environments.

## Laboratory and Field Experiences

1. Work with a partner to determine his individual floating position. Can you, after the position has been found, estimate the locations of the floater's centers of mass and buoyancy? Does the floater's body build support your estimates?
2. Observe the floating position of a partner who is holding the arms to the side. Ask the floater to place the arms overhead and note the new position. Instruct the floater to flex the wrists so the hands are out of water and note the new position. Finally, ask the floater to attempt to float while exhaling. Does this make a difference in his position?
3. Instruct a partner to push off from the side of the pool into a streamlined prone glide and determine the length of the glide. Have the partner repeat the glide but with the hip joints abducted so the legs are spread. What effect does the second position have upon the length of the glide? Which principle of fluid dynamics is being illustrated?
4. Observe a synchronized swimmer perform a crane with one or two full twists and a periscope with twists. Which of the two stunts is more difficult? In which can the twists be executed faster? Why?

5. Using a spring scale, weigh a small piece of wood, a cork, and a piece of metal. Suspend each of these in a beaker of water and reweigh them. Does the comparison of the two weight records confirm that wood and cork float but that metal sinks?
6. As part of their prelaunch training, astronauts are placed in a water environment with weighted belts heavy enough to allow them to position themselves underwater and neither rise nor sink. Consider the consequences of this "zero gravity" simulation and Newton's Third Law, the law of action-reaction. What reaction will the action of swinging a hammer cause? Of pushing or pulling? Of throwing?
7. Place some sand in the bottom of a small bucket and suspend it in a tub of water. Measure the height of the bucket that projects above the surface of the water. Fill the bucket half-full with water and measure its height above the water. Fill the bucket to within a few centimeters of the brim and remeasure its above water height. Finally, completely fill the bucket with water. Do your findings substantiate Archimedes' principle? How do your findings relate to the method by which submarines are maneuvered?

# 18 Applications

In this chapter, an attempt has been made to provide the reader with common movement problems to which solutions are offered. The intent of the several presentations is to place you, the student of kinesiology, in the role of the teacher or coach who must examine critically the literature as well as the movement patterns of your students and athletes and make accurate judgments regarding any kinesiological errors that might be present.

Each problem is stated in paragraph form and is followed by a list of mechanical principles that appear to be relevant. A decision is then made, and each principle is discussed. The problems selected are, by no means, intended to represent all that will be encountered by the teacher or coach. It is hoped, however, that they can be used as bases for generalizations which will afford insight into the solution of other movement problems.

The chapter concludes with a kinesiological analysis of the track start. It is intended to exemplify procedures which, it is hoped, can be generalized to an analytical activity of the student's choice.

## Archery

An archery student has a pronounced tendency to miss to the right of the bull's-eye of the target. The student also evidences some slight instability while shooting by taking a compensatory step after releasing the arrow.

### Application Principle

- Widen the base of support in the direction in which force is to be imparted.

### Decision

The archer is failing to align the feet in a perpendicular direction to the face of the target. The fact that the arrows are hitting right of the bull's-eye suggests that the right foot is out of line and should be moved forward. The compensatory step is required because the reaction force to the release of the arrow is applied at an angle to the base of support rather than perpendicularly through it. A twisting effect is caused, which is followed by the compensatory step to regain balance.

## Badminton

A badminton player is having difficulty clearing the shuttlecock to the back of the court. The difficulty is more pronounced when she attempts to do so while on the run.

### Application Principles

- Forces are vector quantities and can be summed.
- Efficient application of force depends on a firm base of support.
- The more sequential the movement, the more force can be applied to relatively light sports objects.

### Decision

All of the application principles probably apply. Close examination of the player should reveal that her weight is not being shifted forward before she contacts the shuttlecock. She is violating the principle of summation of forces since without forward movement of the body, that force vector is zero and does not contribute to the summation. A worse situation is seen when the player is on the run or backing up when she hits the shuttlecock. The force vector representing the shift of her weight is now acting away from the desired path of the clear and, therefore, is acting in a negative fashion, i.e., the magnitude of the vector must be subtracted from the summation. The player would be well-advised to move into position for the contact, establish a firm base and then move forward into the stroke.

## Basketball

The basketball player is typically advised to impart backspin to the ball when shooting. Is this advice valid?

### Application Principles

- A ball with backspin will tend to rise as it moves through the air.
- A ball with spin will tend to rebound in the opposite direction to that of its contacting surface.
- The more sequential the movement, the more the force that can be imparted.

### Decision

The advice is valid on the basis of the second and third of the principles stated. If the ball strikes either the rim or backboard prior to passing through the hoop, its backspin will deflect it downwardly into the hoop. Equally important is the fact that backspin is imparted to the ball by flexing the wrist rapidly as the ball is released. Additional force is therefore imparted to the ball—some manifesting itself in the ball spin—with the remainder contributing to the increased range of the shooter. The first principle is not relevant because the velocity of the ball is not sufficiently high to cause the ball to rise while in flight.

When landing after the execution of a jump shot, the player must consistently take a step to the side to regain balance. Is this desirable?

### Application Principles

- The line of gravity must intersect the base of support if stability is to be attained.
- Only the projection angle of 90 degrees yields vertical elevation with zero horizontal distance.
- Law of acceleration.

### Decision

The lack of stability of the shooter is not desirable as it places him at a disadvantage as he seeks to move in any direction except toward the balancing step. It will probably not suffice, however, to simply instruct the player to stop taking the sideward step since some error is being committed which causes the loss of balance. Two possibilities are that the player is directing the jump sidewardly rather than upwardly (the second principle), and/or that the player is attempting to shoot from beyond his realistic range and is required to employ inappropriate musculature and body movements in an attempt to accelerate the ball adequately (the third principle).

## Dance

A dancer, while performing the tour jeté, is noted to land with adequate position but covers several centimeters of floor between the takeoff and landing. What error is she committing?

### Application Principles

- The Law of Inertia.
- Only the projection angle of 90 degrees will yield vertical elevation with zero horizontal distance.

### Decision

The law of inertia states that an object will remain in its state of motion until it is acted upon by a force sufficiently large to disturb that state. The vertical force applied to the floor by the dancer is not sufficiently large to completely overcome her horizontal momentum. When she projects her body from the floor, she does so at some angle less than 90 degrees, and as a result covers a certain amount of horizontal distance. Two choices are afforded the dancer; she may change the angle of her vertical force; or she may decrease to zero the horizontal component. The former of the choices is the more preferable since she cannot attain sufficient air time from a "standstill" to complete the turn and land in position. The vertical angle can be decreased effectively by leaning backwardly as the downward thrust is imparted. The two force vectors will then be directed horizontally and at some angle greater than 90 degrees; their resultant should be a vertical one to insure that the dancer's angle of projection is, itself, a 90-degree one.

A dancer cannot hold the arabesque because she continually loses her balance forward. What adjustments can be made to enhance her success?

### Application Principles

- An object will maintain its stability if its line of gravity intersects its base of support.
- Movement of a body part away from the midline causes the center of mass to shift in the direction of the body part.

### Decision

The dancer's line of gravity is falling in front of her supporting foot; compensatory movements must, therefore, be made. Several choices are available and can range from the lowering of the elevated leg to the realignment of the arms to a more sideward position.

## Football

The success of a punt in football is a function of the height and velocity at which it was kicked, and its angle of projection. How will you instruct your punter who has a tendency to kick the ball high but short?

### Application Principles

- As the angle of projection decreases from 90 degrees, the height of projection lessens and the distance covered increases.
- Angular velocity is converted to linear velocity directed along a path tangent to the arc at the point of release.
- The angle of projection should decrease from 45 degrees as the height at which the object is released is increased.

### Decision

The punter should be instructed to allow the ball to drop farther before he contacts it with his foot. The lower point of contact will project the ball at a lower angle and will increase the distance covered by the ball. If all possible distance is to be covered, the point of contact should be such that the tangent to the point is directed at an angle slightly less than 45 degrees.

Is it better to execute a block with the feet on or off the ground?

### Application Principles

- Momentum is the product of mass and velocity.
- Without firm foot contact, reactions of the body to applied forces will be manifested.

### Decision

It is better to execute a block with the feet on the ground, for with firm foot contact, much of the force imparted by the opponent can be transmitted to the ground. If the opponent is large and moving rapidly he will have great momentum, which will be transferred to the blocker. If the blocker's feet are off the ground, he will probably be knocked sideward or backward and his efforts will be largely negated.

## Golf

One of your golf students possesses an effective full swing when she is on a level lie. When faced with a downhill lie, however, she consistantly slices or pushes the ball. You have noticed that she places the ball in front of her back heel regardless of the lie.

### Application Principles

- Efficient application of force requires a firm base of support.
- The angle of incidence equals the angle of rebound.
- The end of a moving lever will describe the arc of a circle with radius equal to the distance between the axis and the arc.

### Decision

We will address the third principle first. Because of this principle, uphill and downhill lies may cause concern that the divot will be taken ahead of or behind the ball, respectively. If this is indeed the case, the results would be devastating. The tendency would be to place the ball forward of normal on an uphill lie and backward of normal on a downhill lie. These adjustments would appear to place the ball in such a position as to allow uninterrupted swings of the club head through its full arc without hitting the ground. To do so, however, would cause impact to be late on an uphill lie and early on a downhill lie.

The second of the application principles now comes to attention. If the ball is hit later than normal, the club head will be rotated to a "closed" facing and the ball will hook. Conversely, a premature hit of the ball will be accompanied by an "open" face of the club head and slicing or pushing will be the result.

At this point, the first application principle becomes important. If the lies are not severe, the golfer can tilt forward or backward slightly in order to achieve a position in which she is perpendicular with the ground. More weight than normal will be placed on the forward or back foot according to the lie; however, if only minimal adjustment is necessary, stability will not suffer significantly. Should the slope of the ground be severe, sufficient adjustment cannot be made. The golfer would then be well advised to aim the ball to allow for a push or slice from a downhill lie or a hook from an uphill lie.

## Gymnastics and Tumbling

A gymnast is unable to complete a full 180-degree twist when performing swivel hips.

### Application Principles

- Velocity of rotation can be increased by shortening the radius of rotation.
- Momentum of one body part can be transformed to another body part.

### Decision

The gymnast is probably committing one of two common errors; either he is failing to extend the hip joints fully as he rebounds from the first seat drop, or he is failing to throw the arms and head upwardly and sidewardly with sufficient force. If the former error is made, the radius of rotation around the vertical axis is elongated and velocity is being slowed, thus disallowing the full 180-degree twist. If the latter error is being made, less than adequate momentum is being generated by the arms and head. Transfer of that momentum to the body will not give the gymnast enough force to execute the twist.

After performing a straddle vault, a gymnast consistently loses balance forward at the landing.

### Application Principles

- The Law of Inertia.
- A body wil remain stable if its line of gravity intersects its base of support.
- Transfer of Momentum.

### Decision

The gymnast is landing in a position of instability either because the trunk is inclined forward or because the center of mass is moving with greater horizontal velocity than can be controlled and reduced to zero by the base of support. Regardless, the fault probably lies in the failure of the gymnast to push appropriately against the horse. From the time of the takeoff to contact with the horse, the gymnast's body is following a curvilinear path which permits forward rotation around the frontal axis. At contact with the horse the legs are higher than the shoulders and are moving under their own forward angular momentum, which they will continue to do until a force large enough to overcome that momentum is applied. That force can only come from the arms and must be strong enough, and directed backwardly enough, to reverse the forward rotation and elevate the shoulders over the feet. The shoulders and trunk will then be provided with backward angular momentum which will transfer to the legs when the upper body becomes vertical. The descent to the landing can then be made with the center of mass more nearly over the feet.

## Jogging

You observe a jogger who extends the elbows every time the arm extends. What would you advise the jogger? On which principle would you base your advice?

### Application Principles

- The shorter the resistance arm, the less force is required to balance a lever.
- For every action there is an equal and opposite reaction.
- It just doesn't look right.

### Decision

It is true that the arm action described above doesn't look right, but this is due, perhaps, to the fact that we haven't seen it often except among inexperienced runners and joggers. One must now wonder why such arm action is not characteristic of topflight performers. The first application principle provides the answer. Whereas the effects of the force of gravity may be enhanced in affecting downward and backward movement of the arm if the elbow is extended, it should be remembered that the elbow flexors must work harder at the end of each backward swing to reflex that joint for the forward swing than would be the case if the elbow were maintained in flexion throughout the backward and forward swings. Efficiency is lost because more energy is required. For distance runners to ignore means of increasing efficiency is to defeat their very purpose—to cover long distances.

Joggers often complain of soreness in the middle of the ball of the foot. The soreness is localized to the tissue below the head of the second metatarsal. What is your recommendation?

### Application Principles

- Velocity of a moving object should be slowed gradually to allow for force absorption.
- The area of force absorption should be as large as possible.

### Decision

The tenderness is caused by the application of force to the metatarsal heads when the foot contacts or pushes off the ground. Joggers who contact the ground with the ball of the foot should be instructed to move the point of contact toward the heel. The metatarsal heads will thus be spared from absorbing force at ground contact. Pushing off the ground may continue to cause a problem in tenderness, however, because the second metatarsal is longer than the first; it is also smaller. If the force of push-off is localized in the second metatarsal, little absorption is possible because of the size of its head. Since this is the case, force will be transmitted to the underlying tissue with tenderness and bruising as the result. Padding of the area will be of help because it will compact with each stride to provide more time to absorb the force of push-off.

## Shot Putting

The best shot putter on your track and field squad is 50 centimeters under the state record. Which of the following principles will provide the best results in helping him achieve a record putt?

### Application Principles

- Range is dependent upon height of release.
- Range is dependent upon angle of projection.
- Range is dependent upon velocity of release.

### Decision

Utopically, time would be available to teach the putter to optimize each of the variables of height, angle, and velocity of release with emphasis being placed on increasing velocity. If the potential record-setting event is only a week or so away, however, you scarcely have time to make but minimal improvements in his release velocity. If a quick check shows he is well extended at release, his release height probably cannot be increased. The remaining variable is angle of release; it may be that an increase or decrease in the angle will achieve the needed 50 centimeters of range.

## Softball and Baseball

A player has become incapacitated because of extreme tenderness in the palm of the glove hand. What adjustments can be made in the technique used to catch the ball?

### Application Principles

- Force absorption is enhanced by lengthening the time over which the force can be absorbed.

### Decision

If the player is a catcher, little can be adjusted except the padding of the glove. The stance required of the catcher makes "giving" movements of the arm considerably more limited than is the case for the other players. If the player is not a catcher, however, he can be coached to elongate the time of force absorption by swinging the arms backwardly in response to the velocity of impact of the ball in the glove, and to position the glove so the ball strikes the webbing or trap between thumb and first finger rather than the palm.

Your right-handed softball pitcher is noted as being somewhat "wild" in that she frequently throws high and low pitches. After close examination, you note that her left shoulder is still well ahead of her right shoulder at the moment of release. What suggestion can you make to improve her accuracy?

### Application Principles

- The more sequential the movement, the more force can be applied to relative light objects.
- An object undergoing angular momentum will travel, when it is released, along a path tangent to its arc at the point of release.

### Decision

The error committed by the pitcher is that of failing to rotate the shoulders completely before the release. Because of the incomplete rotation, she is unable to flatten the arc through which the ball is moving, and therefore is required to time the release very precisely to hit the strike zone. The incorporation of complete shoulder rotation may also increase her velocity since she will be adding a rather large component of force to the sequence of her movement.

## Swimming

While performing the freestyle (crawl), a swimmer is noted to rise and fall with each arm stroke. How can you coach the swimmer to maintain a more horizontal path through the water?

### Application Principles

- Law of action-reaction.
- Water, with its relatively high density, is able to provide for large lifting forces.

### Decision

The swimmer is moving his arms through an entire 180-degree arc beginning with water entry and ending with water release. Arm movement through the initial portion of the arc entails a downward press action, the reaction to which is an upward lift to the head and trunk. Conversely, the final portion of the curve involves an upward press which causes the body to sink. The swimmer should be instructed to omit those portions of the arc by directing the arm extension downwardly at a slight angle so the "catch" will be made lower along the arc. The swimmer should also be instructed to release the water when the hand reaches the vicinity of the front of the thigh. The final segment of the curve will thereby be omitted from the pattern and the inefficient upward press will be eliminated.

## Tennis

When receiving service in the even court, a singles opponent stands several feet behind the baseline in the alley extended. What type of spin should the server impart to the ball?

### Application Principles

- An object in flight to which spin has been imparted will tend to move into the low pressure area created by the spin.
- An object to which spin has been imparted will tend to rebound in the opposite direction from that in which its rebounding surface is moving.

### Decision

If the ball is served with a spin midway between top spin and right-to-left spin,* it will drop and curve away from the receiver while in flight. In addition, the ball will rebound fast and only slightly to the left of normal. Both from the standpoint of ball behavior in flight and when rebounding, a top and right-to-left spin is an appropriate choice.

You have read that when executing a backhand drive, it is more desirable to step diagonally toward the net with the front foot rather than toward the alley line. Do you agree? Why?

### Application Principle

- The more sequential a movement is, the more force can be applied to relatively light sports objects.

### Decision

The sequential movement pattern of a backhand drive begins with forward rotation of the hips and is followed by the shoulders and arm. If the player steps toward the alley with the front foot, the hips will be

*The spin directions of right-to-left and left-to-right are described as being viewed by the hitter.

severely limited in their ability to rotate and the force of the stroke will be impaired. By directing the step of the forward foot diagonally toward the net, the hips will be freer to rotate and will be allowed to contribute more effectively to the stroke.

## The Track Start

A final application of kinesiological principles will be made to the start in track. It is offered as an example of an analysis that can be generalized to other skills in sports and dance. An attempt has been made to include several relevant principles in order to make the example as broad as possible; however, a more practical approach would be to set out a series of questions, the answers to which would reveal necessary movement changes. The questions can arise from a problem that has been observed in a performer, or because a record of a particularly well-skilled athlete is desired, or even from general interest. Regardless of the reason, the analyst should avoid falling into the "data trap." To pose a question such as, "Why is this athlete so successful?" is virtually unanswerable because it offers no clues as to what should be analyzed and why. The analyst can easily be overwhelmed by data that may or may not have anything to do with success and may, indeed, have so few interrelationships that a conclusion cannot be drawn. Far more usable are questions that are directed toward specifics, such as location of the center of mass, determination of angular or linear velocity, calculation of displacement, or noting elapsed time. Knowledge of the principles of kinesiology must obviously be a prerequisite to the forming of meaningful questions.

Figure 18.1. The track start

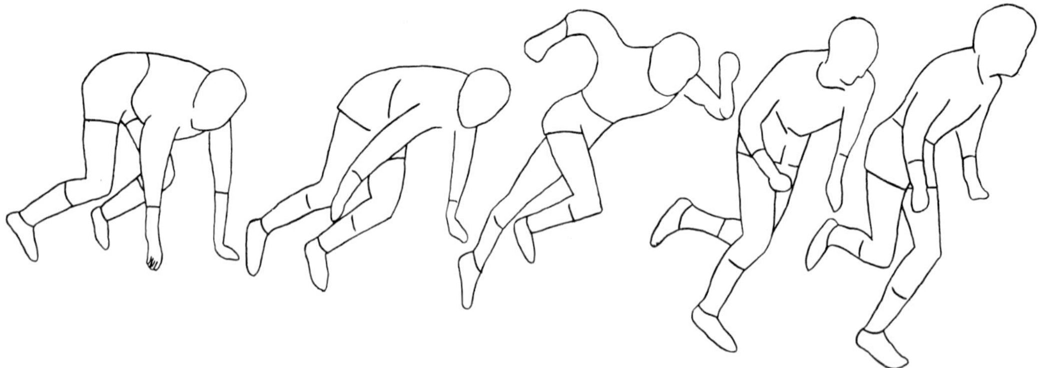

For the most part, the process of answering well-stated questions is a mechanical one that may be time consuming but is certainly not difficult. It is the ability to make accurate conclusions from the results of the analysis that is all-important. If a wrong conclusion is made and the performer is coached to make a change based upon it, the analyst has committed a disservice to all concerned.

Along a more optimistic viewpoint, let us assume that sound conclusions have been made. Before they are superimposed on the athlete, there must be some assurance that any recommended changes can, in fact, be made. The athlete must be physically capable of increasing such factors as strength, flexibility, etc., that are related to improving performance. No amount of coaching in the world will enable a 120-centimeter-tall high jumper to win the national championship or a 50-kilogram shot putter to qualify for the Olympics.

It is particularly during the analysis of athletes who are not possessed of a physical build typically associated with their event that capabilities become increasingly important. That these athletes are successful in the face of high physical odds against them usually means they have already maximized their performance; and, although recommendations can be made that will increase their success, coaches and performers alike will find it difficult if not impossible to enact them.

The analysis that follows has been organized by subheadings to explore principles related to stability, force, friction, linear displacement, velocity and acceleration, angular displacement and velocity, and fluids. Finally, there is a section entitled "Other Forms of Analyses," in which body position and nominal data are discussed. The reader is invited to become fully involved in the analysis by working through the calculations and formulating the graphs.

We will assume that the runner, a female who weighs 50 kilograms, has been filmed from a 90° angle and that the view field includes the first 15 meters of a 100-meter race. Her hip has been marked with an "X" of adhesive tape opposite the joint. The speed of the camera was 60 frames per second.

### **Stability** (fig. 18.2)

What is to be analyzed? The position of the line of gravity while the runner is in the "set" position.

What is the method? Project the film on a piece of graph paper that has been labeled in arbitrary units with the origin in the lower left-hand corner. Complete a stick figure of the runner while she is in "set" position. Using the data from figures 12.6 and 12.8, mark the positions of all segmental centers of gravity and determine their X and Y coordinates. The following data result:

Figure 18.2. Center of mass and line of gravity during the "set" position of the track start

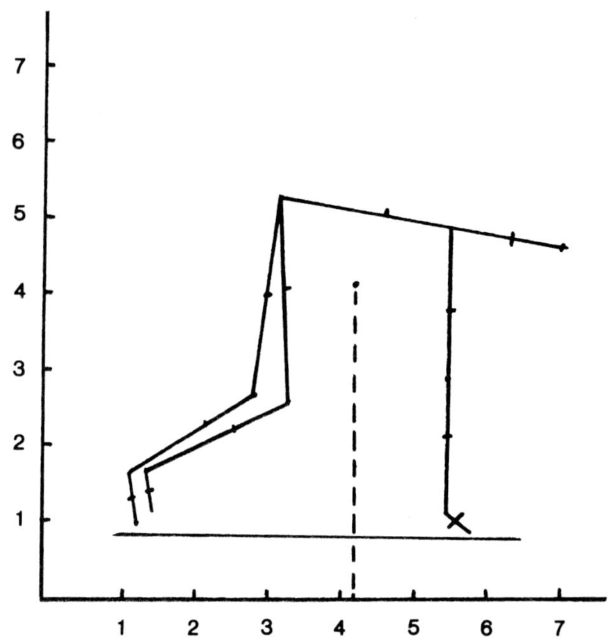


| Segment | X coord. | Y coord. | Segment Weight (Kg.) |
|---|---|---|---|
| Head | 6.3 | 5.0 | 3.65 |
| Trunk | 4.6 | 4.7 | 25.35 |
| Right upper arm | 5.5 | 3.8 | 1.30 |
| Left upper arm | 5.5 | 3.8 | 1.30 |
| Right forearm | 5.5 | 2.1 | .80 |
| Left forearm | 5.5 | 2.1 | .80 |
| Right hand | 5.6 | 1.0 | .35 |
| Left hand | 5.6 | 1.0 | .35 |
| Right thigh | 3.0 | 4.0 | 5.15 |
| Left thigh | 3.3 | 4.1 | 5.15 |
| Right calf | 2.2 | 2.3 | 2.15 |
| Left calf | 2.6 | 2.2 | 2.15 |
| Right foot | 1.2 | 1.3 | .75 |
| Left foot | 1.4 | 1.4 | .75 |
| Total | | | 50 Kg |

Multiply each X coordinate by the weight of the corresponding segment and find a sum. Then, divide it by the runner's weight of 50 kilograms.

$$C.M._X = \frac{(6.3 \times 3.65) + (4.6 \times 25.35) + \ldots + (1.4 \times .75)}{50}$$

$$C.M._X = 4.2$$

Repeat the procedure using the Y coordinates.

$$C.M._Y = \frac{(5.0 \times 3.65) + (4.7 \times 25.35) + \ldots + (1.4 \times .75)}{50}$$

$$C.M._Y = 4.1$$

The center of mass can be located on the graph paper by marking the point represented by X = 4.2 and Y = 4.1. Dropping a horizontal from the center shows that the line of gravity intersects the base of support approximately 65 percent ahead of the feet.

What is the conclusion? Maximum stability would be achieved by aligning the center of mass directly over the center of the base of support. This runner has taken a position that causes the center of her mass to be somewhat forward of the center of the support base. She appears to have made an effective compromise between her need for stability at the start and her desire to become mobile as quickly as possible after the sound of the gun.

### **Force** (fig. 18.3)

What is to be analyzed? The angle of force application to the ground during the start.

What is the method? A line will be drawn through the "X" mark on the hip and the top of the head. It will be assumed that the direction of applied force is parallel to this line. The resulting force vectors will be resolved to show comparisons between backward and downward forces during the start. Five positions will be selected:

Position 1. The first frame that shows observable movement of the runner after the gun is fired.

Position 2. The frame that shows loss of contact between the right (rear) foot and the starting blocks.

Position 3. The frame that shows loss of contact between the left (forward) foot and the starting blocks.

Position 4. The frame that shows loss of contact between the right foot and the ground after the first stride.

Position 5. The frame that shows loss of contact between the left foot and the ground after the second stride.

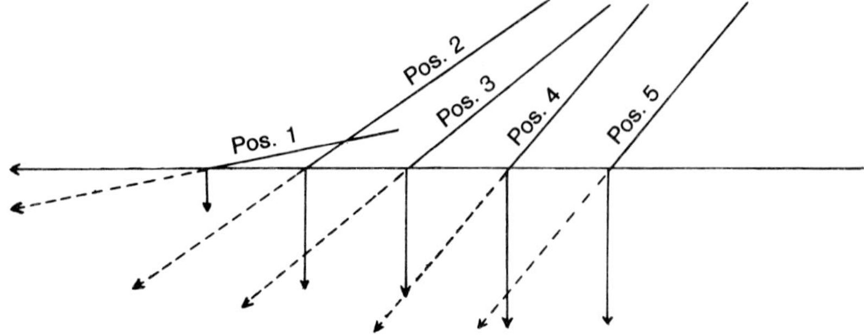


Figure 18.3. Lines of force application

What is the conclusion? The force vectors indicate a gradual change in direction as the runner leaves the starting blocks. These are, in order, approximately 10, 35, 45, 50, and 50 degrees from the right horizontal. As the angle of force application increases, its downward component also increases, but its backward component decreases. Position one shows a great predominance of backward force, which translates into acceleration of the runner from the "set" position. Position two indicates that there has been a drastic increase in force direction; backward force is much less than before and acceleration will be sacrificed. The remainder of the positions show only small changes, which all lead to the more upright posture characteristic of the runner in full stride.

It appears that the major fault occurred at position two. The runner is attempting to become vertical prematurely. A 35-degree angle of force application would be quite acceptable for position 3 as the blocks are left, but is too great for position 2 in which more backward thrust is required.

## Friction

What is to be analyzed? The coefficient of friction between the runner's footwear and the ground at toe-off of the first and second strides.

What is the method? The lines drawn through the hip and the top of the head for positions 4 and 5 as described above will be measured by a protractor. Coefficients of friction will be determined for the two positions. Use of a protractor will verify that the angle of the runner's lean is 50° for both position 4 and 5. These angles are relative to the horizontal, but since the coefficient of friction is the tangent of the angle relative to the vertical, the complement must be calculated.

Complementary angle $= 90° - 50° = 40°$

Coefficient of friction $= \tan 40° = .84$

What is the conclusion? Since most coefficients of friction dealt with in sports and dance range between .2 and 1.0, we can conclude that the runner is well within the range of safety. Her footwear appears to be suited to the track surface and to her performance.

### Linear Displacement, Velocity, and Acceleration

What is to be analyzed? The displacement, velocity, and acceleration of the runner from the sound of the gun through the first three seconds of the race.

What is the method? The adhesive "X" placed on the runner's hip will serve to show displacement of her body. Calculation of center of mass would be a more precise indicator of displacement, but unless a computer program is available, the time required would be too great. And, since center of mass of a running athlete closely approximates the location of the hip joint, no significant error will be incurred by using the "X" marking.

The film is projected on a screen and advanced to the frame that shows the smoke from the starting gun. The counter on the projector should now be set to zero. Every fifteenth frame (15 frames = .25 sec.) will be used to determine the three linear parameters. Suppose the following data have been recorded:

| Time (sec.) | Position (M) | Displacement (M) |
|---|---|---|
| 0 | 0 | 0 |
| .25 | .68 | .68 |
| .50 | 1.38 | 1.38 |
| .75 | 2.73 | 2.73 |
| 1.00 | 4.39 | 4.39 |
| 1.25 | 6.09 | 6.09 |
| 1.50 | 7.61 | 7.61 |
| 1.75 | 8.83 | 8.83 |
| 2.00 | 9.68 | 9.68 |
| 2.25 | 10.17 | 10.17 |
| 2.50 | 10.37 | 10.37 |
| 2.75 | 10.44 | 10.44 |
| 3.00 | 10.58 | 10.58 |

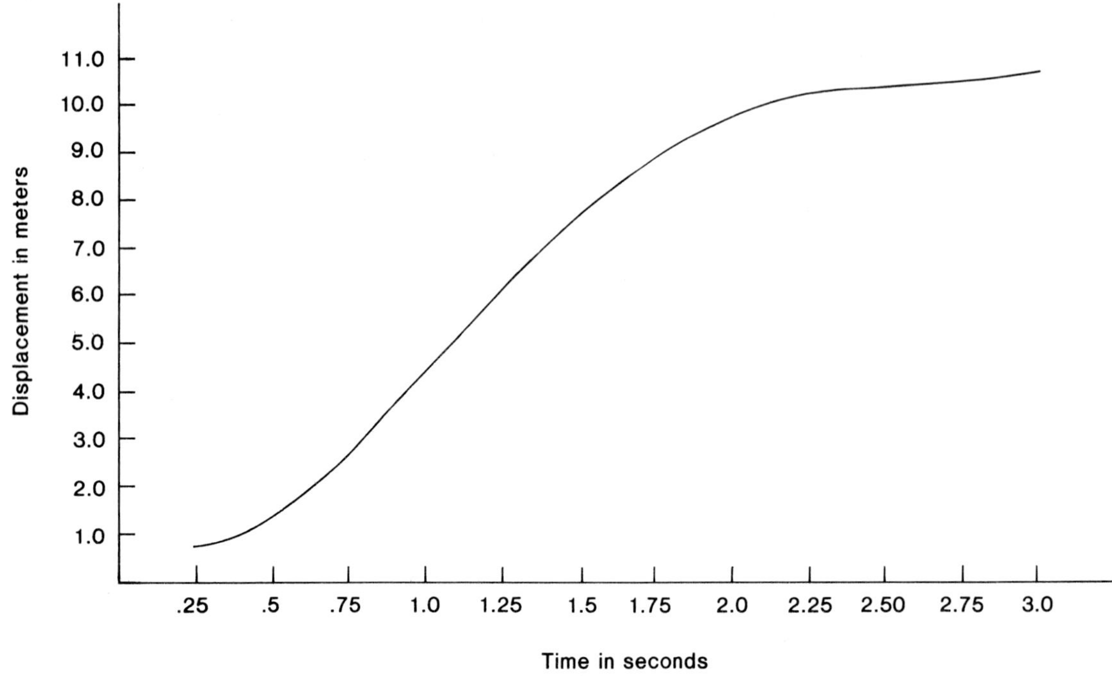


Figure 18.4. Curve of linear displacement data

Since the beginning position of the runner is zero meters, position and displacement data are the same. A graph of displacement data should now be made (fig. 18.4) and, if instantaneous values are of interest, tangents can be drawn at each time point. The rise of the tangent in meters divided by its run in seconds will yield the values of concern. To spur interest in this exercise, the following answers are given. Slight deviations in the students' results and those given here should be excused because of rounding error and graphics error.

| Time (Sec.) | Instantaneous Velocity (rads per sec.) |
|---|---|
| .25 | 11.5 |
| .50 | 12.9 |
| .75 | 14.7 |
| 1.00 | 15.4 |
| 1.25 | 15.0 |
| 1.50 | 13.9 |
| 1.75 | 12.5 |
| 2.00 | 10.9 |
| 2.25 | 9.4 |
| 2.50 | 8.3 |
| 2.75 | 7.9 |

Average velocity can be easily computed from the tabular data given above. During the total time period, 10.58 meters were displaced; average velocity is, therefore,

$$\text{average velocity} = \frac{10.58 \text{ M} - 0 \text{ M}}{3 \text{ sec.}} = 3.53$$

Average acceleration can also be calculated from the presented data. Since average acceleration is equal to:

$$\text{average acceleration} = \frac{\text{final velocity} - \text{initial velocity}}{\text{elapsed time}}$$

and in this example,

$$\text{average acceleration} = \frac{.56 \text{ M/sec.} - 2.72 \text{ M/sec.}}{3 \text{ sec.}} = -.72 \text{ M/sec.}^2$$

since

$$\text{initial velocity} = \frac{.68 \text{ M/sec.} - 0 \text{ M/sec.}}{.25 \text{ sec.}} = 2.72 \text{ M/sec.}$$

and

$$\text{final velocity} = \frac{10.58 \text{ M/sec.} - 10.44 \text{ M/sec.}}{.25 \text{ sec.}} = .56 \text{ M/sec.}$$

What is the conclusion? Average velocity over the first ten and one-half meters is clearly low. Lack of optimum body lean at the start is a contributor as may be lack of strength. Elimination of these faults should increase initial average velocity. Examination of stride rate and length may yield other answers to the problem. Stride length should be such that the center of mass is over the foot when it contacts the ground for each stride. Location of the center of mass at any given time can be accomplished according to the procedures discussed earlier under stability.

The displacement graph indicates that emphasis should be placed on viewing the film at and beyond the 1.75-second mark. The slope of the curve begins to fall off at 1.75 seconds and continues rapidly. For some reason, the runner has failed to maintain her velocity. Examination of the film record for stride length and rate, body lean, head position, etc., will help the analyst determine errors in technique and offer recommendations for change.

The negative average acceleration of .72 meters per second squared shows that the runner, after her initial explosive start, *slowed* an average of .72 meters per second over the three seconds analyzed.

This is a function of her inability to continue the velocity she built up after leaving the starting blocks. Again, examination of the critical frames of film around the 1.75 mark should be illuminating.

### Angular Displacement and Velocity

What is to be analyzed? The displacement and velocity of the right upper arm between the time it begins moving and 10 milliseconds after the opposite foot loses contact with the starting block.

What is the method? Every third frame of the projected film will be analyzed beginning with the frame that shows the first movement of the right arm ($P_0$) and ending 6 frames ($6/60 = 10$ milliseconds) after loss of contact between the left foot and the starting block. For each frame analyzed, a line will be drawn between the shoulder joint and elbow joint. The angular position of each line will be measured from a horizontal line drawn through the shoulder joint.

It has been mentioned before that it is customary to measure angular positions from the right horizontal. Since the camera was placed on the right side of the runner, angular positions will be recorded in a clockwise direction and, therefore, displacements will be negative. For example, suppose the runner being analyzed here began her motion from an angular position of 275 degrees (the shoulder is almost over the elbow). If the position of her upper arm at the time the left foot left the starting block was 150 degrees, the angular displacement would have been 150 degrees minus 275 degrees to equal a negative 125 degrees. Had the camera been located on the left side of the runner, her starting and ending positions would have been recorded as 265 degrees and 390 degrees, respectively, and the displacement of her upper arm would have been 390 degrees minus 265 dgrees to equal a positive 125 degrees. The magnitude of the result is the same; the preceding positive or negative sign simply indicates that, to the viewer or camera, the arm was moving in a clockwise (negative) or counterclockwise (positive) direction.

Displacement and velocity graphs of negative values are often confusing at first sight because we are more used to viewing the results of positive values. If difficulty arises, turn the graph upside down and over so it can be viewed, against a light, from the back of the page. The graph will now appear to be in positive space and may be interpreted more readily.

The following data were recorded from the film of our runner.

| Time (msec) | Position (degrees) | Displacement (degrees) | Displacement (radians) |
|---|---|---|---|
| 0 | 275 | | |
| 5 | 266 | —9 | —.15 |
| 10 | 254 | —21 | —.37 |
| 15 | 239 | —36 | —.63 |
| 20 | 202 | —73 | —1.27 |
| 25 | 158 | —117 | —2.05 |
| 30 | 150 | —125 | —2.18 |
| 35 | 157 | —118 | —2.06 |
| 40 | 206 | —69 | —1.20 |

A graph of the displacement data will now be made with time on the baseline and radians along the Y axis (fig. 18.5).

What is the conclusion? The important issue here is to determine whether the runner's right upper arm reaches its highest point of hyperextension at the moment her left foot loses contact with the starting block. Only if the timing is correct can the right arm be in a position to swing forward into its first stride.

The displacement graph shows that at 30 milliseconds, the right upper arm reached the highest point of hyperextension. If a review of the film shows that the left foot lost contact with the block at 300 milliseconds, the runner's timing is correct. Should this not be the case, however, she and her coach should be informed so that the error can be corrected.

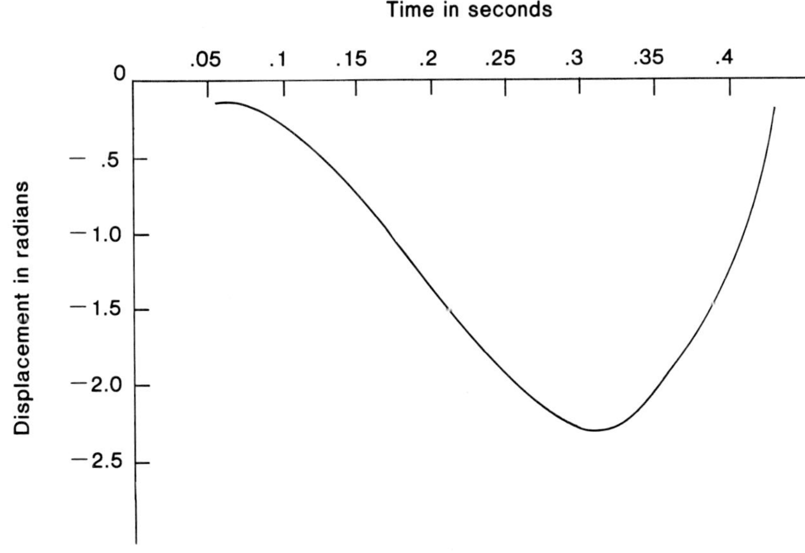


Figure 18.5. Curve of angular displacement data

## Other Forms of Analysis

The analytical examples given above are, by no means, intended to be all inclusive. There are any number of calculations, displacements, velocities, etc., that could be addressed by the analyst in an effort to optimize the performance of the runner. In addition, there are many questions related to performance that need not be answered through mathematics. A simple "yes" or "no" may be quite sufficient. These so-called *nominal* data will answer such questions as, "Is the runner's rear leg completely straight at the moment it leaves the block?" or "Does the runner show observable movement within 15 milliseconds after the gun is fired (the smoke is seen on the film)?" or "Does the head position of the runner suggest that she is looking at a spot down the track rather than at the finish line?" To answer "yes" or "no" to these questions can be as valuable to the analyst as mathematical calculations. If nominal data will suffice as the bases for making recommendations to improve performance, they should be used. To submit such data to rigorous mathematical treatment could be a case of "overkill."

The analyst is frequently aided by tracings or stick figures of the filmed image of the athlete. Knowledge of posture at various time points through the performance can be helpful and, in some cases, may be all that is required to detect movement errors. Interpretation of tracings or stick figures should, of course, be based upon kinesiological principles of efficient movement.

# Bibliography for Part 2

Armbruster, D. A.; Allen, R. H.; and Billingsley, H. S. *Swimming and Diving*. London: Kaye and Ward, Ltd., 1970.

Barham, J. N. *Mechanical Kinesiology*. St. Louis: C. V. Mosby Company, 1978.

Barham, J. N., and Wooten, E. P. *Structural Kinesiology*. Toronto, Ontario: Macmillan Company, 1973.

Broer, M. R. *Efficiency of Human Movement*. 2d ed. Philadelphia: W. B. Saunders Company, 1966.

Bunn, J. W. *Scientific Principles of Coaching*. 2d ed. Englewood Cliffs, N.J.: Prentice-Hall. 1972.

Cochran, A., and Stobbs, J. *The Search for the Perfect Swing*. Philadelphia: J. B. Lippincott Co., 1968.

Cooper, J. M. "Selected topics of biomechanice." Proceedings of the C. I. C. Symposium on Biomechanics, Chicago, The Athletic Institute, 1971.

Cooper, J. M., and Glassow, R. B. *Kinesiology*. 3d ed. St. Louis: The C. V. Mosby Company, 1972.

Counsilman, J. E. *The Science of Swimming*. Englewood Cliffs, N.J.: Prentice-Hall, 1970.

Cousy, B., and Power, F. G. *Basketball Concepts and Techniques*. Boston: Allyn & Bacon, 1970.

Deshon, D. E., and Nelson, R. C. "A cinematographical analysis of sprint running." *Research Quarterly* 35(1964):451-55.

Doherty, J. K. *Modern Track and Field*. Englewood Cliffs, N.J.: Prentice-Hall, 1963.

Dyatchkov, V. M. "The high jump." *Track Technique* 34(1968):1059-75.

Dyson, G. H. G. *The Mechanics of Athletics* London: University of London Press, Ltd., 1970.

Faria, I. E., and Cavanaugh, P. R. *The Physiology and Biomechanics of Cycling*. New York: John Wiley and Sons, 1978.

Featherstone, D. F. *Dancing Without Danger*. Cranbury, N.J.: A. S. Barnes & Co., 1970.

Ganslen, R. V. *Mechanics of the Pole Vault*. 7th ed. Denton, Tex.: 1970.

Gowitzke, B. A., and Milner, M. *Understanding the Scientific Bases of Human Movement*. 2d ed. Baltimore: Williams and Wilkins, 1980.

Groves, R., and Camaione, D. *Concepts in Kinesiology*. Philadelphia: W. B. Saunders Company, 1975.

Hay, J. G. *The Biomechanics of Sports Techniques*. Englewood Cliffs, N.J.: Prentice-Hall, 1973.

Henry, F. M. "Research on sprint running." *Athletic Journal* 6(1952):30.

Hooper, H. O., and Gwynne, P. *Physics and the Physical Perspective*. 2d ed. San Francisco: Harper & Row, Publishers, 1980.

Hopper, B. J. *The Mechanics of Human Movement*. New York: American Elsevier Publishing Company, 1973.

Jensen, C. R., and Schultz, G. W. *Applied Kinesiology*. New York: McGraw-Hill Book Company, 1970.

Kerssenbrock, K. "Analyzing the Fosbury Flop." *Track Technique* 41 (1970):1291-93.

Kirstein, L.; Stuart, M.; Dyer, C., and Balanchine, G. *The Classic Ballet: Basic Technique and Terminology*. New York: Alfred A. Knopf, 1975.

Krause, J. V., and Barham, J. N. *The Mechanical Foundations of Human Motion*. St. Louis: The C. V. Mosby Company, 1975.

Le Veau, B. *Williams and Lessner: Biomechanics of Human Motion*. Philadelphia: W. B. Saunders Company, 1977.

Logan, G. A., and McKinney, W. C. *Kinesiology*. Dubuque, Iowa: Wm. C. Brown Company Publishers, 1970.

margaria, R. *Biomechanics and Energetics of Muscular Exercise*. Oxford: Clarendon Press, 1976.

Mitchell, L. "Some observations on the high hurdles." *Track Technique* 37 (1969):1185-87.

Northrip, J. W.; Logan, G. A.; and McKinney, W. C. *Introduction to Biomechanic Analysis of Sport*. Dubuque, Iowa: Wm. C. Brown Company Publishers, 1974.

Plagenhoef, S. *Patterns of Human Motion: A Cinematographic Analysis*. Englewood Cliffs, N.J.: Prentice-Hall, 1971.

Rasch, P. J., and Burke, R. K. *Kinesiology and Applied Anatomy*. 5th ed. Philadelphia: Lea and Febiger, 1974.

Sweigard, L. E. *Human Movement Potential: Its Ideokinetic Facilitation*. New York: Dodd, Mead and Company, 1974.

Wells, K. F., and Luttgen, K. *Kinesiology*. Philadelphia: W. B. Saunders Company, 1976.

Wooden, J. R. *Practical Modern Basketball*. New York: Ronald Press Company, 1966.

# Index